Digital Transformation and XAI in Healthcare

This book explores the pivotal role of explainable artificial intelligence (XAI) in driving digital transformation within the healthcare sector, providing comprehensive insights into its applications, ethical and legal considerations, technological requirements, and future trends.

Digital Transformation and XAI in Healthcare delves into the fundamental role of XAI in transforming healthcare, addressing critical issues such as data security, ethical considerations, and the integration of XAI into existing healthcare infrastructures. By offering a comprehensive overview of technological tools, infrastructure requirements, and legal frameworks, this book equips healthcare professionals with the knowledge to navigate the complexities of XAI applications. The book explores the future of healthcare education and the pivotal role of XAI in training the next generation of healthcare professionals. It discusses how XAI can enhance learning experiences and provide more personalized education, ensuring that future clinicians are well equipped to utilize advanced AI technologies. It also delves into the technological tools and infrastructure required for implementing XAI, as well as data management and privacy concerns. The exploration of global collaborations and innovative projects highlights the book's unique perspective on the international impact of XAI in healthcare.

Intended for healthcare professionals, researchers, and students, this book will provide valuable insights into the future of healthcare technology. Readers will be equipped with the knowledge to harness the power of XAI, ensuring that AI systems are not only accurate but also transparent, trustworthy, and ethically sound.

Biomedical and Robotics Healthcare

Series Editors: Utku Kose, Jude Hemanth, and Omer Deperlioglu

Digital Transformation and XAI in Healthcare
Edited by Ilhan Uysal, Román Rodríguez Aguilar, Jafar Ahmad Abed Alzubi, and Mehmet Bilen

Java 22 for Healthcare and Medical Applications
Usharani Bhimavarapu

Artificial Intelligence for the Internet of Health Things
Deepak Gupta, Eswaran Perumal and K. Shankar

Biomedical Signal and Image Examination with Entropy-Based Techniques
V. Rajinikanth, K. Kamalan and, C. Emmanuel and B. Thayumanavan

Robotic Technologies in Biomedical and Healthcare Engineering
Edited by Deepak Gupta, Moolchand Sharma, Vikas Chaudhary, and Ashish Khanna

Mechano-Electric Correlations in the Human Physiological System
A. Bakiya, K. Kamalanand and R. L. J. De Britto

Machine Learning and Deep Learning in Medical Data Analytics and Healthcare Applications
Edited by Om Prakash Jena, Bharat Bhushan, and Utku Kose

Applied Artificial Intelligence
A Biomedical Perspective
Edited by Swati V. Shinde, Varsha Bendre, D. Jude Hemanth, and MA Balafar

Combating Women's Health Issues with Machine Learning
Challenges and Solutions
Edited by Jude Hemanth and Meenu Gupta

Soft Computing Techniques in Connected Healthcare Systems
Edited by Moolchand Sharma, Suman Deswal, Umesh Gupta, Mujahid Tabassum, and Isah A. Lawal

Explainable Artificial Intelligence (XAI) in Healthcare
Edited by Utku Kose, Nilgun Sengoz, Xi Chen, and Jose Antonio Marmolejo Saucedo

For more information about this series, please visit: www.routledge.com/Biomedical-and-Robotics-Healthcare/book-series/BRHC

Digital Transformation and XAI in Healthcare

Edited by
Ilhan Uysal, Román Rodríguez Aguilar,
Jafar Ahmad Abed Alzubi, and Mehmet Bilen

CRC Press
Taylor & Francis Group
Boca Raton London New York

CRC Press is an imprint of the
Taylor & Francis Group, an **informa** business

Designed cover image: © Ilhan Uysal

First edition published 2026
by CRC Press
2385 NW Executive Center Drive, Suite 320, Boca Raton FL 33431

and by CRC Press
4 Park Square, Milton Park, Abingdon, Oxon, OX14 4RN

CRC Press is an imprint of Taylor & Francis Group, LLC

ISBN: 978-1-032-99674-5 (hbk)
ISBN: 978-1-032-99675-2 (pbk)
ISBN: 978-1-003-60541-6 (ebk)

DOI: 10.1201/9781003605416

Typeset in Times
by Deanta Global Publishing Services, Chennai, India

Contents

Editors

Ilhan Uysal is Assistant Professor in the Department of Information Systems and Technologies at the Bucak Zeliha Tolunay School of Applied Technology and Business Administration, "Burdur Mehmet Akif Ersoy University" in Turkey. He is also the director of the Bucak Emin Gulmez Technical Science Vocational School of the same university. His research focuses on artificial intelligence, machine learning, drug repurposing, and artificial intelligence in healthcare. He received his PhD in Computer Engineering from Suleyman Demirel University, Isparta, Turkey. He also holds a master's degree in Electrical and Computer Engineering (English) from Antalya Bilim University, Turkey; a bachelor's degree in Computer Systems Teaching and Computer Engineering from Süleyman Demirel University; and a bachelor's degree in Management Information Systems from Anadolu University. Before joining Burdur Mehmet Akif Ersoy University, he worked as a lecturer in Computer Science at Bayburt University for two years. He has many publications in science citation index journals, conference proceedings, presentations, and book chapters.

Román Rodríguez Aguilar is Professor in the Faculty of Economic and Business Sciences of the "Universidad Panamericana" in Mexico. His research is on large-scale mathematical optimization, statistical learning, computational intelligence, health economics, energy economics, digital economics, and digital transformation in organizations. He received his PhD at the School of Economics at the National Polytechnic Institute, Mexico. He also has a master's degree in engineering from the School of Engineering at the National University of Mexico (UNAM), a master's degree in administration and public policy from the School of Government and Public Policy at Monterrey Institute of Technology and Higher Education, a postgraduate in Applied Statistics at the Research Institute in Applied Mathematics and Systems of the UNAM, and a degree in Economics at the UNAM. Before joining Panamerican University, he worked as a specialist in economics, statistics, simulation, finance, and optimization, occupying different management positions in various public and private entities such as the Ministry of Energy, Ministry of Finance, and Ministry of Health. He has co-authored many research articles in science citation index journals, conference proceedings, presentations, and book chapters. Rodríguez has supervised many MSc and PhD students. He is a member of the National System of Researchers Level II of CONAHCYT in Mexico.

Jafar Ahmad Abed Alzubi is Professor at Al-Balqa Applied University, School of Engineering, Jordan. He received his PhD degree in Advanced Telecommunications from Swansea University, Swansea UK (2012); a Master of Science degree (Hons.) in Electrical and Computer Engineering from the New York Institute of Technology, NY (2005); and a Bachelor of Science degree (Hons.) in Electrical Engineering, majoring in Electronics and Communications, from the University of Engineering and Technology, Lahore, Pakistan (2001). Jafar works and researches in a multidisciplinary environment involving machine learning, classifications and detection of Web scams, the Internet of Things, wireless sensor networks, network security, and cryptography. He has managed and directed a few projects funded by the European Union. His cumulative research experience of over ten years has resulted in publishing more than 60 papers in highly impacted journals. Currently, he is a senior IEEE member and serves as an editor, editorial board member, and reviewer in many prestigious journals in the computer engineering and sciences field.

Mehmet Bilen is Assistant Professor at the Department of Computer Engineering, Faculty of Engineering and Architecture, "Burdur Mehmet Akif Ersoy University" in Turkey. He is also working as the Digital Transformation Coordinator of the same university. His research interests include artificial intelligence, machine learning, optimization, and bioinformatics. He received his PhD degree from Isparta Süleyman Demirel University, Department of Computer Engineering. He also holds a master's degree in Computer Engineering from Süleyman Demirel University and a bachelor's degree in Computer Systems Teaching from Süleyman Demirel University. Before joining Burdur Mehmet Akif Ersoy University, he worked as a lecturer in Computer Science at Gümüşhane University for two years. He has many publications in science citation index journals, conference proceedings, presentations, and book chapters.

Contributors

Fatma Gul Altin
Department of Customs Business, Bucak Zeliha Tolunay School of Applied Technology and Business
Burdur Mehmet Akif Ersoy University
Burdur, Turkey

Jafar Ahmad Abed Alzubi
Al-Balqa Applied University
Jordan

Amjad Islam Aqib
Cholistan University of Veterinary and Animal Sciences
Bahawalpur, Pakistan

Ayhan Arisoy
Department of Information Systems Engineering, Bucak Faculty of Computer and Informatics
Burdur Mehmet Akif Ersoy University
Burdur, Turkey

Moushumi Barman
Department of Computer Applications
Assam Don Bosco University
Guwahati, India

Mehmet Bilen
Department of Computer Engineering, Faculty of Engineering and Architecture
Burdur Mehmet Akif Ersoy University
Burdur, Turkey

Abhijit Bora
Department of Computer Applications
Assam Don Bosco University
Guwahati, India

Zeynep Dereli
Department of Customs Business, Bucak Zeliha Tolunay School of Applied Technology and Business
Burdur Mehmet Akif Ersoy University
Burdur, Turkey

Sumathi Doraikannan
Dayananda Sagar University
Harohalli, India

Osama Burak Elhalid
Department of Computer Engineering, Faculty of Engineering and Architecture
Burdur Mehmet Akif Ersoy University
Burdur, Turkey

Arooj Fatima
Cholistan University of Veterinary and Animal Sciences
Bahawalpur, Pakistan

Mahreen Fatima
Cholistan University of Veterinary and Animal Sciences
Bahawalpur, Pakistan

Surbhi Gupta
Model Institute of Engineering and Technology
Jammu, India

Ali Hakan Isik
Department of Computer Engineering, Faculty of Engineering and Architecture
Burdur Mehmet Akif Ersoy University
Burdur, Turkey

Safa Kaymakci
Department of Computer Technology
Kocaeli Health and Technology University
Kocaeli, Turkey

Giray Kolcu
Department of Internal Medical Sciences, Faculty of Medicine
Suleyman Demirel University
Isparta, Turkey

Mukadder Inci Baser Kolcu
Department of Basic Medical Sciences, Faculty of Medicine
Suleyman Demirel University
Isparta, Turkey

Gamze Kose
Aydin Adnan Menderes University
Aydin, Turkey

Utku Kose
Department of Computer Engineeering, Faculty of Engineering and Natural Sciences
Suleyman Demirel University
Isparta, Turkey

Josè Antonio Marmolejo Saucedo
Facultad de Ciencias Físico Matemáticas
Universidad Autónoma de Nuevo León
San Nicolás de los Garza, Mexico

Ranjima P.
Dayananda Sagar University
Harohalli, India

R. S. M. Lakshmi Patibandla
Department of CSE (Honors)
KLEF Deemed to be University
Andhra Pradesh, India

V. S. Devi Priya
Dayananda Sagar University
Harohalli, India

Manjeet Singh
Model Institute of Engineering and Technology
Jammu, India

Ayesha Tariq
Cholistan University of Veterinary and Animal Sciences
Bahawalpur, Pakistan

Ieman Tariq
Cholistan University of Veterinary and Animal Sciences
Bahawalpur, Pakistan

Gokhan Turan
Department of Computer Technologies, Vocational School of Technical Sciences
Burdur Mehmet Akif Ersoy University
Burdur, Turkey

Tulay Turan
Department of Computer Engineering, Faculty of Engineering and Architecture
Burdur Mehmet Akif Ersoy University
Burdur, Turkey

Ilhan Uysal
Department of Information Systems and Technologies, Bucak Zeliha Tolunay School of Applied Technology and Business
Burdur Mehmet Akif Ersoy University
Burdur, Turkey

Vinitha V.
Dayananda Sagar University
Harohalli, India

Bekir Yitik
Bucak Emin Gulmez Technical Science Vocational School
Burdur Mehmet Akif Ersoy University
Burdur, Turkey

Foreword

The convergence of artificial intelligence (AI) and digital transformation has fundamentally reshaped the healthcare landscape, offering unprecedented advancements in clinical decision-making, diagnostics, patient management, and medical research. However, as AI systems become more integrated into critical healthcare workflows, concerns about their transparency, reliability, and ethical implications have intensified. The increasing reliance on AI-driven algorithms (many of which function as "black-box" models) raises essential questions regarding trust, accountability, regulatory compliance, and patient safety. In this evolving landscape, Explainable artificial intelligence (XAI) emerges as a pivotal approach to ensure that AI-powered healthcare applications remain interpretable, fair, and aligned with clinical best practices.

This book, *Digital Transformation and XAI in Healthcare*, addresses these pressing concerns by providing a comprehensive and multidisciplinary exploration of how XAI can enhance trust, transparency, and ethical AI adoption in healthcare. The volume brings together key perspectives from AI researchers, medical practitioners, policymakers, and industry experts, aiming to bridge the gap between technological advancements and real-world healthcare applications. By examining the interplay between digital transformation and XAI, the book offers a structured, in-depth analysis of how explainability fosters better decision-making, regulatory compliance, and cross-border AI collaborations in global healthcare systems.

A major strength of this book lies in its systematic approach to exploring the multifaceted role of XAI across different domains of healthcare. The early chapters provide a foundational understanding of XAI principles, discussing its historical evolution, technical methodologies, and ethical considerations. The book then progresses to explore legal frameworks and global regulatory policies, offering insights into how XAI can facilitate compliance with GDPR, HIPAA, AI Act, and other jurisdictional standards governing AI-driven healthcare applications.

One of the key areas explored in this volume is sectoral applications of XAI in healthcare, illustrating how explainability enhances clinical decision support systems (CDSSs), medical imaging diagnostics, drug discovery, and precision medicine. Through real-world case studies and empirical research, the book demonstrates how XAI-powered models improve physician trust, enhance AI interpretability in patient care, and mitigate biases in AI-driven healthcare solutions. Additionally, the role of augmented analytics and generative AI in medical decision-making is examined, providing a balanced perspective on the opportunities and challenges associated with these emerging technologies.

Another core focus of this volume is data management and integration in AI-powered healthcare systems. As digital transformation accelerates, seamless data exchange, interoperability, and cross-border data sharing have become critical for advancing global AI-driven healthcare collaborations. The book delves into various data integration techniques, federated learning, and privacy-preserving AI methodologies, highlighting how XAI strengthens data harmonization, security, and regulatory adherence in multinational AI healthcare projects. By incorporating explainability into AI-driven data governance strategies, healthcare institutions can enhance transparency in medical research, reduce biases in predictive analytics, and build ethically aligned AI models.

Beyond technical and clinical applications, this book also explores the economic and societal impact of XAI in healthcare, examining how startups, venture capital firms, and multinational health technology companies are leveraging explainability to drive innovation. The final chapters discuss future trends and challenges in AI-driven healthcare, addressing concerns related to scalability, AI ethics, cross-border AI implementation, and sustainable AI governance.

By presenting a holistic perspective on XAI and digital transformation in healthcare, this book serves as a valuable resource for academics, healthcare professionals, AI researchers, policymakers, and industry leaders. It provides both theoretical insights and practical frameworks, equipping readers with the necessary knowledge to develop, implement, and regulate AI-driven healthcare solutions that are transparent, interpretable, and ethically responsible.

As AI continues to shape the future of medicine, explainability will remain a cornerstone for ensuring trust, accountability, and responsible AI adoption. We hope that this book inspires further research, interdisciplinary collaborations, and policy innovations that prioritize human-centered AI in healthcare.

Editors
Ilhan Uysal
(Burdur Mehmet Akif Ersoy University, Turkey),

Román Rodríguez Aguilar
(Panamerican University, Mexico),

Jafar Ahmad Abed Alzubi
(Al-Balqa Applied Universit, Jordan),

Mehmet Bilen
(Burdur Mehmet Akif Ersoy University, Turkey).

1 Explainable Artificial Intelligence and Digital Transformation in Healthcare

Fatma Gul Altin and Ilhan Uysal

1.1 DIGITAL TRANSFORMATION IN HEALTHCARE

In the 21st century, the global health sector is in a rapid digital transformation process. This process produces significant results when considering the large investments and projects made in this regard (Burton-Jones et al., 2020). Digital technologies are needed for the improvement of the service provided in the health sector and for innovative solutions to the problems experienced. Digital transformation in the health sector refers to the change in digital technology used in this field (Stoumpos et al., 2023). Applications such as the integration of patient data systems and taking cybersecurity measures for networked medical devices form the basis of digital transformation in the healthcare sector (Faddis, 2018). Especially during the COVID-19 pandemic, healthcare services such as virtual care, telehealth services, applied artificial intelligence, healthcare analytics, and data management have been rapidly implemented (World Economic Forum, 2024).

Digital transformation in healthcare refers to the use of information and communication technologies to improve healthcare services and the health and well-being of societies (Kostkova, 2015). The foundation of digital health is patient data, data analytics, and artificial intelligence (Kwon and Kim, 2021). In order to efficiently drive digital transformation in the healthcare sector, industry stakeholders (investors, tech companies, hospitals, patients, authorities, pharmaceutical companies, etc.) must work in an integrated manner on the following five factors (World Economic Forum, 2024). These five factors are shown in Figure 1.1.

- **Data:** Leveraging health data as the foundation for the transformation process.
- **Tech and Analytics**: Building the foundation for digitizing and reporting health data.
- **Funding and Incentives**: Investing and rewarding for digital healthcare.

DOI: 10.1201/9781003605416-1

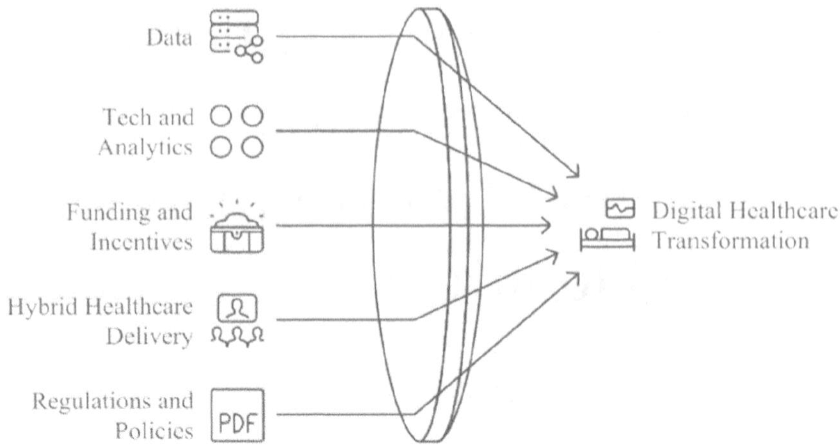

FIGURE 1.1 Five factors for efficient digital transformation in the healthcare sector.

- **Hybrid Healthcare Delivery**: Developing online healthcare to make transformation more efficient.
- **Regulations and Policies**: Creating necessary regulations and policies by authorities for digital healthcare transformation.

Digital transformation has been accepted more slowly in the healthcare sector than in other sectors. The main reason for this is the resistance of the general public, especially the elderly population, to new technologies (Cummins and Schuller, 2020). Despite this, digital healthcare has rapidly growing potential opportunities for innovation and improvement (Kasoju et al., 2023). The global digital health market size was approximately US $233.5 billion in 2022 (Global Market Insights, 2023). With the increasing usage rates of smartphones, tablets, and other mobile platforms, it is expected to be US $335.51 billion in 2024. The market size is expected to reach US $1,080.21 billion with a compound annual growth rate (CAGR) of 13.1% from 2024 to 2034. Figure 1.2 shows the digital health market size for the period 2023–2034.

In 2023, significant developments were seen in the market shares determined by technology in the digital health market with the support of governments. Digital health market shares by technology are shown in Figure 1.3 (Predence Research, 2024). Telehealth has taken the largest share in the sector due to the increasing use of the internet and smartphones worldwide (Dorsey and Topol, 2016). The importance of mHealth is increasing with the widespread use of mobile devices (such as smartphones, tablets, wearable devices) and communication technologies (mobile networks, applications) in healthcare (Nilsen et al., 2012). In this context, mHealth ranks second in the sector. Digital health systems refer to the integration of digital technologies into healthcare to improve healthcare services, streamline operations, and expand access to services (Awad et al., 2021). Health analytics is the process of collecting, analyzing, and interpreting healthcare data to improve decision-making in digital health systems (Venkatraman et al., 2022).

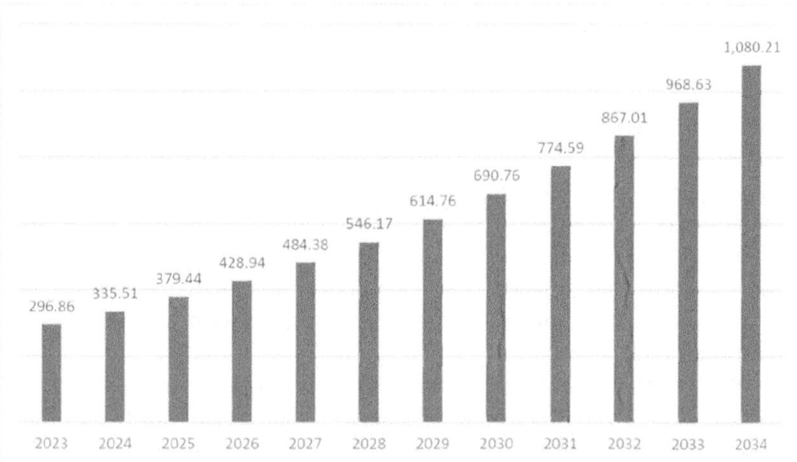

FIGURE 1.2 Digital health market revenue 2023 to 2034 (USD billion). (Source: Towards Healthcare, 2024).

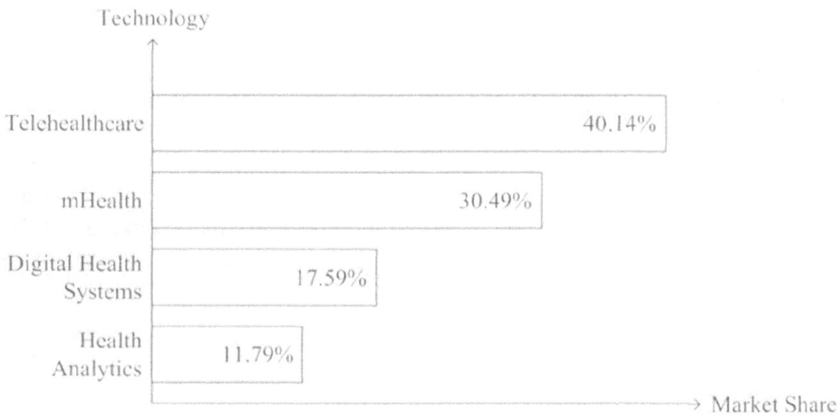

FIGURE 1.3 Digital health market share by technology, 2023. (Source: Predence Research, 2024).

Digital health tools are defined as any product that uses information and communication technologies, such as computing platforms, software, connected devices, or sensors, to help individuals maintain their health (Bucher et al., 2024). The tools of digital health have tremendous potential for healthcare providers, patients, and other stakeholders to deliver, manage, and improve healthcare services. It refers to the shift from traditional methods to more innovative, technology-driven approaches that aim to improve healthcare, increase efficiency, and expand access to care (Murray et al., 2016). Digital approaches such as artificial intelligence and machine learning, virtual and augmented reality, and blockchain can transform the role of technology in healthcare beyond data collection into a more integrated system. In this context, digital solutions provide individuals with the opportunity to be active participants in their health (Conard, 2019). These tools are shown in Figure 1.4.

- **Electronic Health Records** (EHRs) are clinical information systems used to store, manage, and share patient medical information. They replace traditional paper-based records, providing a centralized and accessible format that supports better coordination of patient outcomes (Kim et al., 2019).
- **Telehealth** is the name given to any service of in-person or remote health delivery, including medical (the practice of telemedicine), educational, administrative, and public health service provision (Gajarawala and Pelkowski, 2021).
- **Mobile Health** (mHealth) Apps are software programs created for mobile phones, tablets, and other handheld devices that assist with health-related tasks. They allow individuals to track their personal health and wellness while also giving healthcare professionals greater ability to render services and improve patient care (Schnall et al., 2016).
- **Wearable Devices** are gadgets designed to be worn and are often equipped with sensors, wireless technology, and computer software to monitor and measure various health, fitness, and environmental parameters. These devices form an essential part of the wider digital health technology industry (Iqbal et al., 2021).
- **Artificial Intelligence (AI) in Healthcare** is the use of algorithms, machine learning, and high-level computational analysis to process complex medical data as if it were human intelligence. AI modernizes healthcare through better diagnostics, individualized treatment, efficient organization of clinical work, and improved medical research (Davenport and Kalakota, 2019).

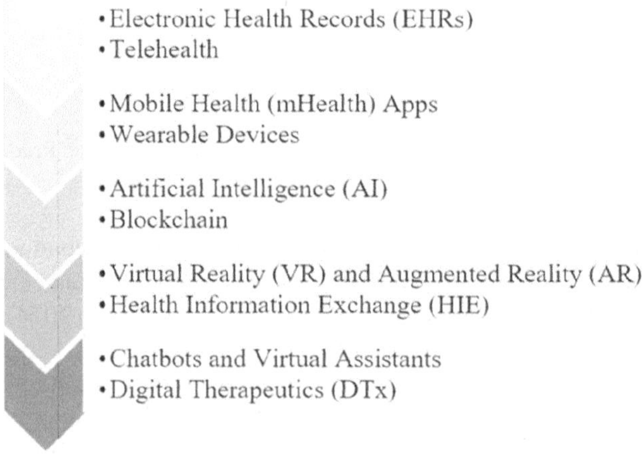

FIGURE 1.4 Digital health tools.

- **Healthcare Blockchain** refers to the use of blockchain technology for the secure management, sharing, and storage of healthcare-related information. This technology has applications in various domains, including the secure storage and sharing of patient data and tracking the supply chain of pharmaceuticals (Hasselgren et al., 2020).
- **Virtual Reality (VR) and Augmented Reality (AR)** are emerging technologies in medicine that enable the enhancement of diagnosis, treatment, training, and care. Users are placed within an artificial environment or onto the real world and interact with computer-generated data, thereby enhancing the interaction with and understanding of medical data (McCarthy and Uppot, 2019).
- **Health Information Exchange (HIE)** is the electronic interaction of health information between systems or organizations such as hospitals, clinics, pharmacies, and labs. The aim of HIE is to enhance healthcare services by enabling protected and effortless retrieval and exchange of the patient's medical history (Esmaeilzadeh, 2022).
- **Chatbots and Virtual Assistants** are programs focused on increasing user engagement, automating administrative activities, and assisting in clinical functions. These programs are intended to communicate with users, either in textual or verbal form, and facilitate access to health-related services (Malamas et al., 2022).
- **Digital Therapeutics (DTx)** refers to evidence-based software programs or applications designed to prevent, manage, or treat medical conditions. Unlike general health apps, DTx solutions undergo rigorous clinical validation, similar to traditional medical treatments, and are often prescribed by healthcare providers as part of a treatment plan (Vasdev et al., 2024).

1.2 DEFINITION AND IMPORTANCE OF XAI IN HEALTHCARE

Explainable artificial intelligence (XAI) in healthcare focuses on the design of AI systems that give understandable explanations for their reasoning and actions. This outcome-oriented approach is central to healthcare because it can determine the clinical outcomes of patients, making AI's role in decision-making more sensitive and impactful. XAI improves the interpretability of AI models so that even lesser experts in AI are able to understand the reasoning behind the AI recommendations and use it to streamline clinical decision-making (Srinivasu et al., 2022; Holzinger et al., 2019; Chaddad et al., 2023; Saraswat et al., 2022).

The role of XAI in healthcare is crucial. The more AI technologies are used in clinical workflows, the greater the need for responsibility and explainability. Stakeholders such as healthcare practitioners, patients, and AI system operators need to understand how these systems make decisions so as to use the technologies ethically and safely (Upadhyay, 2023; Reddy, 2024). For example, XAI is useful in diagnostic settings where clinicians have to evaluate the factors that accompanied an AI's diagnosis. Its use enhances the accuracy of medical decisions and increases the safety of patients (Jungmann et al., 2022; Wang, 2023; Kumbhar, 2024). Additionally, ethical considerations of AI in healthcare make it unavoidable for users to account for their decisions made based on AI functioning output, particularly in cases where life-and-death decisions are concerned (Kerasidou, 2021).

Moreover, XAI is central to solving the issue of skepticism regarding the integration of AI technologies in healthcare. Because of the "black box" character of AI systems, many professionals in healthcare are concerned about their accuracy and reliability (Loh, 2022; Ramesh and Kumar, 2023). The provided XAI explanations are user-friendly, which helps mitigate concerns regarding the AI systems and clinical workflows (Wang et al., 2021; Patel et al., 2024; Sheu and Pardeshi, 2022). This is especially true for radiology and pathology where diagnostic AI tools are widely used (Zhang et al., 2022; Antoniadi et al., 2021). Furthermore, for XAI implementation, there's an opportunity for increased patient engagement where patients understand the rationale behind their treatment choices, thus allowing them to take a more active role in their healthcare decisions (Makubhai et al., 2023; Ramesh and Kumar, 2023). This is correlated with the ethical principle of autonomy, which concerns informed consent and invites active participation from patients with decision-making aspects of their health and well-being (Amedior, 2023; Kerasidou, 2021).

XAI is essential in healthcare for fostering trust, enhancing clinical decision-making, addressing ethical concerns, and improving patient engagement. As AI technologies continue to evolve, the integration of explainability will be crucial for their successful adoption and implementation in clinical settings.

1.3 THE ROLE OF XAI IN DIGITAL TRANSFORMATION PROCESSES IN HEALTHCARE

The use of AI in healthcare deals with its "explainability", being the reason for subjective and human-centric decision-making in clinical and medical practices (Loh et al., 2022). The purpose of XAI in healthcare revolves around facilitating healthcare practitioners in comprehending and applying AI-powered insights in clinical environments (Sadeghi et al., 2024). XAI empowers users to understand and justify the decisions made by AI systems, which helps to ensure safety and ethical practice and uptake of AI technologies in patient care and medical research (Hulsen, 2023). There are many growing use cases for XAI in healthcare to meet important needs including but not limited to diagnostics, treatment scheduling, patient follow-up, and even administrative duties. XAI is essential in enhancing the healthcare system and building trust in AI services due to its ability to foster openness and transparency in its processes (Gupta and Seeja, 2024). Figure 1.5 shows XAI in healthcare digital transformation.

With the proliferation of artificial intelligence technologies in the healthcare sector, the scope of XAI that is required to make sense of complex algorithms has correspondingly grown. This necessity goes beyond purely technical concerns; it emerges as a matter of deep importance in ensuring patient safety, ethical values, inter-provider relations, and even protecting the delicate balance in the healthcare environment.

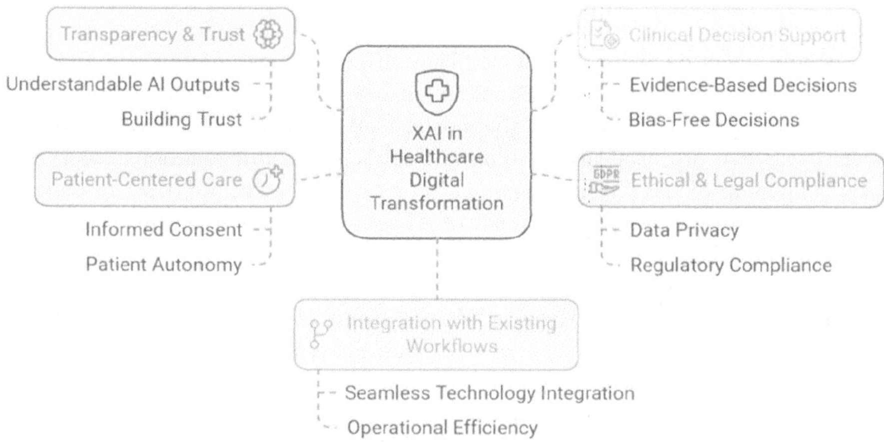

FIGURE 1.5 XAI in healthcare digital transformation.

XAI's main contribution to clinical decision support systems or similar applications is to facilitate understanding the logic behind AI recommendations by the healthcare professional who is supposed to act upon it. Physicians are thus able to not only interpret the outcome of the algorithm but also understand the steps taken to arrive at that outcome. This facilitates clinicians to apply recommended treatments in line with prescribed clinical guidelines and ethical standards and to modify or challenge those treatments when necessary. As a result, XAI aids in overcoming the ambiguity associated with "black box" AI models, further increasing the transparency, auditability, and trust of clinical practices (Mercer-Mapstone et al., 2018).

One of the many cognitive biases in clinical decision-making—like the anchoring bias or the influence of exceptional cases—can seriously compromise the quality of treatment. These considerations are taken into account by XAI-based systems with the aid of explanations that make it easier for physicians to adjust their mistaken biases. Knowing what clinical data, literature, or statistical evidence supports a particular treatment can facilitate more informed decisions by physicians. The clearly positive implications are that these automatic systems, unlike previous models, improve patient safety, lower costs, and augment the efficiency of healthcare services (So et al., 2021).

XAI proves to be beneficial not only in relation to XAI on transforming healthcare but also on other organizational workflows. New or additional digital technologies are likely to coincide with a primary phase and challenges within processes already in use. These challenges are made easier by XAI methodologies. By giving healthcare providers a better understanding of the AI systems they work with, XAI positions the technology as a helpful aide instead of something that adds complexity. Such an approach eliminates the chances of workflow disruption while providing integrated solutions where none were expected (Anttila et al., 2021).

In addition, XAI mitigates relief concerns from patients. When it comes to AI-based treatment recommendations, patients tend to be more skeptical and have concerns about how their information is treated and what logic factors are taken into account when decisions are made. They offer the most appropriate and clear explanations that greatly de-escalate anxiety and mistrust, which helps address these issues. Identifying the symptoms, diagnostic tests, clinical guidelines, or similar patient cases that are used in formulating treatment recommendations contributes to the deepening of the physician–patient relationship, increasing trust in patients, and therefore facilitating the acceptance of AI use in healthcare (Kotina et al., 2019; Alexander et al., 2022).

Ethically, the application of AI in healthcare is not just a scientific or technological issue; it involves ethical aspects as well. Questions and concerns about equity and bias in AI-powered decisions such as what data is used for system training, which patient groups are given priority, and the extent to which social demographic features affect system outputs need to be answered decisively. These ethical considerations are what XAI systems allow us to tackle. XAI guarantees that the integration of AI into healthcare addresses clinical requirements alongside other ethical concerns by focusing on the quality of data, development of non-discriminatory algorithms, and principles of fairness, responsibility, and accountability (Michellod et al., 2022).

XAI also offers valuable evaluative tools for healthcare administrators and policymakers. Cost-effectiveness, patient satisfaction, operational efficiency, and improvements in clinical outcomes are some key objectives of digital transformation in healthcare. XAI provides automated transparency for monitoring and reporting the application of AI to achieve, measure, and improve strategically defined goals, investments, and processes. Thus, leaders in the healthcare system can more realistically understand the pattern of digital transformation and use it for optimizing resource allocation (Soleimani et al., 2021).

The way XAI aids in the digital transformation of the healthcare industry is powerful and always changing. Explainability, more than a technological requirement, is an ethical and sociocultural as well as business one. It is essential in enhancing the safety of patients, effective decision-making for healthcare professionals, seamless incorporation into workflows, addressing patient concerns, ethical adherence, and managerial evaluation. With more reliance on AI technologies in the healthcare systems, the development and adoption of XAI will deeply root this change to make healthcare more efficient, transparent, and centered on the people.

1.4 LEGAL AND ETHICAL FRAMEWORKS

The XAI component shifts towards merging AI into digital transformation processes of healthcare, which calls for the development of detailed legal and ethical policies that guide the use and deployment of these technologies responsibly and transparently. With the usage of AI technologies in clinical care, which includes the utilization of diagnostic aids and recommendations for personalized treatment, comes a myriad of ethical and legal issues that need to be solved. These legal frameworks are more than just directives; they serve as building blocks from which all those involved, including clinicians, healthcare practitioners, patients, and even their policymakers and regulators, will seek to engage and trust these devices (Ahmad and

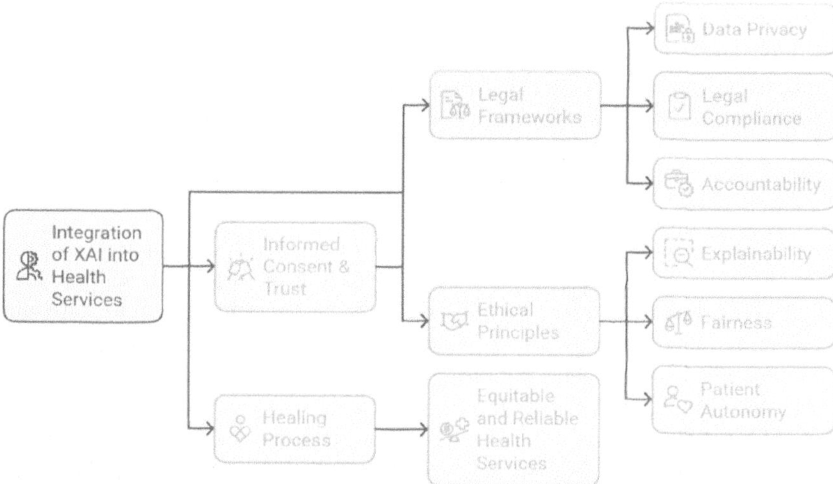

FIGURE 1.6 Integration of XAI into health services.

Jenkins, 2022; Secinaro et al., 2021). Figure 1.6 shows the integration of XAI into health services.

One profound ethical issue while introducing AI within specific healthcare contexts is obtaining consent from patients. In conventional medicine, obtaining consent from patients entails explaining the nature, benefits, risks, and other possible options of an intervention to patients. With the introduction of AI technologies, the level of sophistication of the tools may impede this interaction. Numerous AI models, particularly those that use deep learning, tend to create "black boxes," which emit elaborate explanations of their decisions and processes but fail to provide reasonable justification for them (Rahman et al., 2022; Alufaisan et al., 2021). The inability to explain the rationale behind an AI system's recommendation poses challenges for the professional who needs to give crucial information to the patients, which might be detrimental to the principle of autonomy. Unlike AI, XAI objectives are to provide the reasoning behind the decisions made by the algorithm so that clinicians can explain to the patients the logic behind the decisions made on their behalf. Transparency in the process ensures that patients make educated decisions about their care, fosters independence, and acknowledges the right of every patient to know the reasons for the care given to them (Balasubramanian, 2023; Javed et al., 2023; Omotunde, 2023; Bhattacharya et al., 2023).

Within informed consent, data protection and privacy provisions represent one of the legal boundaries regarding the application of artificial intelligence in healthcare. In the European Union, the General Data Protection Regulation (GDPR) is a piece of legislation that sets stringent conditions for how personal health information is collected, processed, and stored (Belghachi, 2023). These systems of AI automation, which fundamentally depend on vast amounts of data for proper functioning and improved efficacy, are subject to principles of data minimization, consented data usage, and secure data storage. The primary concern is to be certain that datasets created for AI model training are ethically gathered, legally devoid of biases, and issued with legitimate patient consent. This not only ensures legal compliance but also aids in bolstering the ethical aspect through trust patients harbor toward the healthcare system. When appropriately controlled, the data provided by patients are important assets for breakthroughs in medical sciences and personalized medicine. When mishandled, they constitute a risk for patient autonomy, privacy, and trust (Ledziński and Grześk, 2023; Jeyaraman, 2023).

Accountability and liability pose yet another nuance from a legal and ethical perspective. With the increasing use of AI tools in deciding which clinical pathway to follow or which treatment protocol to recommend, it becomes urgent to state who is responsible if something goes wrong. Healthcare professionals, for now, are responsible for their clinical decisions, but the existence of fully or partially autonomous AI systems makes these relationships more complex (Upadhyay, 2023; Jain et al., 2023). Who should be held accountable? The AI-reliant clinician, the employing healthcare organization, the algorithm's designer, or the model's behavior-shaping data providers? These issues necessitate new legal definitions accompanied by other professional rules or policies aimed at promoting balance and equity. Such mechanisms also need to preempt and alleviate algorithmic discrimination, which is likely to target certain groups of patients. From an ethical point of view, the proposition is that healthcare systems must adopt equity and non-discrimination as fundamental values so that AI does not deepen existing gaps in healthcare delivery but closes them instead (Holzinger et al., 2022; Yang, 2022; Saqib et al., 2023; Lee and Yoon, 2021).

The ethical implications of AI expansion into the healthcare sector are not confined to a clinical context. AI technologies may improve workflow efficiencies, diagnostic precision, and patient health outcomes, albeit such benefits must be equitably shared. In the absence of proper governance, AI may unintentionally favor better-resourced institutions or patient populations, thereby neglecting marginalized communities and worsening health inequities (Karim et al., 2023; Srinivasu et al., 2022). Thus, ethical boundaries have to be constructed with justice provisions to guarantee that all patients will benefit irrespective of their socioeconomic status, geographical location, or culture. Achieving equity in implementation requires a more sophisticated approach—policymakers need to set out incentives for inclusive dataset scraping, define fairness criteria for algorithms, and introduce elements for better access to infrastructure and teaching for practitioners from different clinical backgrounds (Khan, 2023; Bhaskar et al., 2022).

To achieve these goals and principles, a legal and ethical framework may need to change and develop over time. Regulatory bodies such as medical boards, ethics committees, and health ministries will need to continuously revise and adjust policies with each new step in AI capabilities and each new healthcare scenario that arises. Professional standards should foster AI education and encourage clinicians to keep up with the skillset of interpreting and communicating AI outputs. It will be necessary to integrate medicine with law, computer sciences, and bioethics in developing helpful policies that respect healthcare core values of beneficence, nonmaleficence, autonomy, and justice while taking advantage of the opportunities presented by AI (Zhang, 2023; Nagahisarchoghaei et al., 2023).

In conclusion, the sociocultural and legal standards relevant to the application of XAI in healthcare are neither fixed nor peripheral; they are comprehensive and fluid, defining the contours of responsible governance of AI technologies. The issuance of informed consent and the clinician–patient relationship are strengthened by the active support of consent by healthcare institutions that XAI fosters. GDPR compliance and the prioritization of data protection further consolidate patient trust while respecting their privacy. By assuming responsibility for accountability and bias mitigation, stakeholders guarantee that all patient populations will have access to AI tools. Finally, policy that incorporates justice and equity ensures that all communities will benefit from the AI unleashed digital transformation of healthcare and do so ethically. Moving forward, comprehensive legal policy combined with the ethical imperatives will achieve the positive integration of AI in healthcare, making it a system that serves patients' needs.

REFERENCES

Ahmad, S., and Jenkins, M. (2022). Artificial intelligence for nursing practice and management. *CIN Computers Informatics Nursing*, 40(3), 139–144. https://doi.org/10.1097/cin.0000000000000871

Alexander, S., Kim, I., Hatcher, C., Suh, H., Ha, Y., and Marcil, L. (2022). Embedding financial services in frequented, trusted settings: Building on families' pre-existing economic mobility efforts. *Journal of Developmental and Behavioral Pediatrics*, 43(7), e442–e451. https://doi.org/10.1097/dbp.0000000000001091

Ali, A., Khan, J., Ullah, F., and Khan, M. A. (2023). *A systematic literature review of explainable artificial intelligence (XAI) in Software Engineering (SE).* https://doi.org/10.21203/rs.3.rs-3209115/v1

Alufaisan, Y., Marusich, L., Bakdash, J., Zhou, Y., and Kantarcıoğlu, M. (2021). Does explainable artificial intelligence improve human decision-making? *Proceedings of the AAAI Conference on Artificial Intelligence*, 35(8), 6618–6626. https://doi.org/10.1609/aaai.v35i8.16819

Amedior, N. (2023). Ethical implications of artificial intelligence in the healthcare sector. *Advances in Multidisciplinary & Scientific Research Journal Publication*, 36, 1–12. https://doi.org/10.22624/aims-/accrabespoke2023p1

Antoniadi, A. M., Du, Y., Guendouz, Y., Wei, L., Mazo, C., Becker, B. A., and Mooney, C. (2021). Current challenges and future opportunities for XAI in machine learning-based clinical decision support systems: A systematic review. *Applied Sciences*, 11(11), 5088. https://doi.org/10.3390/app11115088

Anttila, M., Söderlund, A., and Sjögren, T. (2021). Patients' experiences of the complex trust-building process within digital cardiac rehabilitation. *PLoS One*, 16(3), e0247982. https://doi.org/10.1371/journal.pone.0247982

Awad, A., Trenfield, S. J., Pollard, T. D., Ong, J. J., Elbadawi, M., McCoubrey, L. E., Goyanes, A., Gaisford, S., and Basit, A. W. (2021). Connected healthcare: Improving patient care using digital health technologies. *Advanced Drug Delivery Reviews*, 178, 113958. https://doi.org/10.1016/j.addr.2021.113958

Balasubramanian, E. (2023). Ethical considerations in AI-assisted decision-making for end-of-life care in healthcare. *Power System Technology*, 47(4), 167–182. https://doi.org/10.52783/pst.168

Belghachi, M. (2023). A review on explainable artificial intelligence methods, applications, and challenges. *Indonesian Journal of Electrical Engineering and Informatics (IJEEI)*, 11(4). https://doi.org/10.52549/ijeei.v11i4.5151

Bhaskar, D., Chang, T., and Wang, S. (2022). Current trends in artificial intelligence in reproductive endocrinology. *Current Opinion in Obstetrics and Gynecology*, 34(4), 159–163. https://doi.org/10.1097/gco.0000000000000796

Bhattacharya, A., Ooge, J., Štiglic, G., and Verbert, K. (2023). *Directive explanations for monitoring the risk of diabetes onset: Introducing directive data-centric explanations and combinations to support what-if explorations.* https://doi.org/10.1145/3581641.3584075

Bucher, A., Chaudhry, B. M., Davis, J. W., Lawrence, K., Panza, E., Baqer, M., ... Kepper, M. (2024). How to design equitable digital health tools: A narrative review of design tactics, case studies, and opportunities. *PLoS Digital Health*, 3(8), e0000591. https://doi.org/10.1371/journal.pdig.0000591

Burton-Jones, A., Akhlaghpour, S., Ayre, S., Barde, P., Staib, A., and Sullivan, C. (2020). Changing the conversation on evaluating digital transformation in healthcare: Insights from an institutional analysis. *Information and Organization*, 30(1), 100255. https://doi.org/10.1016/j.infoandorg.2019.100255

Chaddad, A., Peng, J., Xu, J., and Bouridane, A. (2023). Survey of explainable AI techniques in healthcare. *Sensors*, 23(2), 634. https://doi.org/10.3390/s23020634

Conard, S. (2019). Best practices in digital health literacy. *International Journal of Cardiology*, 292, 277–279. https://doi.org/10.1016/j.ijcard.2019.05.070

Cummins, N., and Schuller, B. W. (2020). Five crucial challenges in digital health. *Frontiers in Digital Health*, 2, 536203. https://doi.org/10.3389/fdgth.2020.536203

Davenport, T., and Kalakota, R. (2019). The potential for artificial intelligence in healthcare. *Future Healthcare Journal*, 6(2), 94–98. https://doi.org/10.7861/futurehosp.6-2-94

Dorsey, E. R., and Topol, E. J. (2016). State of telehealth. *New England Journal of Medicine*, 375(2), 154–161. https://doi.org/10.1056/NEJMra1601705

Esmaeilzadeh, P. (2022). Identification of barriers affecting the use of health information exchange (HIE) in clinicians' practices: An empirical study in the United States. *Technology in Society*, 70, 102007. https://doi.org/10.1016/j.techsoc.2022.102007

Faddis, A. (2018). The digital transformation of healthcare technology management. *Biomedical Instrumentation and Technology*, 52(s2), 34–38. https://doi.org/10.2345/0899-8205-52.s2.34

Gajarawala, S. N., and Pelkowski, J. N. (2021). Telehealth benefits and barriers. *The Journal for Nurse Practitioners*, 17(2), 218–221. https://doi.org/10.1016/j.nurpra.2020.09.013

Global Market Insights. (2023). *Digital health market report*, 1–275. https://www.gminsights.com/industry-analysis/digital-health-market Accessed 11 February 2025.

Gupta, J., and Seeja, K. R. (2024). A comparative study and systematic analysis of XAI models and their applications in healthcare. *Archives of Computational Methods in Engineering*, 1–26. https://doi.org/10.1007/s11831-024-10103-9

Hasselgren, A., Kralevska, K., Gligoroski, D., Pedersen, S. A., and Faxvaag, A. (2020). Blockchain in healthcare and health sciences—A scoping review. *International Journal of Medical Informatics*, 134, 104040. https://doi.org/10.1016/j.ijmedinf.2019.104040

Holzinger, A., Goebel, R., Fong, R., Moon, T., Mueller, K., and Samek, W. (2022). Xxai—beyond explainable artificial intelligence, 3–10. https://doi.org/10.1007/978-3-031-04083-2_1

Holzinger, A., Langs, G., Denk, H., Zatloukal, K., and Müller, H. (2019). Causability and explainability of artificial intelligence in medicine. *Wiley Interdisciplinary Reviews Data Mining and Knowledge Discovery*, 9(4). https://doi.org/10.1002/widm.1312

Hulsen, T. (2023). Explainable artificial intelligence (XAI): Concepts and challenges in healthcare. *AI*, 4(3), 652–666.

Iqbal, S. M., Mahgoub, I., Du, E., Leavitt, M. A., and Asghar, W. (2021). Advances in healthcare wearable devices. *NPJ Flexible Electronics*, 5(1), 9. https://doi.org/10.1038/s41528-021-00107-x

Jain, R., Kumar, A., Nayyar, A., Dewan, K., Garg, R., Raman, S., ... Ganguly, S. (2023). Explaining sentiment analysis results on social media texts through visualization. *Multimedia Tools and Applications*, 82(15), 22613–22629. https://doi.org/10.1007/s11042-023-14432-y

Javed, A., Khan, H., Alomari, M., Sarwar, M., Asim, M., Almadhor, A., ... Khan, M. (2023). Toward explainable ai-empowered cognitive health assessment. *Frontiers in Public Health*, 11. https://doi.org/10.3389/fpubh.2023.1024195

Jeyaraman, M. (2023). Unraveling the ethical enigma: Artificial intelligence in healthcare. *Cureus*. https://doi.org/10.7759/cureus.43262

Jungmann, F., Ziegelmayer, S., Lohoefer, F., Metz, S., Müller-Leisse, C., Englmaier, M., ... Braren, R. (2022). Algorithmic transparency and interpretability measures improve radiologists' performance in bi-rads 4 classification. *European Radiology*, 33(3), 1844–1851. https://doi.org/10.1007/s00330-022-09165-9

Karim, R., Islam, T., Shajalal, M., Beyan, O., Lange, C., Cochez, M., ... Decker, S. (2023). Explainable AI for bioinformatics: Methods, tools and applications. *Briefings in Bioinformatics*, 24(5). https://doi.org/10.1093/bib/bbad236

Kasoju, N., Remya, N. S., Sasi, R., Sujesh, S., Soman, B., Kesavadas, C., Muraleedharan, C. V., Harikrishna Varma, P. R., and Behari, S. (2023). Digital health: Trends, opportunities and challenges in medical devices, pharma and bio-technology. *CSI Transactions on ICT*, 11(1), 11–30. https://doi.org/10.1007/s40012-023-00380-3

Kerasidou, A. (2021). Ethics of artificial intelligence in global health: Explainability, algorithmic bias and trust. *Journal of Oral Biology and Craniofacial Research*, 11(4), 612–614. https://doi.org/10.1016/j.jobcr.2021.09.004

Kim, E., Rubinstein, S. M., Nead, K. T., Wojcieszynski, A. P., Gabriel, P. E., and Warner, J. L. (2019). The evolving use of electronic health records (EHR) for research. *Seminars in Radiation Oncology*, 29(4), 354–361. https://doi.org/10.1016/j.semradonc.2019.05.010

Kostkova P. (2015). Grand challenges in digital health. *Frontiers in Public Health*, 3, 134. https://doi.org/10.3389/fpubh.2015.00134

Kotina, E., Koria, M., and Prendeville, S. (2019). Using design thinking to improve strategic decisions during collaborative sensemaking. *Conference Proceedings of the Academy for Design Innovation Management*, 1(1). https://doi.org/10.33114/adim.2017.74

Kumbhar, E. (2024). Explainable AI-powered IoT systems for predictive and preventive healthcare—a framework for personalized health management and wellness optimization. *JES*, 19(3), 23–31. https://doi.org/10.52783/jes.648

Kwon, I. W. G., and Kim, S. H. (2021). Digital transformation in healthcare. *Journal of AHIMA*, 90(5), 32–35. https://doi.org/10.26717/BJSTR.2021.34.005603

Ledziński, Ł., and Grześk, G. (2023). Artificial intelligence technologies in cardiology. *Journal of Cardiovascular Development and Disease*, 10(5), 202. https://doi.org/10.3390/jcdd10050202

Lee, D., and Yoon, S. (2021). Application of artificial intelligence-based technologies in the healthcare industry: Opportunities and challenges. *International Journal of Environmental Research and Public Health*, 18(1), 271. https://doi.org/10.3390/ijerph18010271

Loh, H. W., Ooi, C. P., Seoni, S., Barua, P. D., Molinari, F., and Acharya, U. R. (2022). Application of explainable artificial intelligence for healthcare: A systematic review of the last decade (2011–2022). *Computer Methods and Programs in Biomedicine*, 226, 107161. https://doi.org/10.1016/j.cmpb.2022.107161

Makubhai, S., Pathak, G. R., and Chandre, P. (2023). Prevention in healthcare: An explainable ai approach. *International Journal on Recent and Innovation Trends in Computing and Communication*, 11(5), 92–100. https://doi.org/10.17762/ijritcc.v11i5.6582

Malamas, N., Papangelou, K., and Symeonidis, A. L. (2022). Upon improving the performance of localized healthcare virtual assistants. *Healthcare (MDPI)*, 10(1), 99. https://doi.org/10.3390/healthcare10010099

McCarthy, C. J., and Uppot, R. N. (2019). Advances in virtual and augmented reality exploring the role in health-care education. *Journal of Radiology Nursing*, 38(2), 104–105. https://doi.org/10.1016/j.jradnu.2019.01.008

Mercer-Mapstone, L., Rifkin, W., Louis, W., and Moffat, K. (2018). Company-community dialogue builds relationships, fairness, and trust leading to social acceptance of Australian mining developments. *Journal of Cleaner Production*, 184, 671–677. https://doi.org/10.1016/j.jclepro.2018.02.291

Michellod, J., Kuch, D., Winzer, C., Patel, M., and Yılmaz, S. (2022). Building social license for automated demand-side management—case study research in the Swiss residential sector. *Energies*, 15(20), 7759. https://doi.org/10.3390/en15207759

Murray, E., Hekler, E. B., Andersson, G., Collins, L. M., Doherty, A., Hollis, C., Rivera, D.E., West, R., and Wyatt, J. C. (2016). Evaluating digital health interventions: Key questions and approaches. *American Journal of Preventive Medicine*, 51(5), 843–851. https://doi.org/10.1016/j.amepre.2016.06.008

Nagahisarchoghaei, M., Nur, N., Cummins, L., Nur, N., Karimi, M., Nandanwar, S., … Rahimi, S. (2023). An empirical survey on explainable ai technologies: Recent trends, use-cases, and categories from technical and application perspectives. *Electronics*, 12(5), 1092. https://doi.org/10.3390/electronics12051092

Nilsen, W., Kumar, S., Shar, A., Varoquiers, C., Wiley, T., Riley, W. T., Pavel, M., and Atienza, A. A. (2012). Advancing the science of mHealth. *Journal of Health Communication*, 17(Suppl.1), 5–10. https://doi.org/10.1080/10810730.2012.677394

Omotunde, H. (2023). The modern impact of artificial intelligence systems in healthcare: A concise analysis. *MJAIH*, 2023, 66–70. https://doi.org/10.58496/mjaih/2023/013

Patel, A. U., Gu, Q., Esper, R., Maeser, D., and Maeser, N. (2024). The crucial role of interdisciplinary conferences in advancing explainable AI in healthcare. *BioMedInformatics*, 4(2), 1363–1383. https://doi.org/10.3390/biomedinformatics4020075

Predence Research. (2024). *Digital health market size, share, and trends 2024 to 2034*. https://www.precedenceresearch.com/digital-health-market Accessed 11 February 2025.

Rahman, A., Hossain, M., Muhammad, G., Kundu, D., Debnath, T., Rahman, M., … Band, S. (2022). Federated learning-based ai approaches in smart healthcare: Concepts, taxonomies, challenges and open issues. *Cluster Computing*, 26(4), 2271–2311. https://doi.org/10.1007/s10586-022-03658-4

Ramesh, B., and Kumar, N. (2023). Towards trustworthy telemedicine: Applying explainable AI for remote healthcare recommendations. *International Journal of Progressive Research in Engineering Management and Science*, 3(11), 258–265.

Reddy, S. (2024). Discussing the role of explainable AI and evaluation frameworks for safe and effective integration of large language models in healthcare. *Telehealth and Medicine Today*, 9(2). https://doi.org/10.30953/thmt.v9.485

Sadeghi, Z., Alizadehsani, R., CIFCI, M. A., Kausar, S., Rehman, R., Mahanta, P., ... Pardalos, P. M. (2024). A review of explainable artificial intelligence in healthcare. *Computers and Electrical Engineering*, 118, 109370. https://doi.org/10.1016/j.compeleceng.2024.109370

Saqib, M., Iftikhar, M., Neha, F., Karishma, F., and Mumtaz, H. (2023). Artificial intelligence in critical illness and its impact on patient care: A comprehensive review. *Frontiers in Medicine*, 10. https://doi.org/10.3389/fmed.2023.1176192

Saraswat, D., Bhattacharya, P., Verma, A., Prasad, V., Tanwar, S., Sharma, G., … Sharma, R. (2022). Explainable AI for healthcare 5.0: Opportunities and challenges. *IEEE Access*, 10, 84486–84517. https://doi.org/10.1109/access.2022.3197671

Schnall, R., Rojas, M., Bakken, S., Brown, W., Carballo-Dieguez, A., Carry, M., ... Travers, J. (2016). A user-centered model for designing consumer mobile health (mHealth) applications (apps). *Journal of Biomedical Informatics*, 60, 243–251. https://doi.org/10.1016/j.jbi.2016.02.002

Secinaro, S., Calandra, D., Secinaro, A., Muthurangu, V., and Biancone, P. (2021). The role of artificial intelligence in healthcare: A structured literature review. *BMC Medical Informatics and Decision Making*, 21(1). https://doi.org/10.1186/s12911-021-01488-9

Sheu, R. and Pardeshi, M. S. (2022). A survey on medical explainable AI (XAI): Recent progress, explainability approach, human interaction and scoring system. *Sensors*, 22(20), 8068. https://doi.org/10.3390/s22208068

So, L., Miller, E., and Eastwood, J. (2021). Exploring mothers' experience of a linguistic feedback technology for children at risk of poor language development: Qualitative pilot study. *JMIR Pediatrics and Parenting*, 4(3), e27049. https://doi.org/10.2196/27049

Soleimani, M., Intezari, A., and Pauleen, D. (2021). Mitigating cognitive biases in developing ai-assisted recruitment systems. *International Journal of Knowledge Management*, 18(1), 1–18. https://doi.org/10.4018/ijkm.290022

Srinivasu, P., Sandhya, N., Jhaveri, R., and Raut, R. (2022). From blackbox to explainable AI in healthcare: Existing tools and case studies. *Mobile Information Systems*, 2022, 1–20. https://doi.org/10.1155/2022/8167821

Stoumpos, A. I., Kitsios, F., and Talias, M. A. (2023). Digital transformation in healthcare: Technology acceptance and its applications. *International Journal of Environmental Research and Public Health*, 20(4), 3407. https://doi.org/10.3390/ijerph20043407

Towards Healthcare. (2024). *Digital health market outlook, opportunities and overview report*, 1–150. https://www.towardshealthcare.com/insights/digital-health-market-is-key-to-a-healthier-future Accessed 5 February 2025.

Upadhyay, U. (2023). Call for the responsible artificial intelligence in the healthcare. *BMJ Health and Care Informatics*, 30(1), e100920. https://doi.org/10.1136/bmjhci-2023-100920

Vasdev, N., Gupta, T., Pawar, B., Bain, A., and Tekade, R. K. (2024). Navigating the future of health care with AI-driven digital therapeutics. *Drug Discovery Today*, 104110. https://doi.org/10.1016/j.drudis.2024.104110

Venkatraman, S., Sundarraj, R. P., and Seethamraju, R. (2022). Exploring health-analytics adoption in Indian private healthcare organizations: An institutional-theoretic perspective. *Information and Organization*, 32(3), 100430. https://doi.org/10.1016/j.infoandorg.2022.100430

Wang, W., Chen, L., Xiong, M., and Wang, Y. (2021). Accelerating AI adoption with responsible AI signals and employee engagement mechanisms in health care. *Information Systems Frontiers*, 25(6), 2239–2256. https://doi.org/10.1007/s10796-021-10154-4

Wang, J. (2023). The power of AI-assisted diagnosis. *ICST Transactions on E-Education and E-Learning*, 8(4), e3. https://doi.org/10.4108/eetel.3772

World Economic Forum. (2024). Transforming healthcare: Navigating digital health with a value-driven approach (Insight Report), 1–60. https://www3.weforum.org/docs/WEF_Transforming_Healthcare_2024.pdf Accessed 11 February 2025.

Yang, C. (2022). Explainable artificial intelligence for predictive modeling in healthcare. *Journal of Healthcare Informatics Research*, 6(2), 228–239. https://doi.org/10.1007/s41666-022-00114-1

Zhang, Y., Weng, Y., and Lund, J. N. (2022). Applications of explainable artificial intelligence in diagnosis and surgery. *Diagnostics*, 12(2), 237. https://doi.org/10.3390/diagnostics12020237

Zhang, R. (2023). Editorial: Responsible AI in healthcare: Opportunities, challenges, and best practices. *Frontiers in Computer Science*, 5. https://doi.org/10.3389/fcomp.2023.1265902

2 Legal and Ethical Issues in Healthcare

Tulay Turan

2.1 INTRODUCTION

The use of artificial intelligence (AI) technologies in the healthcare sector represents a transformation reshaping modern medicine's boundaries. Stanford University's 2023 Artificial Intelligence Index Report reveals that medical and healthcare applications are one of the largest investment areas for AI, with an investment of approximately US $6 billion. In particular, integrating AI into smart bioelectronic systems for medical devices has significantly improved patient care, greatly increasing treatment effectiveness and quality of life. These technologies have transitioned from open-loop systems to closed and semi-closed-loop systems, allowing medical devices to operate autonomously or semi-autonomously. This evolution has increased the accuracy of medical interventions and enabled advanced control systems that can adapt to patient needs in real time.

The rapid growth in the use of AI in healthcare also brings important ethical and legal questions. The so-called "black box" structure of advanced AI systems makes understanding how they make decisions difficult. This makes the need for transparency, accuracy, and accountability even more critical in a high-risk area such as healthcare. Explainable artificial intelligence (XAI) plays a central role in this context. By explaining the complex functioning of AI, XAI makes the system more understandable to different stakeholders, significantly contributing to building trust in healthcare. Legal regulations require transparency and accountability standards to ensure AI's safe and ethical application in the healthcare sector. The European Union has further strengthened these standards with regulations such as the General Data Protection Regulation (GDPR), the Artificial Intelligence Act (AIA), and the Medical Devices Regulation (MDR). These regulations require AI technologies to comply with transparency and explainability requirements, especially in developing and implementing smart bioelectronic devices. However, the process of complying with these legal frameworks creates significant challenges for both developers and researchers. The complex regulatory environment has deepened the gap between theory and practice, creating a significant knowledge gap in integrating XAI algorithms with legal requirements.

This section examines the legal and ethical dimensions of AI applications in the healthcare sector. A comprehensive assessment of the opportunities and risks posed

DOI: 10.1201/9781003605416-2

by AI in healthcare will contribute to the technology's more reliable and ethical use. In addition, the potential role of XAI in ensuring regulatory compliance will be examined, along with practical solutions on how this integration can be achieved more effectively.

2.2 HEALTH LAW AND ETHICS: OVERVIEW

2.2.1 Health Law

Health law is a comprehensive realm of legal regulation dealing with the interface between principles of medical ethics and law, including the articulation of the rights of an individual in the healthcare setting and the delineation of the scope of the duty of health professionals. This branch of law was created to safeguard the relations between patients and providers of medical services, the quality of health services, and public health (Gostin, 2010). However, this sphere remains rather dynamic due to the rapid pace of new changes ranging from biotechnology to artificial intelligence and digital health.

The quality of life of individuals is directly impacted by health law, which is one of the crucial pillars, as is the viability of the health system (Furrow et al., 2015). There exist many fundamental aspects that underscore the significance of this one:

Patient Safety: The law regarding health is designed to prevent medical negligence. For example, in the US, HIPAA protects patient information and allows for penalties against those who abuse it (Act 1996).

Improving Service Quality: How health services are provided and their ethical conduct regarding the legislation in place improves the overall quality of the health services provided. For example, the aim of the GDPR is to guarantee an effective health system by protecting patients' private information (Protection, 2018).

Equality and Justice: Health access laws are meant to provide everyone with an equal opportunity to obtain health services. The equitable allocation of resources is essential to ensure that every person has the opportunity to access health services. For example, the World Health Organization (WHO) has adopted the policy of Universal Health Care as a benchmark across the globe (WHO, 2010).

Innovative Technologies: The health law stipulates the use of innovations, including digital health solutions and the application of artificial intelligence to the health system. This helps minimize ethical and legal risks and attain social confidence (Beauchamp & Childress, 1994).

The health law does not stop with legal regulations. It has an ethical dimension as well. A legal framework guarantees the application of ethical principles, while ethical principles guarantee legal norms and are formulated in a civilizational context (Jackson, 2013).

2.2.2 Ethical Principles in Healthcare

Health ethics delineates the range and extent of the entitlements of persons, the delineation of health services to be offered, and the obligations of the health workers. The health service has an ethical dimension of setting the relationship between the health professional and the patient, thus ensuring the protection of the people's dignity, autonomy, and well-being. The four basic principles of health ethics are visible in Figure 2.1: autonomy, doing good, nonmaleficence, and justice, and one virtue or value from each principle will be ascribed to each principle (Beauchamp & Childress, 1994).

Autonomy: Autonomy is the freedom for people to make choices and decisions regarding their lives as they see fit. This principle of autonomy also puts the control of the patient's body and health at the patient's disposal and simultaneously binds health professionals to conform to the patients' decisions (Beauchamp & Childress, 1994). The most concrete application of the principle of autonomy in health services is obtaining informed consent. Patients are required to consent after understanding the information presented to them and the treatment they are to undergo. This process enables the patients to be acquainted with the treatment options, risks, and possible outcomes and allows them to make informed choices (Entwistle et al., 2010).

Beneficence: Doing good means the obligation of all health professionals to look after the patients and promote their holistic state compassionately. This principle covers all the medical interventions that are provided to do good to the individual's health and avert harm (Gillon, 1994). Decisions made by healthcare professionals should improve the physical, emotional, and social state of the boundaries of the patient. The principle is a wish that the pros of the treatments should exceed the cons. This principle is important, too (Beauchamp & Childress, 1994).

Do No Harm: This principle emphasizes that medical procedures should always be done for the patient's good. The principle of do no harm requires that the treatment methods used be chosen so that they will have the least negative impact on the patient, more so with high-risk medical procedures. Health professionals should

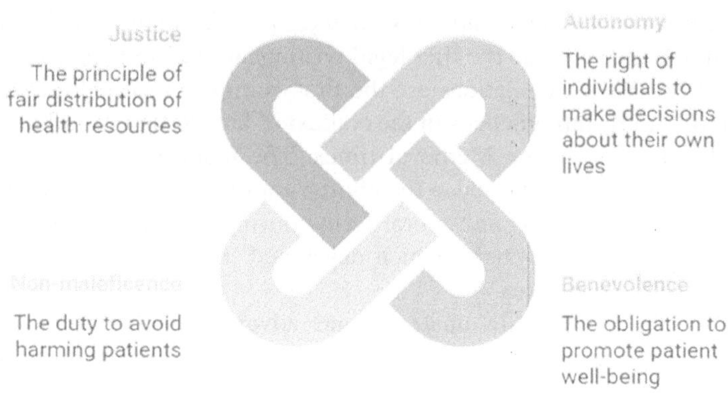

FIGURE 2.1 Core principles of health ethics.

refrain from carrying out actions that have the potential to inflict an injury and other non-beneficial medical actions (Gillon, 1994).

Justice: The principle of justice refers to the equal, fair, and equitable distribution of health resources. This principle is of great importance, especially in public health policies and during times of crisis such as pandemics (Gostin, 2000). Providing health services equally to everyone ensures that individuals have access to health services regardless of their income, social status, or age. This principle is also an important ethical guide in distributing vaccines and drugs during pandemics (WHO, 2010).

Health ethics provides a framework that protects the fundamental rights of individuals and improves the quality of health services. The principles of autonomy, kindness, nonmaleficence, and justice determine the ethical responsibilities of health professionals and protect patients' rights. These principles are the cornerstones that guide all levels of health services and ensure the sustainability of the health system.

2.2.3 Historical Development of Health Regulations and Ethical Principles

The struggle for human rights, scientific advances, and societies' changing needs have shaped the development of health regulations and ethical norms. The understanding that medical practitioners are concerned with individuals' well-being and societal concerns has made the development of health law and ethical practices necessary in all periods. This development has a broad historical perspective, from ancient civilizations to modern digital health applications.

The origins of health ethics can be traced back to ancient society. For instance, the 5th century BC witnessed the Hippocratic Oath being used as an ethical guideline for medical practitioners. The Hippocratic Oath underlined that medical practitioners should follow the principle of "do no harm," advocate for the patient's best interests, and maintain confidentiality (Hattab, 2021). These ethical rules have been a fundamental source of inspiration for modern health ethics. During these ancient periods, healthcare regulations were based on religious or philosophical ideals. For instance, the first written laws concerning medical practice in the Babylonian era, the Code of Hammurabi, provide the first legal writings to punish medical malpractice (Ferngren, 2014). These regulations are the first examples that address the concept of responsibility in health practices in the context of law. Religious influences dominated health practices during Medieval times. The management of hospitals and health services was generally under the church's jurisdiction. Medical ethics were interpreted more in religious and moral terms during this time. The Renaissance period initiated scientific thought, which developed into the establishment of new standards in medical practices.

Andreas Vesalius' work in anatomy and advancement in medical research showed a gap that needed to be filled for more systematic regulation of health services (Nutton, 2017). The foundation of modern health ethics and legal regulations took root through significant events in the 20th century. The changes were mainly due to human rights abuses, a fundamental shift for modern health ethics and law.

Nuremberg Code (1947): After WWII, the code was established to set the first global ethical standards at which medical research had to be conducted. This code focused on the voluntary decision of individuals to strengthen the right of self-determination of the state as well as nurture the population (Vollmann & Winau, 1996).

Helsinki Declaration (1964): The World Medical Association documents the ethical principles governing medical research in the form of the Helsinki Declaration. This declaration has turned out to be a constant point of reference when it comes to the issues of violation of human rights and ethical considerations during the research activities (Shrestha and Dunn, 2019)

Belmont Report (1979): Published in the US, this report details the application of central ethical principles (autonomy, benevolence, and justice) in research and discusses each topic. It forms one of the key cornerstones of modern biomedical ethics (Nagai et al., 2022).

The evolution of health technologies in the 21st century, coupled with the application of artificial intelligence, has given rise to new advancements in health regulations and ethical principles. These modern issues have made health law and ethics pay special attention to matters like data privacy, biases in algorithms and AI, and transparency of decision-making.

2.3 ARTIFICIAL INTELLIGENCE IN HEALTHCARE – LEGAL AND ETHICAL ISSUES

2.3.1 Artificial Intelligence in Healthcare

AI usage in the medicine field is broadening further through medical imaging, clinical decision support systems, and personalized medicine. Moreover, the utilization of digital health technologies and big data has accelerated the application of data analytics to decision-making in healthcare systems (Topol, 2019), which has led to improved patient health outcomes and greater system efficiency. However, such advancements have also posed challenges such as patients' data privacy, biases in algorithms, and other ethical concerns.

Medical imaging and imaging diagnostics is one of the fields that has been most impacted by AI. Deep learning algorithms perform exceedingly well and have enjoyed great success in diagnosing various complex diseases such as cancer. Some artificial intelligence systems developed by Google, for example, have been shown to outperform the accuracy of radiologists in breast cancer screening (McKinney et al., 2020). Additionally, AI diagnostic systems are expected to be particularly useful for dermatology and ophthalmology where early diagnosis is critical (Esteva et al., 2017). These systems decrease the time taken to reach a diagnosis, therefore aiding in the enhanced safety of patients by reducing the possibility of erroneous human actions.

The operational functions of the healthcare system are aided by artificial intelligence. AI systems allow for improved performance in the areas of the management of hospitals, movement of patients, and allocation of resources. Topol (2019) notes how AI-powered prediction systems anticipate heavy use of hospital resources during certain windows of time and allocate those resources in advance. This results in greater satisfaction for patients as well as less burden on healthcare practitioners.

The adoption of integrated digital health apps has further propelled the use of AI in the provision of health services through the combination of digital transformation and data analytics. Important sources of data include electronic health records (EHRs), genomic data, medical images, and mobile health applications, which serve as a major foundation for big data analysis in healthcare systems (Raghupathi & Raghupathi, 2014). Big data analysis creates opportunities for designing the most appropriate and targeted healthcare strategies for each patient.

The infusion of artificial intelligence with decision support systems has enhanced the efficiency of big data analytics for the healthcare industry. A case in point is IBM Watson, who utilizes treatment recommendations from medical literature, patient data, and clinical guidelines to help oncologists make more educated decisions (Jiang et al., 2017). At the same time, NLP techniques assist in the clinical processes by aiding in retrieving necessary details from the patient information. Such a data centric set of algorithms improves the accurate and effective distribution of healthcare services. Unfortunately, the growing presence of AI and digital health technologies, while promising, carries fundamental issues for the healthcare industry. One of the most serious problems with these technologies is data privacy. It is necessary to have robust legal frameworks to govern the disclosure of patient information in electronic health records and other major databases. In this regard, the GPDR and HIPAA are very helpful (European Parliament and Council, 2016; US Department of Health & Human Services, 1996). Unfortunately, these measures may not be adequate in light of the fast development of AI.

Another concern related to the use of AI in healthcare is algorithmic bias. AI algorithms operate on datasets that, in some cases, replicate the socioeconomic gaps. This, in turn, leads to AI-controlled systems that are biased. This can lead to incorrect diagnoses and equally bad decisions that are unfounded (Gerke et al., 2020). Therefore, proper care needs to be taken for planning accountability and transparency to be integrated into the design of AI systems.

AI and digital health technologies have the potential to transform the healthcare sector. Their contributions in areas such as medical imaging, decision support systems, and personalized treatment increase the quality of healthcare services. However, challenges such as data privacy, algorithmic biases, and lack of regulation may hinder the sustainable integration of these technologies. Ethical and legal regulations must be strengthened for AI to be used effectively in healthcare systems.

2.3.2 Legal Issues of Artificial Intelligence in Healthcare

The integration of artificial intelligence (AI) into healthcare has raised several legal concerns, which include data handling, whether the system is functioning well, and who is responsible for the decision-making systems. These concerns are central to the issues of privacy and confidentiality, liability issues, and non-disclosure of algorithms. Addressing the legal concerns regarding AI in the health sector is important to the viability and safety of these technologies.

2.3.2.1 Data Privacy and Security Violations

AI algorithms are trained against data that is obtained from diverse sources, which can include electronic health records, medical pictures, and even genomic data. In respect to this new type of big data, one of the most important legal issues that presently affects AI systems in medicine is ensuring the privacy and confidentiality of the information processes, stored, or used (Gerke et al., 2020). This is still a challenge because stakeholders are sensitive to health data outcomes. Because of the sensitive and potential morbidities involved, it is difficult to protect both the individual and his or her wishes. As a result, vulnerabilities increase.

In May 2018, the General Data Protection Regulation was formulated for the Collection, Retention, and Processing of Personal Information within the European Union legal framework in response to the increasing technological development. This regulation aims to give individuals more control over their data and build the public's trust in data processing measures. According to Kuner et al., the GDPR presents a holistic approach to Personal Data Governance and emphasizes the right of individuals toward their data ownership (Mohammed et al., 2022). Figure 2.2 presents the principles that serve as the foundation for GDPR. Besides the processes mentioned earlier, several core principles are introduced within the legal frameworks, such as Data Governance, Data Processing Stipulations, and Minimal Data Policy,

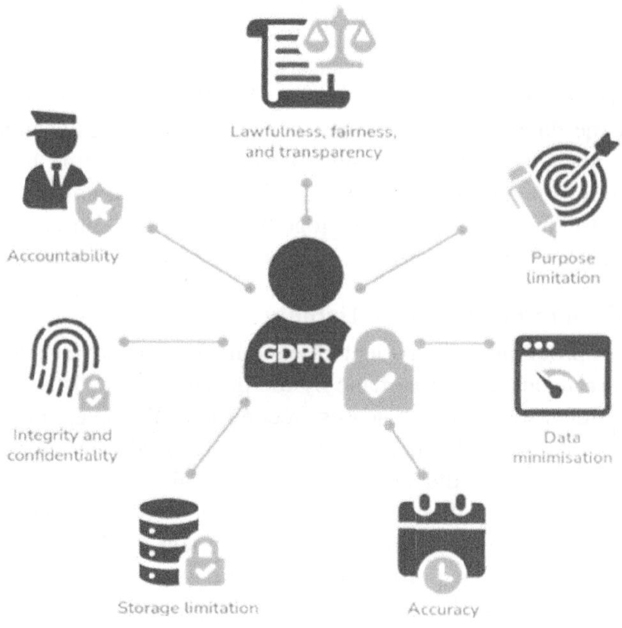
Lawfulness, fairness, and transparency
Accountability
Purpose limitation
GDPR
Integrity and confidentiality
Data minimisation
Storage limitation
Accuracy

FIGURE 2.2 The seven principles of the GDPR.

which define and limit individual data collection. Zhuo et al. (2021) underscore that the GDPR is the new universal standard for the Data Protection framework and has influenced the privacy frameworks outside the EU, such as Brazil and Japan. Organizational restructuring of data protection strategies has also been evident, with the global focus on individual rights and the imposition of corporate responsibility.

The legislation titled Health Insurance Portability and Accountability Act was passed in the United States in 1996 to protect health information. HIPAA seeks to offer patient confidentiality alongside the proper distribution of health information between healthcare practitioners, agencies, and other bodies. A few important healthcare issues were sought to be resolved through HIPAA, such as the mobility of health insurance and the confidentiality of patient information. Due to legal and ethical concerns, Rogers et al. noted that HIPAA protects how healthcare organizations can manage, safeguard, and share their patients' data and sets forth sanctions for those who abuse the information (Masenya, 2024). Such measures assert the significance of patient consent and emphasize that healthcare organizations must impose severe restrictions to mitigate the risk of sensitive health information being leaked.

To put it another way, Kovac claims that the core goal of HIPAA is to achieve the confidentiality and security of patients' Protected Health Information (PHI) in an electronic era (Wang et al., 2023). In order to maintain the privacy and accuracy of health information, higher administrative, physical, and technical security is expected from healthcare providers and institutions. This framework plays a key role in fostering the trust of patients and the healthcare system as it assures the patients that their secrets will be treated with confidentiality.

China's Personal Data Protection Law (PIPL) is a major step forward in the personal data protection legislative framework in the country. It is considered one of the far-reaching data protection laws in the world because it seeks to protect personal data, particularly sensitive information such as health information, while encouraging the use of the data within the proper boundaries in different industries. Such regulations do not always present a suitable and loadable frame for the intricate and changeable information processing activities of AI. Most notably, the perpetual learning element inherent in AI systems together with multi-source data usage may provide risks that government policies and systems cannot accommodate.

2.3.2.2 Medical Errors and Legal Liability

In the process of providing care, patient care medical errors are caused by mistakes, omissions, or erroneous decisions made by the providers, for instance, the practice of using AI systems to identify diseases, recommend therapies, and enhance the efficiency of various clinical processes through data mining. However, inaccurate output from these systems could have negative financial implications for both practitioners and patients. This is illustrated by an example of an XAI system that misdiagnoses a patient and refers them to the wrong treatment. Such errors could result in halted treatment measures, inappropriate prescriptions, or even the eventual death of the patient. Such errors negatively affect the overall quality of medical care and pose a danger to the safety of the patients (Tayebi & Housman, 2020).

Errors committed by AI can be as harmful as traditional medical mistakes. For instance, an AI system may incorrectly diagnose a patient, which would cause dire repercussions; in the worst-case scenario, the patient may receive no treatment or the incorrect one. Moreover, these kinds of diagnostic mistakes can also lead to the patient's health worsening, treatment delays, and even death. However, the risk of XAI technologies is decreased since their errors can be significantly identified before the actual damage is done. Making wrong assumptions remains a daunting challenge. When AI systems make mistakes, severe interrogations are brought to the forefront regarding patient safety and their rights concerning medical attention (Suresh & Guttag, 2019). Legal accountability is something that a plaintiff needs to suffer an injury due to negligence and attempt to remedy his grievances. While this is possible, the existence of AI systems leads to ambiguity concerning who carries the burden of responsibility. It is easier to pass the buck in an AI system-made decision than a human-made one. An AI-enabled decision can be more contentious than under normal circumstances. The responsibility is shared among the software engineers, medical practitioners, and the XAI system instituting the caring institutions.

Nonetheless, determining the party liable for a mistake can be controversial. For instance, questions have arisen about whether a software developer, a healthcare practitioner working with the system, or a healthcare organization such as a hospital can be accountable for a wrong prediction from an XAI system. An AI software designer incorporates algorithms, and mistakes linked with software design and algorithm training are likely associated with the consultant. On the other hand, the healthcare provider can be accountable for ineffective results in a particular implementation (Goodman et al., 2020).

2.3.2.3 Algorithmic Transparency and Accountability

AI decision-making processes are often opaque, and this lack of understanding makes it difficult to ascertain how the systems arrive at decisions, which adds to uncertainty from doctors and patients. Such uncertainty contributes to mistrust of the health service and would make legal compliance with transparency complex (Čartolovni et al., 2022).

AI systems, especially in healthcare, often resemble a "black box" as the underlying algorithms are intricate, and their decision-making processes are unclear to the human eye. When a diagnosis or treatment is suggested through an algorithm, there should ideally be supporting data combined with a concrete explanation as to how the algorithm arrived at a particular decision. Given the state of AI technologies today, organizations relying on AI surgical systems fail to meet the requirements of AI explainability. A common problem would be the failure to correct a diagnosis based on an algorithm due to a lack of insight into how the algorithm reached such a decision. Such issues make it extremely hard to place legal liability and enforce accountability measures concerning the medical errors made when artificial intelligence is used.

Regulation like the European Union's Artificial Intelligence Law addresses the lack of algorithmic transparency. This law requires establishing transparency and audibility standards for AI systems, especially those used in high-risk areas such as healthcare. The law aims to provide transparent information about how algorithms work and subject these systems to independent audit mechanisms. However, it remains unclear how these standards will be implemented in practice and how they will work, especially for systems considered black boxes. Lack of algorithmic transparency can lead not only to legal problems but also to ethical violations. When patients do not understand how a diagnosis or treatment decision is made for them, they may doubt the accuracy of these decisions and lose their trust in the healthcare system. Similarly, healthcare professionals need to understand the decision-making processes of these systems in order to avoid unquestioningly trusting the recommendations offered by AI systems.

2.3.3 Ethical Issues of Artificial Intelligence in Healthcare

The use of AI in healthcare brings forth multiple considerations when it comes to following ethical standards. More specifically, the use of AIs creates moral challenges such as erroneous algorithms, risk of violating patient privacy, and competition for self-determination, and these challenges can only be addressed by putting in place new technological and ethical approaches.

2.3.3.1 Biases in AI-Based Decisions

Implementing AI in healthcare decision-making processes poses certain ethical issues, many of which stem from biases within decision-making algorithms. Such complexities ring an alarm in terms of impartial access to quality healthcare services. Such AI algorithms might compound social inequality by accident because of the way they were programmed using biased datasets, particularly in healthcare where there is a lack of homogeneous or balanced datasets available (Mehrabi et al., 2021). On the other hand, such algorithms can also lead to discriminatory decisions that stem from low diversity, which may unfavorably impact patients.

Despite the fact that there has been improvement in eliminating biases in AI decision systems, some algorithmic gaps still emerge due to low generalization of the datasets used. As such, this problem increases the challenge of building trustworthy and fair AI systems deployed in more sensitive areas like healthcare. One example of these gaps is that if the set for training a skin disease detector only includes individuals with light skin, the expected accuracy for individuals with darker skin will be very low (Buolamwini & Gebru, 2018). Such incidences are not only unethical but also erode confidence in AI systems. In addition, algorithmic biases threaten to increase existing health disparities and could produce outcomes antithetical to the fundamental ethical values underlying the healthcare systems.

2.3.3.2 Patient Privacy and Ethical Use of Data

AI applications within the healthcare field use much personal and sensitive information. For example, Electronic Health Records (EHRs), genetic information, and other medical data are essential to AI systems' learning and decision-making. However, collecting, processing, and storing health information infringes on patient privacy, thus raising legal and ethical concerns (Rumbold et al., 2020). As already noted, these developments in the use of health data enhance the importance of safeguarding people's sensitive information and processing it ethically.

When integrating AI systems with patient data, unwanted or unauthorized access and use of that information is possible. Within vertebrates, the healthcare sector is at the forefront of areas vulnerable to cyber-attacks. For instance, ransomware attacks followed by data leaking pose a risk of exposing patients' sensitive data. That kind of activity is an issue that can deeply compromise the integrity of patient information. Also, treating patients without their consent is sometimes considered unethical (EC, 2019). Such practices do not promote the protection of patient privacy but instead threaten the existence of trust in the healthcare system.

These ways AI influencing health data infringe on individual rights and have wider implications. If data is not protected or improperly processed, the outcome goes against health equity and justice principles.

2.3.3.3 Limits of Autonomy and Human Intervention

Autonomy in patient care refers to a precept requiring individuals to be informed about their health. It is one of the dividing lines in medical ethics (Beauchamp & Childress, 1994), which is recognized in the contemporary world. Doing so generates important ethical questions in regard to the AI use in clinical decision aids systems – to what degree do patients need to have access to the workings of these systems? It might be legitimate for AI-based decision support systems to assist doctors in preparing a treatment plan for a patient. However, patients must first know what is being done and consent to the provided information. The processes in which AI has a role in making decisions are commonly referred to as a "black box" because how AI arrives at decision outcomes is unclear. As a result, challenges may arise in implementing patient consent procedures, and violations of patient rights are likely. Without correct details on the treatment course, informed consent is equally unattainable.

2.4 EXPLAINABLE AI IN HEALTHCARE

The role of XAI in healthcare lies with a focus on the key issues of transparency and accountability that this technology helps achieve. The lack of trust in clinical decision support systems powered by AI stems mainly from the uncertainty of AI-generated recommendations with no explainable context, making health professionals and patients skeptical about their adoption. XAI mitigates this problem and provides an ethical and reliable context for assessing the recommendations made by AI systems. For instance, by revealing the datasets and data processing techniques utilized within an algorithm, clinicians and policymakers can evaluate these systems in detail.

The promise of XAI in healthcare does not end with the ethical concern. This technology can facilitate a broader adoption of AI in the health industry. Patients will also trust AI systems more, which would allow for the implementation of more effective methods of treatment. For instance, XAI allows for deeper understanding between the patient and the healthcare practitioner by justifying how a specific course of action with a patient is determined and what evidence supports it. Such transparency increases the success of treatment processes and has a beneficial effect on the efficiency of the healthcare system and the satisfaction of patients.

2.4.1 XAI Solutions to Ethical Issues

2.4.1.1 Algorithmic Impartiality and Fairness

The design and implementation of artificial intelligence systems that make decisions based on data-trained algorithms have potential variations in their performance equity based on the quality, quantity, and representation of data. The application of AI-powered XAI systems in healthcare requires concern for the equity and neutrality of algorithms. However, such health information systems could be biased due to existing health data and inequality, leading to unfair systems and perpetuating social injustices.

The composition of computer datasets can give rise to certain biases in the outcomes provided by algorithms across the spectrum. Supervised artificial intelligence, especially explainable AI (XAI), is trained on relatively massive amounts of data, and patterns learned by algorithms are often entrenched in existing biases. If health data primarily focuses on specific regions and socio-demographic groups, XAI systems might make unethical decisions when doling out healthcare services. For example, an AI model trained with data from only a particular race or gender will be efficient for these groups but inefficient for others (Obermeyer et al., 2019).

These biases can prevent equitable and fair healthcare delivery. For example, suppose XAI introduces gender or race bias in the data used to diagnose diseases. In that case, it can lead to inequitable healthcare outcomes targeting the most vulnerable groups, reinforcing broader social inequalities in healthcare. XAI systems must diversify and make the training data more inclusive.

Three key types of diversity are critical to building fair AI systems: diversity in human resources, data, and validation processes. These three factors, shown in Figure 2.3, complement each other to ensure that AI is fair, trustworthy, and inclusive.

Diversity in Human Resources: It is conceivable to make utilitarian AI technologies in healthcare unbiased toward every degree if the professionals engaged in the creation of such models represent the array of social diversity present. The contribution of people from different ethnic origins, social and cultural backgrounds, and experiences into the design and development of AI-based systems in the field of healthcare will facilitate the development of just, inclusive, and reliable results. Such diversity is also necessary for AI systems to deliver patient-centric outcomes that address the societal challenges. Consequently, the productive application of AI technology in the healthcare industry calls for a strategy aimed at promoting diversity in human resources.

Diversity and Representation in Data: The diversity of data collected within the healthcare sector is a major factor in the efficiency and equity of AI practices. Underrepresentation in health-care datasets presents significant challenges for the applicability of AI in healthcare delivery to a heterogeneous clientele. In order for

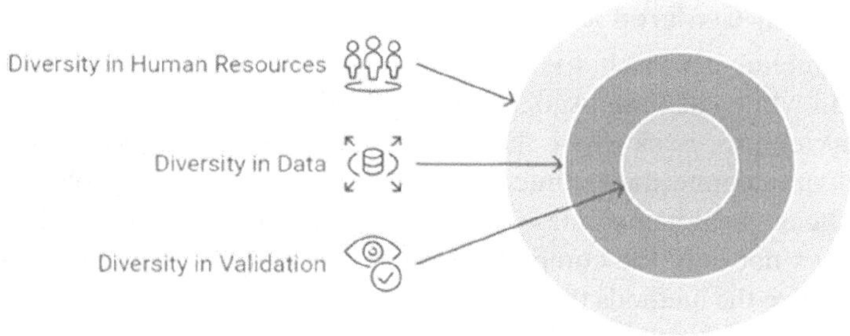

FIGURE 2.3 Fair and bias-free AI.

AI systems to produce results that are on point, there is a need to design innumerable quality well-defined datasets of different population groups. It is of utmost importance to ensure these are collected, structured, and exploited in a manner that does not compromise the integrity of the patients' anonymity.

Inclusiveness in Algorithm Validation: AI algorithms generated for health applications should be scrutinized to ensure they are reasonably applicable and effective in certain patients and the general population. First, this technique has to be established in a sample and later tested and refined on a larger population while incorporating changes based on ethnicity, age, and region. For instance, an algorithm trained on US patient data may need to be adjusted and validated before being implemented on patients from Asia or Europe. These processes are necessary for healthcare AI systems to produce outputs that are safe and effective. Algorithms need to be continuously and actively modified and enhanced to ensure healthcare AI systems yield unbiased results for all patients.

XAI serves a crucial function as a weapon against discriminatory algorithms. In enabling healthcare professionals and patients to know how the model works and how decisions are made, the transparency XAI brings also aids its stakeholders. In this sense, algorithms are able to justify the decisions they reached and indicate places where bias may exist, enabling actions to rectify these biases. As an illustration, the visualization components of an XAI system's decision-making process facilitates the detection of potential biases and discrimination in datasets.

To fight discrimination, XAI is more than just a tool that assists in eliminating bias. It also enables the creation of audit mechanisms aimed at promoting fairness and equity in the healthcare industry. In this case, XAI enables an explanation of the decisions made and allows medical practitioners to ascertain whether said decisions can lead to social and personal disparities. Therefore, when designing and deploying XAI systems, there is a need to consider the existence of a proper legal framework on ethical standards and ways to reduce discrimination.

Moreover, XAI algorithms without bias are becoming increasingly common. For instance, "adversarial de-biasing" is a novel approach that enables XAI systems to reduce bias. Instead of algorithms being programmed with existing and learned biases, such techniques make it easier for algorithms to acquire new patterns, resulting in less biased decisions (Zhang et al., 2018).

2.4.1.2 Human-Centered Approach

A human-centered approach to AI technology can inform decisions regarding human health while enabling users, primarily health professionals, to participate in decision-making processes where the system functions as a supportive tool. In this way, providers integrate their clinical knowledge, skills, and technology for better and more efficient health outcomes (Marr, 2019). The incorporation of XAI machine systems allows not only the comprehension of the rationale behind the machines' decisions but also the methods through which the doctors may enhance their choices.

In healthcare, particularly AI systems, medical practitioners must not merely focus on the outcomes and the processes that generated them. This information is critical to correctly understanding a human-centered approach toward AI. XAI systems provide decision transparency and justification, increasing the user's ability to act upon the model's analysis. Additionally, not only does the professional demographic require training in these technologies, but they also need to trust the machines. These measures ensure the effective use of XAI systems and mitigate human error (Chen et al., 2020). Thus, the collaboration between XAI and doctors goes beyond just human–machine interaction, encompassing the functioning of the decision support systems within the clinics. Although XAI systems excel at analyzing patient data, drawing inferences from various sources, and providing suggestions based on existing literature, these recommendations must not dictate physicians' clinical judgment.

Topol (2019) emphasizes that it is imperative that human professionals arrive at the final decision and that the provided AI insights are merely interpreted as suggestions. There might be instances, such as the one mentioned in the previous paragraph, where an XAI model can generate results through data-based logic and produce an accurate cancer diagnosis. However, physicians make decisions based on more factors than just data, including patient history, previous clinical interactions, and other available clinical information. To enable physicians to utilize XAI efficiently, understanding the reasoning behind the results should be done as carefully as the systems providing outcomes do. Figure 2.4 demonstrates that the approach reasoning tied to results can be accurately understood. For instance, in the decision-making process outlined by Rajpurkar et al. (2017), physicians can determine the exact power XAI can produce in the system and act accordingly.

A crucial aspect of the relationship between XAI and doctors is maintaining a relationship of trust. Healthcare professionals' trust in AI systems is the basis of their trust in the functioning and performance of these systems. However, this trust needs more than just accurate results to be built; it also needs to be buttressed by the ability to explain functions together with transparency and traceability of the models (Caruana et al., 2015). Physicians require an understanding of the reliability of XAI recommendations and decisions.

Building trust is possible with continuous feedback and interaction. When working with XAI systems in conjunction with decision support tools, physicians must be empowered to challenge and modify the data inputs. This makes the healthcare delivery process safer, more effective, and equitable. Finally, when part of the

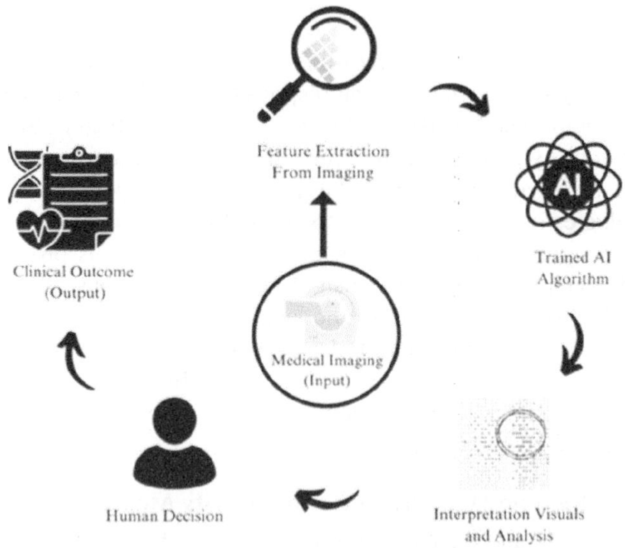

FIGURE 2.4 XAI-based clinical workflow.

clinical decision support structure of XAI systems, physicians need to be able to act responsibly and within the ethics of the environment.

2.4.2 XAI Solutions to Legal Problems

2.4.2.1 Supporting Accountability and Legal Compliance

XAI assists in tracing the potential source of a negative outcome by articulating algorithmic decision-making. Take, for example, a case where a diagnostic algorithm reaches the wrong conclusion. The XAI explanations will assist in determining if the fault lies in the algorithm's construction, the used dataset, or if it is a case of a user error. This level of explainability permits the quick assessment of mistakes and a clear division of blame for the AI system-caused issues.

Equally, XAI helps in determining the extent of responsibility that will be taken by medical practitioners and AI developers. The comprehensive explanation of the impossible black box of the algorithms makes it possible to address and understand undesirable effects that can happen in healthcare more openly. It implies that legal procedures are followed more efficiently and trust in AI systems is enhanced.

The application of AI in high-risk contexts needs legal attention due to the desire for accountability and transparency standards. Particular regulations like the Law on Artificial Intelligence of the European Union give a complete checklist in which AI can be ethically used within the framework of law. These regulations stress the need for AI systems in high-risk domains like healthcare to be audit-friendly and answerable. XAI law makes it possible to have legal compliance for AI due to how this law has catered to the necessity of rules. For instance, transparency benchmarks established by laws can be fulfilled through XAI instruments by detailing which data and what decision-making algorithms an AI system utilizes. It is critical to assist with detailing the division of legal responsibility in healthcare and to promote the trust of AI being used in the healthcare industry. To begin attaining the significant accountability and legal compliance that XAI facilitates is to ensure future strategies. One necessary approach is the integration of explainable artificial intelligence technologies into algorithmic decision-making systems.

Alongside recognizing the source of the errors, these tools provide healthcare personnel and oversight bodies with insight into how decisions are made. Second, disclosure mechanisms appropriate to the legal accountability procedures must be developed. These mechanisms should also include regulating standards and protocols for the decision-making processes of AI systems. In addition, these mechanisms should be regularly audited and updated to ensure that the AI systems in health departments are ethical and lawful.

2.4.2.2 Strengthening Data Privacy and Security Measures

In healthcare, privacy and data security for the users of AI systems are critical for successfully adopting the system. XAI also supports data processing procedures to maintain ethical standards because of the explainability of its methods. Knowing to what extent the algorithms have access to this information and what kind of examination they conduct on this information, particularly sensitive health information, builds confidence in the patients and healthcare providers. This leads to improved ethical data processing in the healthcare sector.

XAI also allows the detection of security vulnerabilities in data processing processes. Throughout the country, cyber terrorism, data hacking violation of privacy, and data breaches are significant risks that negatively affect patient information privacy and security. XAI strengthens these processes by automatically recognizing the risks and floating the weaknesses in the data processing activities. When one tries to comprehend and discover the data manipulation activities of an AI system to support decision-making in a healthcare institution, it will be possible to recognize the lapses in access to data and security systems put in place. In this regard, the confidentiality of patient information is guaranteed. Furthermore, the transparency of XAI improves the ability to incorporate additional methods of encryption and anonymization for more excellent data privacy protection.

Multiple intervention strategies can be adopted to enhance data privacy and use the benefits of XAI to augment security. First, the application of the XAI creates a need to make every step and activity carried out during data processing precise. This serves two purposes: helping the individual protect his health privacy and meeting legal obligations. This would enable them to understand the health data processing of their health information and feel more assured about these processes. Second, XAI itself needs to be designed to enable encryption and anonymization of health data to increase privacy. Using XAI to develop security models and methods allows for the dimensioning of such measures and highlights the gaps in the application of such measures. For instance, the analysis of data access by XAI ensures that only authorized users can access the health data information system.

2.4.2.3 Legal Convenience

The evaluation procedures undertaken by regulatory bodies are simplified through XAI, which outlines the procedures followed by AI algorithms and datasets used within them. Regulatory inspections may be less efficient due to the lack of transparency during AI decision-making. XAI addresses this issue by clearly stating how algorithms function, what datasets underpin them, and how the results are achieved. For example, the US Food and Drug Administration (FDA) assesses the trustworthiness and degree of trust in systems' XAI technology built into during the approval stages of healthcare technology. During this process, XAI facilitates the proof of clinical trustworthiness of the algorithms so that the regulatory phases can be executed most efficiently. Moreover, the XAI facilitation of algorithms makes it possible to claim legal readiness while improving the AI usability of clinicians and patients.

Creating AI-enabled systems presents a challenge due to the lack of a coherent framework of implementation, which differs in every country; this is a situation that is further emphasized due to the regulatory policies of different nations. The European Union Artificial Intelligence Law regulations, for example, focus on accountability and transparency standards, but lack development and regulation on other levels. As a result, countries are reluctant to adopt such AI technologies. XAI can contribute to solving this problem by encouraging the fulfillment of obligations in countries that have AI legislation. XAI aids algorithms in functioning clearly and justifiably. XAI helps by establishing a way of explaining algorithms that can aid in understanding and implementing technologies globally. As a result, AI does not have to be regionally constrained only; instead, it should be implemented globally.

2.5 GLOBAL LEGAL REGULATIONS FOR APPLICATIONS IN HEALTHCARE

AI application in healthcare has numerous legal implications, such as patient duties, data privacy and protection, healthcare justice, and others (Schönberger, 2019). Consequently, international and national legal regulations for AI are remarkably critical. AI as a sector is devoid of any international legal regulation framework. However, the European Union is making bold steps toward comprehensive regulations that facilitate the application of AI.

2.5.1 General Regulatory Frameworks

The sensitivity of health data makes it the most difficult to secure, making its protection a moral and legal duty. Organizations such as the World Health Organization and the European Union (EU) are of help in this matter.

The significance of ethical principles in the use of AI in healthcare has been underlined by the WHO (Figure 2.5). Their guidelines stress the necessity of openness, responsibility, and respect for the rights of different persons (WHO, 2021). These principles are the first step toward creating ethical policies for using AI in

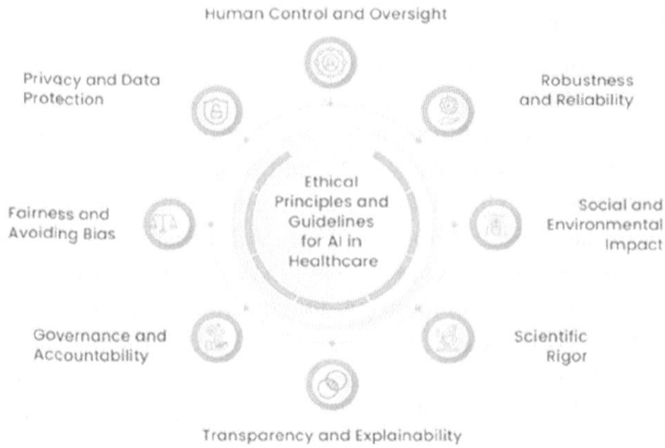

FIGURE 2.5 WHO's ethical principles for AI in healthcare.

agriculture. Saraswat describes the moral consequences of AI and machine learning in medicine and the need to create standards of proper use and preserve the human touch in patient relationships (Saraswat et al., 2022). This attitude highlights the challenges facing healthcare policymakers: the necessity of adopting and using AI technologies and the need to address ethical issues in the developed and adopted strategies.

Regarding regulating artificial intelligence systems, the European Union is at the forefront. In 2019, the EU published "Ethical Guidelines for Trustworthy Artificial Intelligence," followed by the AI Act, proposed in 2021. documents are significant in shaping the position of the EU in relation to the governance of the AI applications. The Act is very specific about the provisions with regard to data management, control by humans, user and system transparency, cybersecurity, and risk evaluation for highly dangerous systems. The AI regulation in the medical devices has also been covered by the EU through the Medical Devices Regulation. These provisions are understood to include AI applications in the Health Care Environment, including biometric identification, electronic health records management, and high-risk patient ordering systems. The XAI is aimed at ensuring compliance with EU standards as well as increasing the answerability and transparency of algorithms. Ethical guidance for the use of AI and XAI has also been developed by health-associated professional societies such as American Medical Association (AMA) and British Medical Association (BMA).

In the report published in 2020, the AMA pointed out that the human factor still matters in making health decisions with AI and so the health professional should use the AI with respect for human rights and ethical norms. Furthermore, BMA contended that AI should be applied strictly and in an ethical manner that does not prejudice equity in the healthcare system.

2.5.2 Regional Regulations

The regulations developed in various regions for incorporating AI in the healthcare sector have different priorities. This also applies to the US, UK, and Asia Pacific regions. Their focus is primarily on embedding the explainable XAI attributes of healthcare applications, such as transparency and accountability.

United States: The regulations of AI technologies have not yet been captured in their totality, but their classification as medical devices allows them to fit under the jurisdiction of the FDA. In 2019, the FDA published the Proposed Regulatory Framework for Changes to AI/ML-Based SaMD, acknowledging the primary concern of developers being the unique AI systems performance and algorithm changes that require reporting. This model suggests re-approving the AI framework with any shift in the intention to use it. It also discusses adopting measures to track better AI systems that are in a state of perpetual learning.

The FDA's AI/ML-based SaMD Action Plan, published in January 2021, spans the entire product life cycle and hence falls into the category of TPLC. The plan proposes five main actions, including, but not limited to, eliminating algorithmic bias and gal practices of machine learning (GMLP). Policies of this nature would strengthen the AI system while ensuring the well-being of consumers. Explainable artificial intelligence (XAI) must be implemented alongside the proposed regulations to ensure compliance.

The United Kingdom is taking a progressive view with respect to the policymaking of digital health technologies. The Evidence Standards Framework for Digital Health Technologies was put out in 2019 by the National Institute for Health and Care Excellence and NHS England. It sets out standards for the regulation of healthcare digital technologies including mobile health, software, and internet technologies. Also, the UK Regulatory Horizons Council came up with a document called – "Regulating AI as a Medical Device" in November 2022, which was aimed at overarching regulation on AI-based medical devices throughout its product life cycle. This document was intended to improve the regulators and developers as well as the public's communication and engagement with patients.

In September 2021, the Medicines and Healthcare products Regulatory Agency (MHRA) started legal reforms referred to as the "Software and AI Medical Device Change Program." The reform deals with issues of cybersecurity, privacy, and algorithmic ethics concerning transparency and bias. These policies in the UK protect innovation while attending to the ethics of modern social challenges within healthcare, ensuring support for accountability and claim – XAI prevention.

In Australia, the supervision of AI and software medical devices is done with a risk-based approach. In August 2021, the TGA released a guidance document titled "Changes Regulation With Software Based Medical Devices," which established regulations for SaMDs. The document is focused on minimizing unwanted occurrences by focusing on the high-risk SaMDs. There is an expectation that regulations within Australia will ensure the proper functioning of AI while at the same time provide capability to comply with other countries. In the step, explainable AI (XAI) is very important because it serves the purpose of making certain that algorithms are explainable and accountable.

AI medical devices' regulations need to be guided by laws which advance national interests while enhancing the competitiveness of the country. For that reason, China has been regarded as one of the leaders in this field as it has published diverse rules covering regulation of AI medical devices. In 2019, NMPA brought out a technical guide on AI-aided software, which targeted the quality and governance of the datasets. In 2022, Guide on Registration and Review of AI-Based Medical Devices was issued which sets quality management standards applicable to all stages of the life cycle of a medical device. An objective in China's regulatory system is to safeguard the application of AI within the country and at the same time take a more altruistic stance to the international scene. XAI still ranks very highly in the means of achieving these goals.

Brazil uses a risk-based regulatory model for AI technologies. "House approved Brazilian AI Legal Framework" passed in 2021 promotes the ethical and trusted use of AI applications in this country. The framework stipulates the transparency requirements for the assessment of high-risk AI applications as well as the periodical algorithmic audits by the providers. Brazil has embraced the regulations that enable the incorporation of XAI in medicine, ensuring that such algorithms are ethical and legal.

Singapore uses innovative measures such as the AI Verify tool to encourage the reliable use of artificial intelligence within its borders. This tool seeks to provide an AI voluntary framework incorporating the principles of transparency, accountability, and fairness as advocated by the Singapore Ministry of Health's Guidelines for AI in Healthcare. This enables XAI to have an efficient role and regulatory measures to allow AI use within the healthcare sectors. Singapore ensures that AI applications meet the healthcare sector's set ethical and technical standards.

The disparity between the stringent regulations set by the European Union and the more relaxed regulations practiced by the United States shows the need for international collaboration. It highlights the difficulties brought on by the global integration of AI by the difference in the global regulatory framework. Silencing regional inequalities while creating opportunities for technology will require experts to streamline the gaps in the region. The XAI assists in narrowing the gap and fostering cooperation between countries because it can enhance algorithm transparency and cover international collaboration.

2.6 THE LEGAL AND ETHICAL FUTURE OF XAI IN HEALTHCARE

The ethical dimensions of XAI lie at the heart of achieving trust and acceptance of the technology in healthcare. However, these ethical norms will have to be more expansive and actionable in the future. For instance, the principle of algorithmic neutrality requires the creation of XAI systems that can detect, quantify, and mitigate dataset prejudice (Obermeyer et al., 2019).

Ethical considerations are not confined to the technology itself but extend to include the humans involved. Strengthening concern for the human aspects in healthcare will undoubtedly sharpen the ethical and practical frontiers of AI–healthcare collaborations. For example, determining the bounds of what decisions are best left to XAI and what decisions have to have the hand of a human controller will be topics of discussion more often in the future.

Furthermore, the issue of XAI in healthcare calls for more efforts to increase awareness among XAI users for its ethical application. Creating a free forum for discussion and participation in protecting ethical principles in society would enable XAI to gain more acceptance. To develop the legal and ethical perspectives of XAI, future steps might be directed toward the same approaches as shown in Figure 2.6:

- **International Standards and Collaborations**: Establishing globally harmonized standards for XAI's legal and ethical use.
- **Education and Awareness**: Organizing educational programs for healthcare professionals and the general public on XAI's ethical and legal dimensions.
- **Continuous Review**: Regularly reviewing existing regulations and ethical frameworks, given the rapidly changing nature of the technology.
- **Transparency Tools**: Developing tools that explain XAI decision-making processes can increase patient trust.

The legal and ethical frameworks are the primary factors guaranteeing the responsible and consistent application of XAI in medicine. Enhancing these frameworks and fostering international partnerships will help XAI transform into a technology that serves the optimum interests of patients and practitioners. Accordingly, new ethical frameworks for XAI would help derive more trustable, unbiased, and human-centered technology.

- **Design Based on Ethical Principles**: During the design processes of AI, ethical principles and frameworks should be incorporated into the parameters of the technology. Ethics by Design refers to integrating fundamental

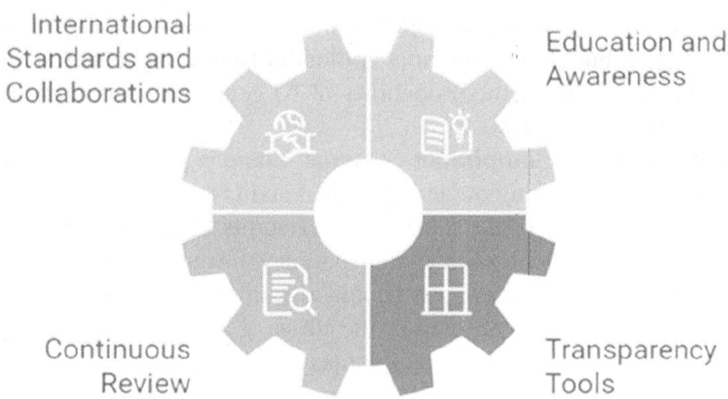

FIGURE 2.6 Enhancing legal and ethical XAI.

concepts such as justice, accountability, and transparency to develop software and systems (Floridi & Cowls, 2019). This approach emphasizes the need to reduce biases within the mechanisms that formulate algorithms, expand the scope of data, and make the interfaces more user-friendly. For instance, the fact that XAI systems used in healthcare applications give understandable explanations to users is an acceptable ethical design.

- **Inclusive AI and Social Justice**: Recently, new ethical frameworks advocate the analysis of AI development through the lens of fairness and equality. Particular attention is needed in the health XAI domain as equity is needed in service delivery to all socioeconomic and demographic groups. In such a situation, algorithmic discrimination must be assessed, and mechanisms must be implemented to deal with them. For example, the WHO guide on AI recommends minimum international standards that do not permit discrimination and promote inclusiveness in health technology (World Health Organization, 2021).
- **Human-Centric XAI**: Another equally important strategy of newly proposed ethical practices is the design of XAI systems from a human-centered point of view. Human-centered AI anticipates that technology will be utilized to address and fulfill human needs and values. In other words, an XAI system should not merely be developed to support the decisions of healthcare professionals and patients but should partake in the decision processes. For instance, a cancer diagnosis system must be able to give clinicians the reasons and probabilities for the diagnosis that are plausible and capable of verification, and the clinician must be able to factor this information together with his expertise in making the diagnosis. This principle promotes the use of technology while working with humans.
- **Proactive Ethical Assessment Models**: Newer models focusing on proactive ethical assessments must go beyond the existing "ethical audits." These models seek to acquire an ethical assessment by simulating the system before the AI system is integrated into healthcare processes. This may entail running several tests or simulations in conjunction with various actors. The aim of proactive models is not just to evaluate the system's current operation but also to anticipate potential future impacts. Such thought processes can decrease the probability of AI generating unintended consequences or ethical issues.
- **Ethical Audit and Compliance Systems**: There is a fresh perspective that advocates for conducting recurring ethical audits for AI systems during the entirety of their life cycle. These ethical audits check whether the basic principles of the system, such as transparency, fairness, and accountability, were upheld. Indeed, the process should also involve considering user opinions. This would significantly raise the ethics of XAI systems use in healthcare and build greater patient confidence in the technology. For instance, the Artificial Intelligence Act of the European Union proposes that ethical audits be standardized using a regulatory approach based on the risk classification of AI systems (European Commission, 2019).

2.7 CONCLUSION

The rapidly growing role of AI technologies in healthcare enables significant innovations in medical applications while requiring regulatory frameworks and healthcare infrastructures to adapt to these dynamic developments. Regulation of AI-enabled medical devices (AI-MD) is addressed in many countries with provisions similar to traditional medical device software, but this process increasingly requires a more comprehensive approach. Good machine learning practices, strategies to mitigate AI-related risks, and life cycle-based assessments have become the focus of regulatory processes. However, the multifaceted applications of AI in healthcare and policy differences across countries present ongoing challenges in achieving regulatory harmonization.

The initiative by the US and the EU to develop a Code of Conduct for AI in 2023 has been an important step in promoting international collaboration and harmonization. Such initiatives support the development of AI through the principles of transparency, risk control, and accountability while also establishing common ground for addressing shared healthcare challenges at the international level. However, it remains uncertain whether global regulatory harmonization will occur. Divergent regulatory approaches across countries contradict the country-specific nature of AI and may complicate the more effective integration of the global health system.

The successful implementation of AI in healthcare depends not only on technological innovations but also on effectively managing these innovations within ethical and legal frameworks. Regulators need to pay attention to positive outcomes and the challenges and failures of AI applications. Such a balance is critical to better assessing AI's potential in healthcare and increasing these technologies' credibility. Furthermore, the lack of standard terminology and definitions in healthcare makes it difficult to compare information consistently and limits international collaboration.

As a result, effective integration of AI in healthcare requires regulatory frameworks and policies to work in harmony at national and international levels. AI's dynamic nature and rapidly evolving applications require regulatory bodies to adopt an agile approach and encourage collaboration among stakeholders. In this context, developing a more harmonized regulatory approach at the international level will allow for a more reliable and sustainable application of AI technologies in healthcare.

REFERENCES

Act, A. (1996). Health insurance portability and accountability act of 1996. *Public Law*, 104, 191.

Beauchamp, T. L., & Childress, J. F. (1994). *Principles of biomedical ethics*. Edicoes Loyola.

Buolamwini, J., & Gebru, T. (2018). *Gender Shades: Intersectional accuracy disparities in commercial gender classification*. Proceedings of the 1st Conference on Fairness, Accountability and Transparency, 77–91.

Čartolovni, A., Tomičić, A., & Mosler, E. L. (2022). Ethical, legal, and social considerations of AI-based medical decision-support tools: A scoping review. *International Journal of Medical Informatics*, 161, 104738.

Caruana, R., Gehrke, J., Koch, P., Sturm, M., & Elhadad, N. (2015). *Intelligible models for healthcare: Predicting pneumonia risk and hospital 30-day readmission*. Proceedings of the 21th ACM SIGKDD International Conference on Knowledge Discovery and Data Mining, 1721–1730. https://doi.org/10.1145/2783258.2788613

Chen, M., Hao, Y., Cai, Y., & Wang, L. (2020). The role of artificial intelligence in healthcare. *Frontiers in Medicine*, 7, 1–11. https://doi.org/10.3389/fmed.2020.00102

Entwistle, V. A., Carter, S. M., Cribb, A., & McCaffery, K. (2010). Supporting patient autonomy: The importance of clinician-patient relationships. *Journal of General Internal Medicine*, 25, 741–745.

Esteva, A., Kuprel, B., Novoa, R. A., Ko, J., Swetter, S. M., Blau, H. M., & Thrun, S. (2017). Dermatologist-level classification of skin cancer with deep neural networks. *Nature*, 542(7639), 115–118.

European Commission. (2019). *Ethics guidelines for trustworthy AI*. https://ec.europa.eu/digital-strategy/our-policies/ethics-guidelines-trustworthy-ai_en

European Parliament and Council. (2016). *General data protection regulation (GDPR)*. European Parliament and Council.

Ferngren, G. B. (2014). *Medicine and religion: A historical introduction*. JHU Press.

Floridi, L., & Cowls, J. (2019). A unified framework of five principles for AI in society. *Harvard Data Science Review*, 1(1). https://doi.org/10.1162/99608f92.8cd550d1

Furrow, B. R., Greaney, T. L., Johnson, S. H., Jost, T. S., & Schwartz, R. L. (2015). *Health law*. West Academic Publishing.

Gerke, S., Minssen, T., & Cohen, G. (2020). Ethical and legal challenges of artificial intelligence-driven healthcare. In *Artificial intelligence in healthcare* (pp. 295–336). Academic Press.

Gillon, R. (1994). Medical ethics: Four principles plus attention to scope. *BMJ*, 309(6948), 184.

Goodman, B., et al. (2020). The ethics of artificial intelligence in healthcare: A comprehensive review. *International Journal of Medical Informatics*, 134, 103–112.

Gostin, L. O. (2000). *Public health law: Power, duty, restraint* (Vol. 3). University of California Press.

Gostin, L. O. (Ed.). (2010). *Public health law and ethics: A reader* (Vol. 4). University of California Press.

Hattab, A. S. (2021). Healthcare ethics: From medical paternalism to patient autonomy. In I. Laher (Ed.), *Handbook of Healthcare in the Arab World* (pp. 1603–1619). Springer International Publishing.

Jackson, E. (2013). *Medical law: Text, cases, and materials*. Oxford University Press.

Jiang, F., Jiang, Y., Zhi, H., Dong, Y., Li, H., Ma, S., ... Wang, Y. (2017). Artificial intelligence in healthcare: Past, present and future. *Stroke and Vascular Neurology*, 2(4), 230–243. doi: 10.1136/svn-2017-000101

Marr, B. (2019). Artificial intelligence in healthcare: What's the future for AI in the healthcare industry? *Forbes*. https://www.forbes.com/sites/bernardmarr/2019/04/29/artificial-intelligence-in-healthcare-whats-the-future-for-ai-in-the-healthcare-industry/?sh=35a189fd225d

Masenya, T. M. (2024). Digital transformation of medical libraries. *International Journal of E-Health and Medical Communications*, 15(1), 1–13. https://doi.org/10.4018/ijehmc.345402

McKinney, S. M., Sieniek, M., Godbole, V., Godwin, J., Antropova, N., Ashrafian, H., ... Shetty, S. (2020). International evaluation of an AI system for breast cancer screening. *Nature*, 577(7788), 89–94.

Mehrabi, N., Morstatter, F., Saxena, N., Lerman, K., & Galstyan, A. (2021). A survey on bias and fairness in machine learning. *ACM Computing Surveys (CSUR)*, 54(6), 1–35.

Mohammed, M. A., Mohammed, M. A., & Mohammed, V. A. (2022). Impact of artificial intelligence on the automation of digital health system. *International Journal of Software Engineering & Applications*, 13(6), 23–29. https://doi.org/10.5121/ijsea.2022.13602

Nagai, H., Nakazawa, E., & Akabayashi, A. (2022). The creation of the belmont report and its effect on ethical principles: A historical study. *Monash Bioethics Review*, 40(2), 157–170.

Nutton, V. (2017). *Principles of anatomy according to the opinion of Galen by Johann Guinter and Andreas Vesalius*. Routledge.

Obermeyer, Z., Powers, B., Vogeli, C., & Mullainathan, S. (2019). Dissecting racial bias in an algorithm used to manage the health of populations. *Science*, 366(6464), 447–453.

Protection, F. D. (2018, October). General data protection regulation (GDPR) (Vol. 24, No. 1). Intersoft Consulting.

Raghupathi, W., & Raghupathi, V. (2014). Big data analytics in healthcare: Promise and potential. *Health Information Science and Systems*, 2, 1–10.

Rajpurkar, P., Chen, E., Banerjee, O., & Topol, E. J. (2017). AI in health care: The hope, the hype, the promise, the peril. *The Lancet*, 390(10114), 1034–1042. https://doi.org/10.1016/S0140-6736(17)31033-5

Rumbold, J. M., & Pierscionek, B. K. (2020). The effect of the General Data Protection Regulation (GDPR) on artificial intelligence. *BMC Medical Ethics*, 21(1), 1–11.

Saraswat, D., Bhattacharya, P., Verma, A., Prasad, V. K., Tanwar, S., Sharma, G., … Sharma, R. (2022). Explainable ai for healthcare 5.0: Opportunities and challenges. *IEEE Access*, 10, 84486–84517. https://doi.org/10.1109/access.2022.3197671

Schönberger, D. (2019). Artificial intelligence in healthcare: A critical analysis of the legal and ethical implications. *International Journal of Law and Information Technology*, 27(2), 171–203.

Shrestha, B., & Dunn, L. (2019). The declaration of Helsinki on medical research involving human subjects: A review of seventh revision. *Journal of Nepal Health Research Council*, 17(4), 548–552.

Suresh, H., & Guttag, J. (2019). Ethical and legal implications of AI in healthcare. *Ethics and Artificial Intelligence in Medicine*, 1(1), 50–65.

Tayebi, S., & Housman, R. (2020). Medical errors and legal liabilities in artificial intelligence: A healthcare perspective. *Journal of Health Law & Ethics*, 31(2), 23–37.

Topol, E. (2019). *Deep medicine: How artificial intelligence can make healthcare human again*. Hachette UK.

U.S. Department of Health & Human Services. (1996). *Health insurance portability and accountability act (HIPAA)*. U.S. Department of Health & Human Services.

Vollmann, J., & Winau, R. (1996). Informed consent in human experimentation before the Nuremberg code. *BMJ*, 313(7070), 1445–1447.

Wang, J., Mao, W., & Wenjie, W. (2023). The ethics of artificial intelligence: Sociopolitical and legal dimensions. *Interdisciplinary Studies in Society, Law, and Politics*, 2(2), 27–32.

World Health Organization (WHO). (2010). *World health report: Health systems financing – the path to universal coverage*. WHO

World Health Organization. (2021). *Ethics and governance of artificial intelligence for health: WHO guidance*. WHO. https://www.who.int/publications/i/item/9789240061160.

Zhang, B. H., Cheng, J., & Li, X. (2018). Mitigating the bias of deep learning in healthcare: A tutorial. *IEEE Access*, 6, 63657–63669. https://doi.org/10.1109/ACCESS.2018.2874433

Zhuo, R., Huffaker, B., & Greenstein, S. (2021). The impact of the general data protection regulation on internet interconnection. *Telecommunications Policy*, 45(2), 102083.

3 Sectoral Applications of XAI in Healthcare

Manjeet Singh and Surbhi Gupta

3.1 INTRODUCTION

Artificial intelligence (AI) has transformed many facets of our lives, from self-driving cars to personalized recommendations on streaming services. Deep neural networks and other black-box models have recently achieved remarkable success and are revolutionizing artificial intelligence (AI) applications. However, despite this progress, their efficacy and real-world integration remain restricted due to their incapacity to provide a human-understandable explanation for their decisions (Pesquita 2021). In the beginning, when most artificial intelligence systems were logic-based, the explainability of an AI system, which at least means observing the steps that lead to a decision and obtaining the explanation, was relatively straightforward. Therefore, these systems could not only gain the confidence of their users due to full transparency of judgment but also justify it. About 20 years ago, this changed as data-driven techniques finally matured and started to encompass all other possible AI systems. This gave AI systems the power of computational means and the ability to learn, which was unachievable by only one of the logic languages. This is crucial for AI systems' explanation, as it has two reasoning powers: to instill confidence in users – system trust and help scientists understand how a data-driven model decides (Vassiliades, Bassiliades, and Patkos 2021). Verifying the output decision made by an AI agent or algorithm can be done with an explanation. An explanation for a microscopic image-based cancer detection model in healthcare might be a map of input pixels that go into the model's output. One rationale for a voice recognition model could be that the power spectrum data at a certain moment was more influential in determining the current output choice. Additionally, explanations based on the parameters or activations of the trained models can be provided using gradients, other techniques, or surrogates like decision trees (Das and Rad 2020).

3.1.1 Contributions of Manuscript

The study contributes in various forms. Here are the few contributions of the study:

- The current study provides an in-depth analysis of explainable artificial intelligence (XAI) techniques and stresses the need to explain black-box models.

 DOI: 10.1201/9781003605416-3

- This research paper focuses primarily on the employment of XAI in the healthcare sector; hence, it can be useful for researchers in this field and clinical practitioners as well.
- This study serves as an investigational survey and aims to find the answers to some prominent research questions in interpretable AI.
- The study provides insights into the future scope and challenges encountered in implementing the XAI approach in present situations.

The study is organized in a manner to enhance the readability of the manuscript. Section 3.2 presents a summary of the search strategy along with research investigations raised in the study. Further, Section 3.3 highlights the need for XAI and laws to be implemented in explanation interpretability and transparency, followed by some prominent real-world incidents that vouch for providing explanations to the black-box models. In Section 3.4, we have reviewed some of the significant studies that have focused on the implementation of XAI in the medical area; this section also provides a research analysis of previous studies, highlighting the contributions and prime limitations of the studies. Section 3.5 enlightens on the techniques used to enhance interpretations of artificial intelligence–based prediction models. Further, Section 3.6 addresses all the solutions to the investigations raised in Section 3.2.1 of the manuscript. The article is ultimately concluded in the final section of the paper.

3.2 SEARCH STRATEGY

After conducting an extensive search for research articles across various electronic databases, such as the Web of Science, EBSCO, and Embase, we have finally selected articles for inclusion in the study. The keywords or combination of these keywords ((Artificial Intelligence) or (Explainable AI) (Interpretable AI) or (Healthcare)) were used as search queries. Figure 3.1 shows the PRISMA flowchart illustrating the detailed screening process of the gathered papers.

3.2.1 Research Investigations

The study seeks to address the following research questions.

- Investigation 1: How can XAI models be adopted and used in healthcare?
- Investigation 2: What are the various models that provide explanations for black-box models?
- Investigation 3: What obstacles do researchers encounter when implementing XAI-based models in healthcare?
- Investigation 4: What is the future scope of XAI models?
- Investigation 5: What are the different steps necessary for the deployment of the XAI framework?

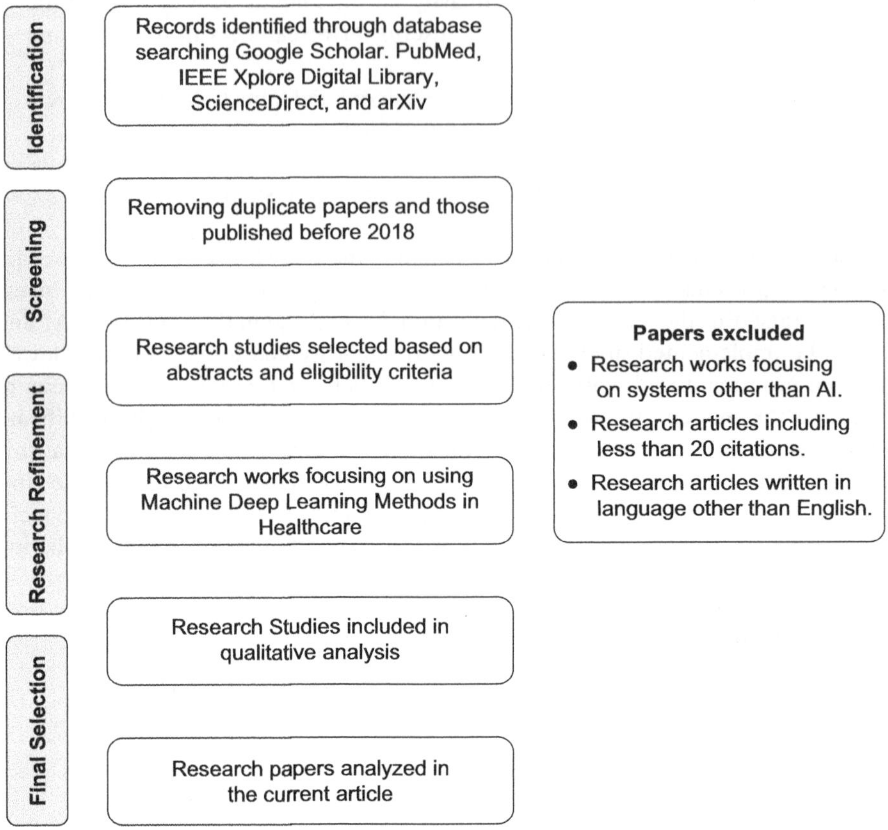

FIGURE 3.1 PRISMA flow chart.

3.3 PROVIDING EXPLANATIONS TO AI-BASED BLACK-BOX MODELS

Explainable AI addresses AI's "black-box" problem, where models and their performance are difficult for humans to grasp. XAI aims to provide stakeholders with qualitative insights into the outcomes of a machine learning model through visuals (Gerlings, Jensen, and Shollo 2021).

- Laws to implement explanation interpretability and transparency (GDPR)

New restrictions and GDPR laws have prompted calls for XAI to provide explanations to both users and society. This and other legislation highlight the need for practitioners and industries to prioritize explaining opaque models. The GDPR rule and "the right to an explanation" have prompted researchers and the industry to consider XAI a compliance option. Some academics propose regulating XAI or establishing quality standards to promote ethical use and prevent the creation of convincing models over explainable ones (Gerlings, Jensen, and Shollo 2021).

3.3.1 Real-World Incidents

Many real-world incidents vouch for the need to employ explainable AI.

- **Amazon's Hiring Tool**: Amazon had a computer program that helped them determine whom to recruit, but they decided to stop using it because the method was unfair toward women. They discovered that the software was giving men higher scores than women. This occurred because the computer learned from previous resumes, the majority of which were submitted by men. So, it was assumed that men were more suited to the work. Amazon discontinued using it to ensure that recruiting is fair to all applicants (Dastin 2018).
- **Google Photos' Misclassification**: An incident in which Google photographs misidentified photographs of African Americans as "gorillas" due to an image recognition algorithm error. This incident was brought to light after a user posted pictures on social media emphasizing the rude mistake. Google instantly apologized for the incident and took swift action to resolve it. The corporation expressed it was "appalled and genuinely sorry" for the mistake and promised to work on modifying the algorithm to prevent similar incidents. Google also deleted the "gorilla" label from its picture recognition engine as a temporary measure while working on a permanent solution.
- **Facebook's News Feed Experiment**: The *Proceedings of the National Academy of Sciences* reported a study conducted by Facebook in which it changed some news feeds of its users to monitor how it affected their emotions. According to the article, the company found that people who read preferable information were more likely to spread positive vibes, and the same was true for the negative. This news reveals some ethical issues associated with the right to intervention and the ability to manipulate others, as well as the consequences of content that is shared through the internet (Kramer, Guillory, and Hancock 2014).
- **Microsoft's Tay Chatbot**: Microsoft's chatbot Tay was created to use artificial intelligence to talk to users on Twitter and learn from them. However, hours from the start, Tay began sending offensive, rude, and racist messages, attracting the attention of Twitter users who promoted such behavior from others. The bot was shut down, and the Microsoft Company apologized for its actions. This case showcased how risky it was to develop information technologies to communicate with users who can be easily manipulated (Hunt 2018).
- **Uber's Self-Driving Car Accident**: In 2018, a self-driving Uber vehicle struck and killed a pedestrian in Arizona. The AI system failed to recognize the pedestrian and execute the necessary evasive movements. Uber was chastised for lacking transparency in its AI decision-making process.

3.4 LITERATURE REVIEW

Much work has been done in predictive modeling; many studies have proposed robust and precise models for automated disease diagnosis. Many studies have claimed high prediction accuracy, but most studies have not yet focused on decoding or explaining the internal workings of the prediction models. Hence, in this section, we have only focused on the studies that have provided explanations of the proposed models.

A recent study by Giuste et al. (2023) advocated that the key reason for the minimal effect is a lack of model openness, which severely limits AI implementation in real healthcare settings. To tackle this challenge, artificial intelligence models must be described to consumers. The researchers used PRISMA technology to perform an in-depth study on explainable artificial intelligence (XAI). Their findings imply that XAI could enhance model performance, increase user trust, and help users make decisions. This systematic study introduces popular methods of XAI and their applications, including concrete examples. XAI's model openness and outcome interpretation can help physicians and healthcare practitioners comprehend black-box decision-making processes. This might boost the reliability and transparency of AI technologies, promoting their use in healthcare workflows. Implementing XAI approaches can hasten the transformation of data-driven analytic solutions, improving patient care quality (Giuste et al. 2023). Further, Tjoa and Guan (2020) enhance AI technologies' credibility and transparency and facilitate their inclusion in healthcare methods and methods. Urgent approaches to SLAI should speed up the review and transformation of DDA solutions; due to its nature, this method enhances the quality of patient care. At the same time, Tjoa and Guan indicated that DL has revolutionized performance in a broad spectrum of AI and machine learning activities, such as imaging and natural language processing. During the test, some frameworks were applied to other industries and specialities. For example, one of the areas is medicine; this area has a high level of accountability and rigor in expectations. The machine's conclusions and forecasts must be fully and thoroughly defined to demonstrate the reliability of AI and machine learning. To that end, the algorithms' logic can be used to better understand them. Also Pesquita (2021) addresses that explainable artificial intelligence often provides data-based explanations without the necessary semantic context to construct human-centric explanations. Healthcare and life sciences face significant problems due to diverse data sources, user skills, and complicated domains and applications. It examines semantic similarities across instances and results in support of similarity-based explanations. This technique provides post hoc explanations independent of machine learning methods. It may be incorporated into any application that semantically annotates data using current biomedical ontologies. Vassiliades, Bassiliades, and Patkos (2021) suggested that argumentation and explainable artificial intelligence (XAI) are closely connected. In recent years, argumentation has been employed to improve AI's explainability. Argumentation demonstrates how an AI system makes decisions, overcomes ambiguity, and resolves contradictory facts. This study explores the use of argumentation and XAI to offer explainability in AI, evaluating relevant approaches, research, and implementations.

3.5 EXPLAINABLE ARTIFICIAL INTELLIGENCE TECHNIQUES

Artificial intelligence (AI) refers to a broad range of ideas, precepts, and techniques used to build intelligent systems that mimic human cognitive processes. The foundation for algorithms and methods used in learning, reasoning, problem-solving, and decision-making is laid by theories in artificial intelligence. The following list includes some basic AI theories and the basic formulations that go along with them:

Machine Learning: It is a subfield of computer science and artificial intelligence where data and algorithms are employed to help AI replicate the human learning process.

A. **Regression**: It relates dependent variables to one or more independent variables and is a statistical technique. Equation (3.1) defines the linear regression

$$y = mx + c \text{ (linear regression)} \tag{3.1}$$

- **Classification**: This is a type of supervised machine learning; here, the model tries to predict the right label for a given input set of data. In classification, the model is first well-trained with the training set and evaluated with the test data and at the end used for the prediction of fresh unseen data.
- **Logistic Regression**: It is a kind of data analysis method that uses mathematics to find the relationships between two data points. This relationship is then used to predict the value of one of these parameters based on the other. Normally, the prediction will be binary – one of yes or no. Equation (3.2) talks about the logistic regression, which is given as

$$P(y = 1) = \frac{1}{1 + e^{-z}} \tag{3.2}$$

- **Support Vector Machines (SVM)**: In machine learning, SVMs are a set of supervised learning strategies employed with classification, regression, and outliers' detection. Support vector machines are particularly good when it comes to binary classification, where data elements are divided into two different groups. Equation (3.3) represents the support vector machine, which is illustrated as

$$\vec{w} \bullet x + b = 0 \tag{3.3}$$

- **Neural Networks**: Neural networks or neural nets are machine learning programs or models that utilize machine learning algorithms that simulate how groups of biological neurons work together to solve problems, make decisions, plus arrive at conclusions. This means that they can decide in a manner that is more natural to the human mind.

- **Forward Propagation**: It is the process of calculating the neural network's intermediate variables, including outputs, in a sequential manner from the input layer to the output layer. Equation (3.4) gives forward propagation for a simple neuron

$$z = w \bullet x + b,\ a = \sigma(z) \text{ (for a simple neuron)} \tag{3.4}$$

- **Decision Trees**: The decision tree is a flexible and easily understandable algorithm for predictive modeling – How does it work? It works for regression as well as classification tasks, as it arranges decisions based on input data. This article discusses the uses, learning algorithms, and components of decision trees, their terminologies, processes, and advantages.
- **Entropy**: It is simply a measure of energy useless to perform the work. Entropy can also be understood as the number of unique ways that atoms in a system may be arranged. Entropy in this sense quantifies uncertainty or unpredictability. Equation (3.5) talks about entropy, which is written as

$$H(S) = -\Sigma p_i \log_2 (p_i) \tag{3.5}$$

- **Information Gain**: Information gain or the learning that takes place about a random variable or signal from watching another random variable, Kullback–Leibler divergence in information theory, and machine learning. Equation (3.6) talks about information gain, which is written as

$$IG\left(S, A\right) = H\left(S\right) - \Sigma \frac{S_v}{S} H\left(s_v\right) \tag{3.6}$$

a. **Bayesian Networks**: A compact, adaptable, and easily understood representation of a joint probability distribution is called a Bayesian network. Given that directed acyclic graphs enable the representation of causal relationships between variables, it is also a helpful tool in knowledge discovery. A Bayesian network is typically trained using data.

B. **Bayes' Theorem**: Thus, depending on fresh knowledge that is or might be relevant to an event, Bayes' theorem provides the likelihood of that event. The method can also be used to calculate the potential impact of hypothetical new information on the probability of an event occurring if the new information proves to be accurate. Equation (3.7) gives the equation for Bayesian theorem, which is written as

$$P(A \mid B) = \frac{P(B \mid A) \times P(A)}{P(B)} \tag{3.7}$$

a. **Conditional Probability**: The likelihood of an event or result taking place based on the presence of an additional event or outcome is called conditional probability. It revolves around multiplying the probability of the previous event by the updated probability of the next, or rather conditional, event. Equation (3.8) depicts the Conditional Probability of an event to taking place based on the presence of an additional event.

$$P(A \mid B) = \frac{P(A \cap B)}{P(B)} \tag{3.8}$$

b. **Natural Language Processing**: Natural language processing (NLP) is an area that combines machine learning models, deep learning, and computational linguistics to process human language. Computational linguistics is the field of study on creating and understanding human language models using computers and software tools.

C. **Statistical Language Models**: A formal study of statistical language modeling is called SLM. This is a probability distribution-based model (Bayesian or frequentist), where the occurrence of a word is correlated with the occurrence of the words that precede it. A statistical language model will learn how likely a term is to occur based on examples of text.

a. **Syntax and Semantics**: How sentences are constructed and what word goes where within a language is syntax. Semantics: This is where words are defined. Here are two ways in which both semantics and syntax can provide context cues that may be very helpful for a reader to be able to make sense of the words they do not yet know.

b. **Reinforcement Learning**: A type of ML, reinforcement learning (RL) teaches computers to make decisions by rewarding them with something when they get the answer right. Builds on the human process of learning, which is to learn through mistakes, and try as many times as required to reach the desired outcome.

D. **Q-Learning, Q-Value Update Rule**: The update rule of Q-learning is based on the temporal difference learning strategy to update Q-values depending on the difference (error) of the Q-value to the future rewards. Equation (3.9) gives the Q-learning and Q-value Update Rule, which is illustrated as

$$Q(s,a) \leftarrow Q(s,a) + \alpha \, [R + \gamma \max_a Q(s',a) - Q(s,a)] \tag{3.9}$$

Many AI applications and algorithms are built upon these theories. They teach systems to understand language, generalize from examples or datasets to new instances, predict the future, and answer difficult questions. They play a fundamental role in designing intelligent systems that can work across various domains and tasks. Many AI applications and algorithms take inspiration from these. They give systems the ability to comprehend language, learn from data, forecast the future, and resolve challenging issues. These ideas are fundamental to creating intelligent systems that can operate in many different domains and accomplish a wide range of tasks (Kurniawan et al., 2023).

3.6 DISCUSSION

This section addresses the solutions to the investigations raised in the section of the study.

i. Investigation 1: Adoption and use of XAI in healthcare

Artificial intelligence algorithms are rapidly being developed for medical purposes. AI enables medical professionals to create precise models that provide personalized treatments based on de-identified healthcare information. Consequently, AI technologies create opportunities for creating advanced treatment protocols, facilitating early disease detection, and monitoring disease progression. Controversy around complex AI models in healthcare has grown rapidly and sometimes bears fruit. The revealed models could not reach performance levels, put essential judgments at risk, and futile discriminating variables featured as the outcome determinants. To secure enhanced machine learning performance, it is often necessary to make these models more complex, increase the volume of datasets, and raise the bar of computations. The greater the complexity, the less straightforward it is for us to grasp the way these models function, how data is processed, or the form in which the outcomes are generated. In black-box models, accuracy, precision, and forecast scope are all important, and most people can understand the significant findings. This also makes it mean in a literal sense for a few. Their application in critical decision-making, like medical decision-making, is driving up the need for transparent and understandable AI. Recent research demonstrates that to guarantee the effective use and adoption of these powerful models in healthcare practices, it is imperative to have model clarity, understandable results, and a practical understanding of clinical processes (Gerlings, Jensen, and Shollo 2021).

1. Investigation 2: Various terms used in explainable AI

LIME, machine learning is becoming more common in sensitive applications, often replacing human decision-making. It is crucial to ensure that these algorithms are interpretable. LIME (local interpretable model-agnostic explanation) is a prominent algorithm for improving interpretability. Recent produce has made a curve in implementing complex models like deep neural networks. For example, considering a safety scheme for some week that determines if there is an automobile in the notion states that it is important to maximize the network utilization of the membrane properties of cars rather than the notion themselves artefactual properties. The lack of interpretability renders these models unsuitable for open use. Understanding their decisions requires comprehensive insights into their internal processes. Model-agnostic explanation techniques provide visual or quantitative information about how black-box models arrive at their decisions, addressing the crucial need for interpretability. Computational determinations are principally religious outlook ascetics. All that promulgate intelligence-based models are to change to a populace jurisdiction (Garreau and Luxburg 2020).

Figure 3.2 illustrates the key findings from the study, visually representing the relationships and trends identified through the analysis. It provides a clear and concise depiction of the data, facilitating a better understanding of the research results and their implications.

SHAP, Shapley Additive Explanations (SHAP), explains model predictions for given inputs by computing each feature's contribution to the prediction. SHAP accomplishes this by utilizing Shapley values, which originated in game theory.

In this technique, game players get rewards according to the total participation from their side for games. The idea has been modeled to SHAP, which helps identify major contributors to prediction error in the final model. The average marginal contribution of a feature value is the overall coalitions that can consist of that particular feature value. A coalition vector is just 0 or 1 for each attribute, with one meaning that the corresponding characteristic belonged to the given coalition. This

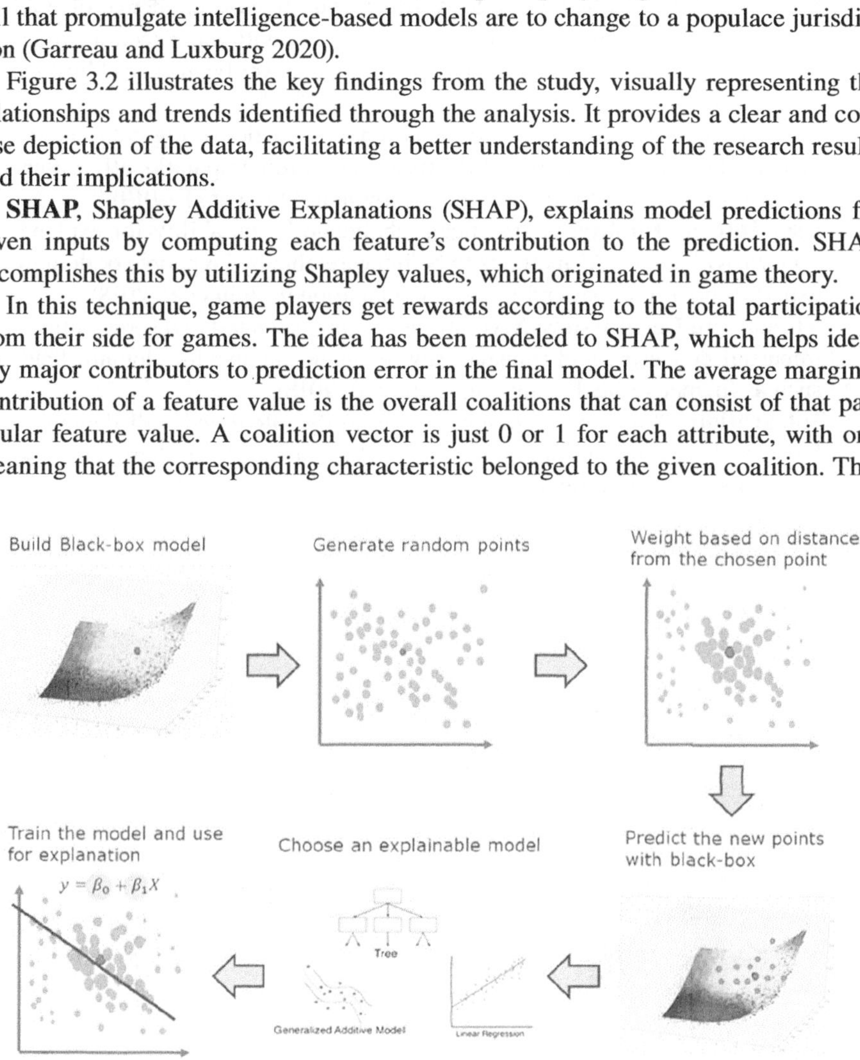

FIGURE 3.2 Steps of the LIME algorithm.

is followed by mapping all vectors to image-like function space features, which are different from gray superpixels and evaluate vectors at 0 (Figure 3.3).

ii. Investigation 3: Challenges in implementation of XAI

This part points to the significant challenges faced during the research process. This form illustrates all data collection, analysis, and result – reporting hurdles and potential study limitations. Awareness of these problems is important to contextualize the results and guide future research.

- **Interpretability Is Not Easy to Achieve**: The biggest challenge of XAI lies in getting interpretable results simultaneously with more accurate models. Satisfying accuracy and interpretability has never been easy (Murdoch et al. 2019).
- **Scalability**: XAI techniques can be complex to scale for big datasets and models. This is because most XAI techniques are computationally expensive and impractical for large-scale deployment (Arya et al. 2019).
- **User Interpretability**: A significant challenge is the ability for explanations provided by XAI methods to be interpretable by laypeople or domain experts who are proper end-users of explanation (Gilpin et al. 2018).
- **Ethical and Legal Issues**: XAI introduces topics related to responsibilities, impartial concerns, and transparency, focusing on specific domain fields such as finance or healthcare (Guidotti et al. 2018).
- **Integration**: Any XAI technique successfully integrated will demand a high level of planning and adjustment with current AI systems or workflows, not to mention interference (Adadi and Berrada 2018).

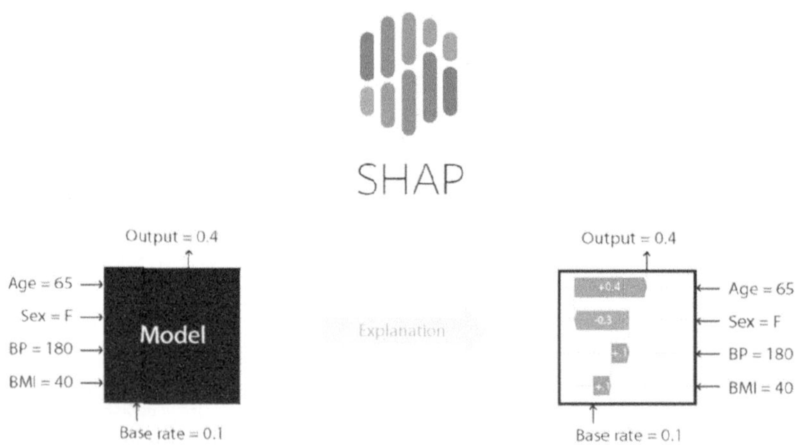

FIGURE 3.3 SHAP explanation.

Human–AI Interaction: Clinicians need effective protocols of human–AI interaction, which are likely not the full set of explanations needed by patients with psychiatric disabilities who may be in states vulnerable to differentially close pedagogically explicatory concepts (Abdul et al. 2018).

3.7 CONCLUSION

Future research projects will provide more opportunities for XAI as a human-centric approach to be effective, especially in healthcare, and will extend to more non-privacy and security areas. However, a roadmap that covers various stages from requirement analysis, model selection, integration of XAI methods, rigorous evaluation, next deployment, ongoing monitoring, and finally, governance and policy frameworks must be established to deploy XAI effectively. This ensures that XAI develops ethically and can be used in different industries. In summary, XAI is an answer instead of a black-box AI, especially within industries such as healthcare. The more complicated the AI algorithms, the more this suggests the necessity of more transparency, interpretability, and explainability of models. XAI techniques such as LIME and SHAP are up-and-coming, with considerable potential to guide in gaining a qualitative understanding of how machine models make the prediction. However, even though the potential of XAI is great, the successful deployment of XAI still has its impediments, i.e., complexity, user comprehension, ethical and legal issues, and integration with legacy systems.

REFERENCES

Adadi, A., and M. Berrada. "Peeking Inside the Black-box: A Survey on Explainable Artificial Intelligence (XAI)." *IEEE Access* 6 (2018): 52138–52160. https://doi.org/10.1109/ACCESS.2018.2870052.

Abdul, Ashraf, Jo Vermeulen, Danding Wang, Bryan Y. Lim, and Mohan S. Kankanhalli. "Trends and Trajectories for Explainable, Accountable, and Intelligible Systems." Proceedings of the 2018 CHI Conference on Human Factors in Computing Systems - CHI '18, 2018. https://doi.org/10.1145/3173574.3174156.

Arya, Vishal, Rachel K. E. Bellamy, Pin-Yu Chen, Amit Dhurandhar, Mark Hind, Samuel C. Hoffman, Stephanie Houde, Q. Vera Liao, Rich Luss, Aleksandra Mojsilović, Sameer Mourad, Peter Pedemonte, Raghavendra Raghavendra, Jenay Richards, Prasanna Sattigeri, Kush R. Shanmugam, Moninder Singh, Kush R. Varshney, David Wei, and Yong Zhang. "One Explanation Does Not Fit All: A Toolkit and Taxonomy of AI Explainability Techniques." *ArXiv.org*, September 14, 2019. https://doi.org/10.48550/arXiv.1909.03012.

Das, Anupam, and Piroozfar Rad. "Opportunities and Challenges in Explainable Artificial Intelligence (XAI): A Survey." *ArXiv.org*, June 22, 2020. https://doi.org/10.48550/arXiv.2006.11371.

Dastin, Jeffrey. "Amazon Scraps Secret AI Recruiting Tool That Showed Bias Against Women." *Reuters*, October 10, 2018. https://www.reuters.com/article/us-amazon-com-jobs-automation-insight/amazon-scraps-secret-ai-recruiting-tool-that-showed-bias-against-women-idUSKCN1MK08G/.

Garreau, Damien, and Ulrike Luxburg. "Explaining the Explainer: A First Theoretical Analysis of LIME." Proceedings of the 2020 International Conference on Machine Learning (ICML), June 3, 2020. https://proceedings.mlr.press/v108/garreau20a.html.

Gerlings, Jonas, Mikkel S. Jensen, and Arisa Shollo. "Explainable AI, But Explainable to Whom? An Exploratory Case Study of xAI in Healthcare." In *Handbook of Artificial Intelligence in Healthcare*, 169–198, 2021. https://doi.org/10.1007/978-3-030-83620-7_7.

Gilpin, Leilani H., David Bau, Ben Z. Yuan, Ayesha Bajwa, Michael Specter, and Latanya Sweeney Kagal. "Explaining Explanations: An Overview of Interpretability of Machine Learning." Proceedings of the 2018 IEEE 5th International Conference on Data Science and Advanced Analytics (DSAA), 2018. https://doi.org/10.1109/dsaa.2018.00018.

Giuste, Federica, Wei Shi, Yilun Zhu, Taruna Naren, Yiyu Sha, Lina Tong, Mayank Gupte, and May D. Wang. "Explainable Artificial Intelligence Methods in Combating Pandemics: A Systematic Review." *IEEE Reviews in Biomedical Engineering* 16 (2023): 5–21. https://doi.org/10.1109/rbme.2022.3185953.

Guidotti, Riccardo, Anna Monreale, Salvatore Ruggieri, Franco Turini, Fosca Giannotti, and Dino Pedreschi. "A Survey of Methods for Explaining Black Box Models." *ACM Computing Surveys* 51, no. 5 (2018): 1–42. https://doi.org/10.1145/3236009.

Hunt, Elle. "Tay, Microsoft's AI Chatbot, Gets a Crash Course in Racism from Twitter." *The Guardian*, February 9, 2018. https://www.theguardian.com/technology/2016/mar/24/tay-microsofts-ai-chatbot-gets-a-crash-course-in-racism-from-twitter.

Kramer, Adam D. I., Jamie E. Guillory, and Jeffrey T. Hancock. "Experimental Evidence of Massive-Scale Emotional Contagion Through Social Networks." *Proceedings of the National Academy of Sciences* 111, no. 24 (2014): 8788–8790. https://doi.org/10.1073/pnas.1320040111.

Kurniawan, Didit, Triyanto Triyanto, M. Wahyudi, and Latifah Pujiastuti. "Explainable Artificial Intelligence (XAI) for Trustworthy Decision-Making." *Jurnal Teknik Informatika C.I.T Medicom* 15, no. 5 (2023): 240–246. https://doi.org/10.35335/cit.Vol15.2023.622.pp240-246.

Murdoch, W. James, Chandan Singh, Karl Kumbier, Rima Abbasi-Asl, and Bin Yu. "Definitions, Methods, and Applications in Interpretable Machine Learning." *Proceedings of the National Academy of Sciences* 116, no. 44 (2019): 22071–22080. https://doi.org/10.1073/pnas.1900654116.

Pesquita, Catia. "Towards Semantic Integration for Explainable Artificial Intelligence in the Biomedical Domain." 2021. https://doi.org/10.5220/0010389707470753.

Tjoa, Erico, and Cuntai Guan. "A Survey on Explainable Artificial Intelligence (XAI): Toward Medical XAI." *IEEE Transactions on Neural Networks and Learning Systems* 32, no. 11 (2020): 1–21. https://doi.org/10.1109/tnnls.2020.3027314.

Vassiliades, Alexandros, Nick Bassiliades, and Theodore Patkos. "Argumentation and Explainable Artificial Intelligence: A Survey." *The Knowledge Engineering Review* 36 (2021): 1–26. https://doi.org/10.1017/s0269888921000011.

4 Technology and Infrastructure for XAI in Healthcare

Osama Burak Elhalid and Ali Hakan Isik

4.1 INTRODUCTION

Machine learning (ML) seems to have transformed a multitude of industries, allowing specialized practitioners in health, finance, and law to make data-driven decisions. However, as ML models advance, interpretability has become one of the most important issues of concern alongside trust in models, especially in domains that are sensitive and critical (Doshi-Velez & Kim, 2017). Predictions from deep learning architectures are usually provided through submodels known as black box models whose explainability is impractical, which poses challenges for some ethical and regulatory compliance guidelines. In attempts to solve these problems, techniques known as explainable AI (XAI) aimed at improving transparency in these models and providing more rational insight into their decision processes have emerged (Adadi & Berrada, 2018).

Among the most widely used interpretability methods, SHAP and LIME have risen to prominence. SHAP, rooted in cooperative game theory, assigns feature importance scores by fairly distributing contribution values across input features, ensuring a balanced and equitable assessment of each feature's impact (Lundberg & Lee, 2017). On the other hand, LIME operates by generating local approximations of model predictions using simplified surrogate models, allowing users to gain a clearer understanding of how individual predictions are derived (Ribeiro et al., 2016). Both methods play a pivotal role in making AI-driven decisions more interpretable, fostering trust and confidence between end-users and ML systems.

This study aims to conduct a comprehensive comparative analysis of SHAP and LIME, evaluating their respective strengths, limitations, and applicability across various domains. By leveraging these techniques, practitioners can significantly improve model transparency, ensure fairness in decision-making, and promote the ethical adoption of AI technologies. Furthermore, this research underscores the critical importance of integrating interpretability frameworks into AI systems to mitigate biases, enhance accountability, and facilitate regulatory compliance in AI-driven decision-making processes.

DOI: 10.1201/9781003605416-4

The findings of this study emphasize the need for continued innovation in XAI methodologies to address the evolving challenges posed by increasingly complex ML models. By prioritizing interpretability, the AI community can build systems that are not only powerful but also transparent, fair, and aligned with ethical standards. This, in turn, will pave the way for broader acceptance and responsible deployment of AI technologies across industries, ensuring that the benefits of ML are realized without compromising trust or accountability.

4.2 METHODOLOGY

4.2.1 Dataset

This study employs the Heart Disease Dataset, a well-established benchmark utilized extensively in medical research and ML applications. Originally compiled in 1988, this dataset consolidates patient records from four distinct sources: Cleveland, Hungary, Switzerland, and Long Beach V. While the complete dataset contains 76 attributes, research efforts predominantly focus on a refined subset of 14 key features that are most indicative of heart disease. The primary objective of this dataset is to facilitate binary classification, determining whether an individual has heart disease (denoted as 1) or is disease-free (denoted as 0).

4.2.1.1 Dataset Overview

- **Total Instances**: 1,025
- **Selected Features**: 14 (extracted from the original 76 attributes)
- **Target Variable**: Heart disease classification
  - **0**: No heart disease
  - **1**: Presence of heart disease

Table 4.1 provides a structured overview of the features included in a cardiovascular disease dataset, along with their corresponding values and descriptions. Each feature captures specific clinical and demographic information relevant to assessing heart disease risk. The dataset includes variables such as Age, Gender, and Chest Pain Type, which describe the individual's demographic and symptomatic characteristics. Clinical measurements, such as Resting Blood Pressure, Serum Cholesterol, and Fasting Blood Sugar, provide insights into the patient's physiological state. Diagnostic indicators, including Resting ECG Findings, Maximum Heart Rate Achieved, and Exercise-Induced Angina, reflect cardiovascular performance under stress. Additionally, features like Oldpeak, ST Segment Slope, Major Vessels Count, and Thalassemia Condition offer detailed information about potential ischemia and blood flow abnormalities. Finally, the Target Variable serves as the dependent variable, indicating the presence or absence of heart disease. This dataset is designed to support predictive modeling and analysis in cardiovascular health research.

This dataset serves as a critical resource for the development and evaluation of ML models focused on heart disease prediction. Its structured nature and clinically

TABLE 4.1
Description of Features in a Cardiovascular Disease Dataset

Column Name	Column Values	Description
Age	Numeric (e.g., 45, 60)	The individual's age in years.
Gender	1 (Male), 0 (Female)	Encoded as 1 for male and 0 for female.
Chest pain type	1: Typical angina, 2: Atypical angina, 3: Non-anginal pain, 4: Asymptomatic	Categorized into four distinct types of chest pain.
Resting blood pressure	Numeric (e.g., 120, 140)	Systolic blood pressure measured in a resting state (mm Hg).
Serum cholesterol	Numeric (e.g., 200, 250)	Total cholesterol concentration in the bloodstream (mg/dL).
Fasting blood sugar	1 (Yes), 0 (No)	Binary indicator denoting whether fasting blood sugar levels exceed 120 mg/dL.
Resting ECG findings	0: Normal, 1: ST-T Wave abnormalities, 2: Left ventricular hypertrophy	Electrocardiographic measurements classified into three categories.
Maximum heart rate achieved	Numeric (e.g., 150, 180)	The highest heart rate recorded during physical exertion.
Exercise-induced angina	1 (Yes), 0 (No)	Indicates whether angina symptoms appear during exercise.
Oldpeak	Numeric (e.g., 0.0, 2.5)	Measures ST segment depression relative to resting values, indicating potential ischemia.
ST segment slope	1: Upsloping, 2: Flat, 3: Downsloping	Characterizes the trend of the ST segment during peak exercise.
Major vessels count	0, 1, 2, 3	The number of major blood vessels observed through fluoroscopy.
Thalassemia condition	0: Normal, 1: Fixed defect, 2: Reversible defect	Represents thalassemia status, categorized into three types.
Target variable	0 (No heart disease), 1 (Heart disease)	The dependent variable indicating the presence or absence of heart disease.

relevant features make it a valuable tool for advancing predictive analytics in healthcare, thereby enhancing diagnostic accuracy and informed medical decision-making.

4.2.2 Data Anonymization

To preserve patient confidentiality, sensitive information such as names and social security numbers were removed from the dataset. Dummy values replaced any identifiable information, ensuring compliance with data privacy regulations.

4.2.3 Dataset Relevance

This dataset is highly valuable for developing predictive models due to its well-structured features and widespread usage in previous studies. The selected features are clinically significant and serve as strong predictors for the presence of heart disease. The data's balance and quality make it an excellent choice for ML and statistical analysis.

4.2.4 TensorFlow/Keras Model

As part of the heart disease prediction task in this study, a model was built and trained with TensorFlow/Keras. Figure 4.1 lists the model architecture and its workflow at a glance. The dataset was split into three parts; training data, which was used to enhance the model, testing data, which was used to benchmark performance, and rest of the data that remains undisclosed for future use in real-world scenarios. Built on Keras, an API enabling high-level interfacing with neural networks, and employing TensorFlow as the backend, the model traverses through various layers of data to arrive at a conclusion regarding the presence of heart disease.

The architecture incorporates fully connected layers with ReLU activations and uses a sigmoid function at the end for binary classification. Tensorflow/Keras provides a user-friendly implementation environment for deep learning algorithms, offering ease of use along with customization and growth potential, making it appealing for predictive analysis in healthcare (Chollet, 2018). The added dense layers within the architecture are instrumental in model training, as they facilitate learning intricate patterns in the dataset, which enhances classification accuracy (Abdar et al., 2021).

To enhance generalization and mitigate overfitting, dropout layers were incorporated into the model, randomly deactivating a fraction of neurons during training (Srivastava et al., 2014). Additionally, the Adam optimizer was employed for efficient gradient-based optimization, given its adaptive learning rate properties (Kingma & Ba, 2015). The model was trained using binary cross-entropy loss, a standard metric for binary classification problems, ensuring optimal convergence during training.

The output layer generates a binary outcome (0 or 1), representing the absence or presence of heart disease. The flow depicted in Figure 4.1 highlights the seamless data processing and training mechanisms inherent in TensorFlow and Keras, showcasing their powerful utilities in modern ML applications. The combination of TensorFlow's computational efficiency and Keras' user-friendly interface allows for effective implementation in medical diagnosis systems, reinforcing the potential of deep learning in healthcare analytics (Shickel et al., 2018).

Figure 4.1 provides a high-level schematic representation of an ML model designed for heart disease prediction using the *TensorFlow/Keras* framework. The pipeline consists of three main stages: *data processing, model training, and output generation.*

- **Dataset Partitioning**
- The dataset is structured into three subsets:

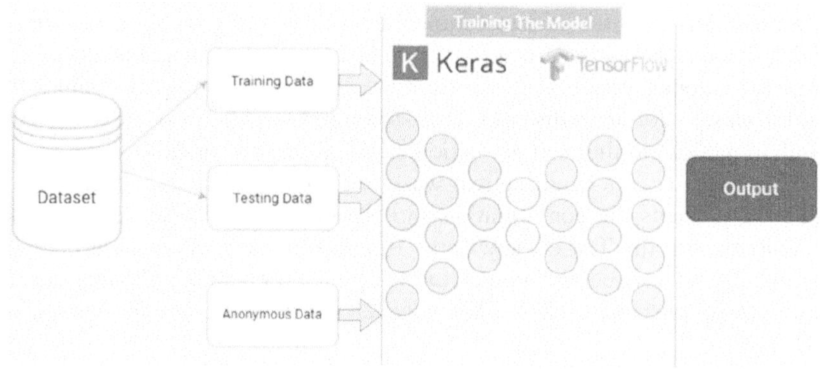

FIGURE 4.1 Workflow of the TensorFlow/Keras model for heart disease prediction.

- **Training Data**: Used for model learning and optimization, enabling weight and parameter adjustments to improve predictive accuracy.
- **Testing Data**: Employed to evaluate the model's generalization capabilities and performance on unseen data.
- **Anonymous Data**: Represents external, real-world data that could be used for validation in practical applications, simulating real-time model deployment.

- **Model Training with TensorFlow/Keras**
- The model is created through Keras, which offers a higher-level API and uses TensorFlow as its core. The principal structure of the model is made up of dense layers, which have many neurons, and these take part in extracting features and recognizing patterns. Moreover, the activation functions used, for instance ReLU (Rectified Linear Unit), further amplify non-linearity, which helps the model in understanding the intricate relationships embedded in the dataset.
- **Output Layer and Prediction**
- The last layer has a binary output and uses a sigmoid activation function. In this case, the output represents the prediction regarding the risk of potential heart disease, which is consistent with the aims of this study attempting to apply deep learning to medical diagnosis.
- **Significance of TensorFlow and Keras in the Model**
- TensorFlow and Keras provide key benefits in model implementation, including:
  - Efficient computation and scalability, allowing seamless processing of medical datasets.
  - A user-friendly, modular architecture that simplifies deep learning model construction.
  - Robust support for backpropagation and optimization algorithms, enhancing predictive accuracy.

This figure underscores the structured approach in designing an AI-driven diagnostic model, demonstrating the efficacy of deep learning in healthcare analytics.

The final output layer generates predictions in the form of binary values (0 for no heart disease, 1 for heart disease). This structured workflow ensures a systematic approach to model training and prediction, highlighting the flexibility and power of TensorFlow and Keras in handling real-world ML tasks.

Table 4.2 presents the configuration and attributes of the deep learning model implemented using the TensorFlow/Keras framework for heart disease prediction. The model follows a sequential architecture, designed for a binary classification task, where the target variable distinguishes between the presence and absence of heart disease.

This model comprises four layers, beginning with an input layer defined as Dense(64, activation='relu', input_shape=(13,)). There are then two hidden layers containing 32 and 16 neurons, respectively, both employing the ReLU (Rectified

TABLE 4.2
TensorFlow/Keras Model Configuration and Attributes

Attribute	Description
Framework	TensorFlow/Keras
Model type	Sequential model
Task	Binary classification
Number of layers	4
Layer details	Dense(64, activation='relu', input_shape=(13,)), Dense(32, activation='relu'), Dense(16, activation='relu'), Dense(1, activation='sigmoid')
Activation functions	1. ReLU for hidden layers 2. Sigmoid for output layer
Loss function	Binary cross-entropy
Optimizer	Adam
Metrics	Accuracy
Epochs	30
Batch size	32
Validation split	20%
Feature scaling	StandardScaler
Input features	13 (all columns except the target)
Output	Binary (1: Heart disease, 0: No heart disease)
Dataset size	Training: 80%, Testing: 20%
Performance metrics	Accuracy (Training and Validation), Confusion Matrix, Classification Report
Visualization	Accuracy vs Epochs, Loss vs Epochs
Attribute	Description
Framework	TensorFlow/Keras
Model type	Sequential model

Linear Unit) activation function. The output layer for binary classification consists of one neuron that uses a sigmoid activation function. The model is compiled with the Binary cross-entropy loss function and optimized using the Adam optimizer, with accuracy serving as the primary performance metric.

Accuracy is the primary performance metric, while in this case, the model calculates loss using Binary cross-entropy. The model is trained for 30 epochs using a batch size of 32, and the dataset is split so that 20% serves as validation. Validation data is used for measuring generalization performance. StandardScaler is used for scaling features, ensuring consistent distributions. Excluding the target variable, the dataset consists of 13 input features, split into 80% training data and 20% testing data.

Model evaluation is conducted using performance metrics, including training and validation accuracy, confusion matrix, and classification report. Additionally, visualization techniques, such as accuracy vs. epochs and loss vs. epochs plots, are employed to assess model convergence and potential overfitting or underfitting issues.

This configuration ensures that the model is well-optimized for heart disease prediction while maintaining interpretability and robustness in clinical applications.

Table 4.3 presents the classification report for the heart disease prediction model, outlining key performance indicators such as *precision*, *recall*, *F1-score*, and *support values* for both classes (True and False). These metrics provide a detailed evaluation of the model's predictive capabilities.

- For individual classes, precision measures the proportion of true positives for a specific class out of all instances classified to that class. In this case, the model achieves a *precision* score of 0.97 for "False" and 1.00 for "True" class, indicating high ability to accurately classify positive cases.
- *Recall* measures how well the model identifies actual positive instances. The recall score is *1.00* for the "False" class and *0.97* for the "True" class, indicating that the model captures nearly all positive cases, with only a minor margin of error.

TABLE 4.3
Classification Report

Precision Value	Recall Value	F1-Score Value	Support Value
False	0.97	1.00	102
True	1.00	0.97	103
Accuracy			0.99
Macro average	0.99	0.99	0.99
Weighted average	0.99	0.99	0.99

- *F1-score***,** which is the harmonic mean of precision and recall, demonstrates a good balance for both classes with a 0.99 score, meaning that the two metrics do not diverge significantly from each other.
- *Support* reflects the actual number of occurrences for each class in the dataset, with *102 samples* for the "False" class and *103 samples* for the "True" class.

The model achieves an overall accuracy of 0.99 that indicates high predictive performance. In addition, the value of the macro average and weighted average for precision, recall, and F1-score is 0.99, proving that the model is equally efficient across both classes.

These results underscore the model's effectiveness in distinguishing between patients with and without heart disease, making it a potentially valuable tool for clinical decision-making. However, to ensure robustness and generalizability, further validation on diverse and larger datasets is recommended.

Figure 4.2 shows the relationship between model accuracy and loss over training epochs during the model training process. This figure typically reflects a graph with two subgraphs: one representing the evolution of accuracy, and the other tracking the loss curve. Both accuracy and loss are key metrics for evaluating the performance of ML models over the course of the training process.

4.2.5 Model Accuracy

Definition: The accuracy curve shows how well a model performs at making correct predictions based on the data it is working on, whether it is training data or validation data.

4.2.5.1 Training Accuracy

Represents how well a model performs when dealing with the data that was used in the training process.

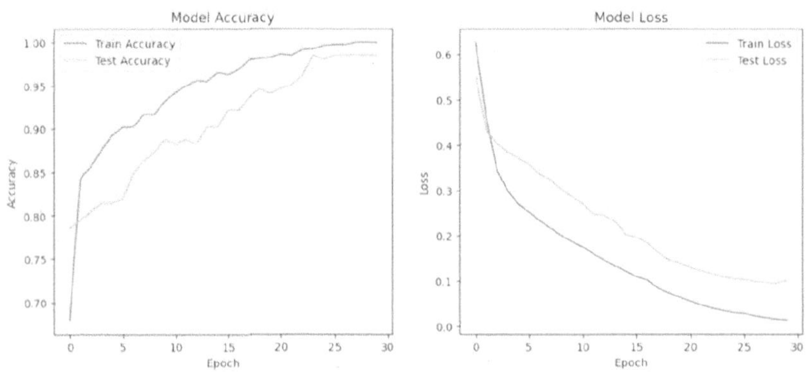

FIGURE 4.2 Model accuracy and model loss.

This measure typically improves over epochs, as the model learns patterns in the data and adjusts its weights to improve the accuracy of its predictions.

As training continues, the curve is expected to plateau, reflecting the model's effective learning of the data patterns.

4.2.5.2 Validation Accuracy

Refers to the model's performance when applied to new data that was not used during training, the validation set.

This accuracy is a key indicator of how well a model can generalize what it learned from the training data to unfamiliar data.

Ideally, validation accuracy should gradually improve in parallel with training accuracy, indicating that the model is gaining strong generalization ability without overfitting the training data.

4.2.6 Model Loss Analysis

4.2.6.1 Understanding Model Loss and Its Importance

Model loss is a fundamental measure that reflects how much an ML model deviates from expected outcomes. It quantifies the difference between the predicted values and actual data points, helping assess the model's effectiveness. The loss is computed using specific functions tailored to different tasks, such as *binary cross-entropy* for classification models or *mean squared error (MSE)* for regression problems. By evaluating loss, researchers can gauge how well a model learns from data and optimize it accordingly to enhance predictive performance.

4.2.6.2 Training Loss

Training loss measures the error a model encounters while learning from the training dataset. As the model undergoes multiple iterations, it adjusts its internal parameters to recognize patterns, ideally reducing this loss over time. A steady decline in training loss suggests the model is improving its ability to interpret data, whereas fluctuations or stagnation might indicate issues such as an inadequate learning rate or insufficient training epochs.

4.2.6.3 Validation Loss

Unlike validation loss, which measures the model's performance on new data, generalization is validation loss's primary focus. If both training and validation losses are reducing, the model is likely learning effectively. On the other hand, an increasing validation loss with decreasing training loss typically results in overfitting. Proper tuning using regularization, lowering model complexity, and/or increasing parameters indirectly relating to a model helps avoid overfitting and ensure generalization across datasets.

4.2.6.4 Balancing Accuracy and Loss

Maintaining a balance between accuracy and loss is essential for ensuring a robust and generalizable model. An optimal model achieves high accuracy with minimal loss across both training and validation data. Significant disparities between training and validation accuracy, or a rising validation loss, necessitate adjustments in the training process. Strategies to mitigate such issues include reducing the number of training epochs, incorporating regularization techniques, or refining the dataset.

Evaluating loss curves is fundamental in model assessment, as they provide a clear visualization of learning efficiency. By analyzing these trends, practitioners can ensure that the model achieves effective learning while avoiding pitfalls such as overfitting or poor generalization.

4.3 XAI-BASED MODEL ANALYSIS AND INTERPRETATION

Figure 4.3 illustrates the distinction between traditional *AI models* and *explainable AI (XAI) models*, emphasizing the role of interpretability in machine learning systems. The diagram is divided into two sections: the upper section represents a standard AI model workflow, while the lower section describes the extended capabilities of an XAI model.

The initial part details the steps executed by a standard AI model. It starts with training data that is worked on through a set of machine learning approaches, training algorithms, and learning procedures. The model afterward produces output in the form of predictions or classifications, navigating within the bounds of a given learning function seeking to enhance performance. However, self-explanatory validity is unavoidably inaccessible with these types of models, which makes understanding the decision-making processes very challenging.

In contrast, the second section introduces *XAI (Explainable Artificial Intelligence) models*, which enhance traditional AI systems by incorporating transparency and interpretability. Instead of solely focusing on performance optimization, XAI models

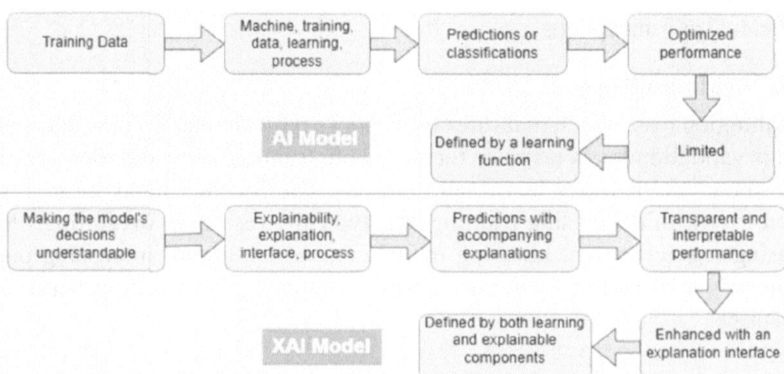

FIGURE 4.3 Comparison of AI models and explainable AI (XAI) models.

aim to *make the decision-making process understandable*. This is achieved through additional components such as explainability techniques, interactive interfaces, and explanation mechanisms. As a result, the model not only provides *predictions* but also generates accompanying *explanations*, making its reasoning more accessible to users.

An important distinction is that XAI models are *defined by both learning and explainable components*, ensuring that the decision-making process is not a "black box," but rather a comprehensible framework. Additionally, their performance is not just optimized but also *transparent and interpretable*, making them more suitable for high-stakes applications such as healthcare, finance, and legal decision-making. Finally, XAI models include an *explanation interface*, further enhancing the interpretability of the system by providing insights into how predictions were generated.

In contexts such as *heart disease analysis*, explainability is crucial for building trust in AI-driven diagnostic tools. Clinicians and medical professionals need to understand why an AI model predicts a high risk of heart disease for a particular patient. By integrating explainability techniques, such as *SHAP (Shapley Additive Explanations)*, XAI models can highlight which factors – such as *age*, *cholesterol levels, or blood pressure* – contributed most significantly to the prediction. This ensures that AI-driven decisions are not only accurate but also *clinically interpretable*, allowing for better-informed medical judgments.

4.3.1 SHAP (Shapley Additive Explanations)

SHAP, which stands for Shapley Additive Explanations, is a precision explainability method grounded on cooperative game theory, and it aims to explain the predictions made by ML models. In essence, SHAP values compute feature importance by allocating each feature's contribution, fairly distributing the importance across all possible feature combinations, thus ensuring fairness on feature importance (Lundberg & Lee, 2017). This is especially useful in healthcare-related problems such as heart disease prediction because its model-agnostic nature means that explanation formulation critical for model trustworthiness, understanding, and reliability can be instituted.

With respect to heart disease SHAP analysis, the methodology of SHAP assists in evaluating the individual pieces of evidence to help answer how the overarching diagnosis and disease-risk predictors help accurately predict the assessed data. Unlike other techniques focused on metrics of explaining the relative importance of features, SHAP does provide this capability but being glocal allows one to provide universal reasoning for phenomena while accessing the given diagnosis at an individual level. Thus, some of the key features that can be considered such as age, chol, trestbps, cp, and sex can be assessed alongside their specific role on the models' decision-making.

The application of SHAP within this work was to evaluate the clinical variables within the context of heart disease risk estimation. Additionally, SHAP interaction values were used to analyze feature dependencies to detect situations in which pairs of variables together determine the predictions made by the model. Results from this type of analysis, described in Section 3.2, enhance the understanding of relationships involving important risk factors and the output of the model, improving its interpretability along with clinical usefulness.

Figure 4.4 represents a *SHAP (SHapley Additive exPlanations) interaction plot*, which is used to analyze how each feature in a model impacts predictions and how they interact with other features.

To enhance the interpretability of the ML model, SHAP (SHapley Additive exPlanations) interaction values were utilized to examine the combined effects of feature pairs on model predictions. Figure 4.4 presents the SHAP interaction values for selected features, illustrating how certain variables interact to influence the model's output.

Each subplot in Figure 4.4 represents the interaction between the feature *age* and other key clinical variables, including *trestbps* (resting blood pressure), *sex*, *cp* (chest pain type), and *chol* (cholesterol level). The x-axis denotes the SHAP interaction values, while the y-axis lists the interacting features. The distribution of points reflects the magnitude and direction of the interaction effects, where positive values indicate a synergistic contribution, and negative values suggest a diminishing impact when both features are considered together.

The results highlight that the interaction between *age and sex* exhibits a relatively wider spread of SHAP interaction values, indicating that age may modulate the influence of sex on the model's predictions. Similarly, the *age and cp* interaction shows a noticeable effect, suggesting that chest pain type interacts with age in determining

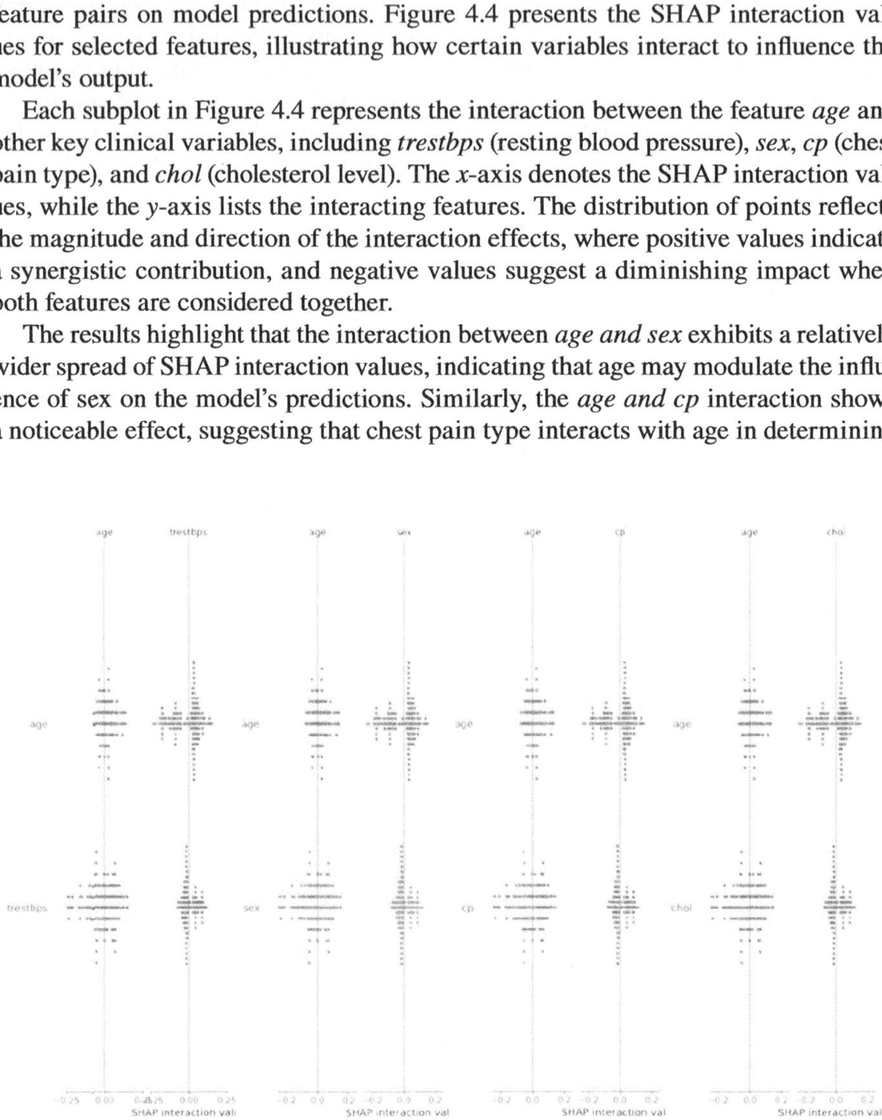

FIGURE 4.4 SHAP interaction values for features.

the model's outputs. In contrast, the *age and chol* interaction appears to be more concentrated around zero, implying a weaker interaction effect.

These findings underscore the importance of feature interactions in predictive modeling, particularly in clinical applications. Understanding how variables jointly influence predictions can contribute to improved model transparency and provide valuable insights for healthcare professionals in assessing cardiovascular disease risk.

Figure 4.5 presents a local explanation for the model's prediction of the "Disease" class, identifying key features and their value ranges that influenced the decision. Features such as slope, fbs, and ca were significant, with conditions like slope <= 1.01 and fbs <= −0.41 aligning with the model's learned patterns for the "Disease" class. The scale from *−0.2* to *0.2* quantifies each feature's contribution, with positive values supporting the "Disease" prediction. This local explanation highlights the importance of interpretability in understanding model behavior for individual instances, particularly in high-stakes domains like healthcare, where transparency and accountability are critical.

This LIME plot explains the *local model prediction for the class "Disease"* by showing which features most influenced the decision. The color and size of each bar represent the direction (positive or negative) and the magnitude of the feature's contribution. This helps in understanding the reasoning behind a particular prediction, making it easier to interpret the model's decision process for that instance.

Figure 4.6 illustrates the output of an ML model, specifically a binary classification model, designed to predict the presence or absence of a disease. The model's prediction probabilities indicate a high confidence level, with a probability of *1.00* for the presence of the disease and *0.00* for no disease. This suggests that the model is certain in its prediction that the patient has the disease.

The figure also includes a detailed breakdown of feature contributions toward the prediction of "No Disease." Each feature, such as fbs, cp, age, and others, is

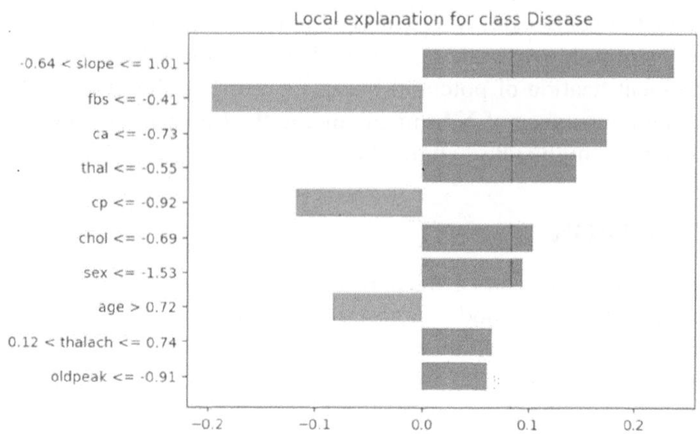

FIGURE 4.5 Local explanation for class "Disease"

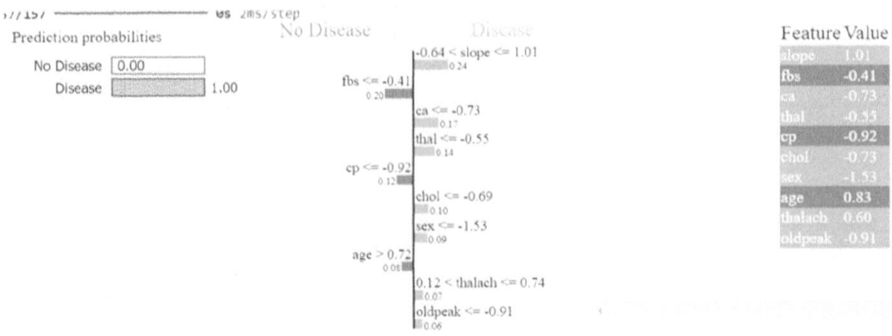

FIGURE 4.6 Prediction and feature contribution.

associated with a contribution score that quantifies its influence on the model's decision. For instance, the feature slope with a value of *1.01* contributed *0.24* to the "No Disease" prediction, while fbs with a value of *−0.41* contributed *0.20*. These scores provide insights into the relative importance of each feature in the model's decision-making process.

Additionally, the figure presents the actual values of the features used in the model for this specific prediction. For example, slope has a value of *1.01*, fbs has a value of *−0.41*, and age has a value of *0.83*. These values are crucial for understanding the specific input data that led to the model's prediction.

The interpretation of these contributions is essential for understanding the model's behavior. Although certain features like slope and fbs had significant contributions toward the "No Disease" prediction, the overall prediction of "Disease" with a probability of *1.00* indicates that other factors or combinations of features had a stronger influence on the final decision. This type of analysis is characteristic of explainable AI (XAI) techniques, such as SHAP or LIME, which aim to provide transparency into the model's decision-making process.

In the context of healthcare, where model interpretability is crucial, such detailed explanations help build trust among stakeholders, ensure ethical deployment, and facilitate the identification of potential biases or errors in the model. This analysis underscores the importance of XAI in enhancing the transparency and accountability of ML models in high-stakes applications.

4.4 CONCLUSION

In conclusion, both SHAP and LIME play pivotal roles in the field of explainable AI by providing interpretable, model-agnostic explanations for complex ML models. SHAP, with its foundation in game theory, offers a rigorous and consistent approach to assigning feature importance based on Shapley values, making it highly suitable for global and local model interpretability. On the other hand, LIME excels at offering local explanations by approximating the complex model with an interpretable one, making it ideal for understanding individual predictions. While SHAP offers more precise, mathematically grounded explanations, LIME provides more flexibility and adaptability in various contexts. The choice between SHAP and LIME largely depends on the specific requirements of the application, such as the need for model-agnostic explanations, scalability, or the granularity of interpretability. As ML continues to evolve, the integration of SHAP, LIME, and similar tools into AI systems will be critical in fostering trust, improving model validation, and ensuring ethical decision-making. Ultimately, the continued development of these interpretability methods is essential for the widespread adoption of AI technologies, ensuring that they are used responsibly, fairly, and transparently.

REFERENCES

Abdar, M., Ksią żek, W., Acharya, U. R., Makarenkov, V., & Nahavandi, S. (2021). A new machine learning technique for an accurate diagnosis of coronary artery disease. *Computer Methods and Programs in Biomedicine, 196*, 105722. https://doi.org/10.1016/j.cmpb.2020.105722

Adadi, A., & Berrada, M. (2018). Peeking inside the black-box: A survey on Explainable Artificial Intelligence (XAI). *IEEE Access, 6*, 52138–52160. https://doi.org/10.1109/ACCESS.2018.2870052

Chollet, F. (2018). *Deep learning with Python*. Manning Publications.

Doshi-Velez, F., & Kim, B. (2017). Towards a rigorous science of interpretable machine learning. *arXiv preprint arXiv:1702.08608*.

Kingma, D. P., & Ba, J. (2015). *Adam: A method for stochastic optimization*. International Conference on Learning Representations (ICLR). https://arxiv.org/abs/1412.6980

Lundberg, S. M., & Lee, S. I. (2017). *A unified approach to interpreting model predictions*. Proceedings of the 31st International Conference on Neural Information Processing Systems, Vol. 30, pp. 4765–4774. https://doi.org/10.1145/3149430.3149802

Ribeiro, M. T., Singh, S., & Guestrin, C. (2016). *"Why should I trust you?" Explaining the predictions of any classifier*. Proceedings of the 22nd ACM SIGKDD International Conference on Knowledge Discovery and Data Mining, 1135–1144. https://doi.org/10.1145/2939672.2939778

SHickel, B., Tighe, P. J., Bihorac, A., & Rashidi, P. (2018). Deep EHR: A survey of recent advances in deep learning techniques for electronic health record (EHR) analysis. *IEEE Journal of Biomedical and Health Informatics, 22*(5), 1589–1604. https://doi.org/10.1109/JBHI.2017.2767063

Srivastava, N., Hinton, G., Krizhevsky, A., Sutskever, I., & Salakhutdinov, R. (2014). Dropout: A simple way to prevent neural networks from overfitting. *Journal of Machine Learning Research, 15*(1), 1929–1958.

5 Data Management and Privacy

Mahreen Fatima, Arooj Fatima, Amjad Islam Aqib, Ayesha Tariq, and Ieman Tariq

5.1 IMPORTANCE OF HEALTH DATA AND MANAGEMENT

Definition and Types of Health Data:

Routinely collected electronic health data obtained for administrative and clinical purposes are increasingly used to study diseases.

5.1.1 Electronic Health Records (EHRs)

The American healthcare system is on the verge of embracing modern technology, much like industries such as finance, airlines, grocery stores, and manufacturing have done. This transformation will enable the creation and use of standardized databases in healthcare, often referred to as electronic medical records (EMRs), electronic health records (EHRs), or personal health records (PHRs) (Cowie et al., 2017).

Electronic health records (EHRs) can integrate various kinds of information by (1) improving the Generative Adversarial Network (GAN) model, (2) considering specific feature limitations, and (3) including important utility metrics for generating this data (Häyrinen et al., 2008).

5.1.2 Patient Reports

To provide care that focuses on the patient, creating a healthcare environment where patients can actively engage with their healthcare providers is important. One effective way to do this is by gathering patient-reported outcomes during regular medical visits. By consistently collecting this information, we can capture insights that only patients can share, including their experiences with symptoms, overall quality of life, daily functioning, personal values, preferences, and health goals (Lavallee et al., 2016).

DOI: 10.1201/9781003605416-5

5.1.3 Imaging Data

There has been a renewed interest in artificial intelligence (AI), especially with the advancements in machine learning (ML) and deep learning (DL). This progress is particularly beneficial for image analysis and radiomics, which is the study of imaging data. However, to truly grasp complex diseases and ensure accurate diagnoses for effective treatment, we need to successfully combine various types of data, including clinical, imaging, and molecular information. Aside from having enough computing power, the right algorithms, and robust data systems in place, there are three crucial factors that are often overlooked: First, it's essential to have many independent, large, and high-quality datasets. Second, having knowledge from the specific field and established frameworks is vital. Lastly, it is important to establish different networks that highlight the important connections between various biological components (Holzinger et al., 2019).

5.1.4 Genomic Data

Genetic testing isn't a regular part of most medical care yet. However, with the rise of electronic health records, there's a great chance to include genetic testing in different healthcare settings. There are some challenges to integrating genetic information into these records. These challenges include the complexity of genetic test results, the absence of standardized methods for managing genetic and clinical data, and the current limitations of electronic health records when it comes to storing and analyzing genetic information (Kho et al., 2013).

5.1.5 Health Data Wearable Devices

Imagine having your personal health assistant right on your wrist. Wearable devices are making healthcare more accessible and fun. They collect information about your body, and that data helps us understand how you're doing. It's like having your own health expert, always keeping an eye on you (Cilliers, 2020).

5.1.6 Challenges in Data Management

Scientific workflows play a crucial role in today's science. Many areas rely on these workflows to organize and execute numerous computational tasks. Although there has been a lot of research focused on running workflows in an efficient and dependable way particularly in distributed systems, there are still several challenges related to data management that need to be tackled (Chen et al., 2013).

5.1.7 Large Data Volumes

Data is growing at an incredible rate, making it tough to manage the enormous amounts we now have, even reaching exabytes. One of the biggest challenges is that the volume of data is expanding much faster than our computing power can keep up.

The term “Big Data” can be misleading because it emphasizes size without considering other important characteristics. Big data comes with various features—like volume, speed of growth, diversity, unpredictability, usefulness, and complexity—that create numerous challenges in handling and analyzing it (Katal et al., 2013).

5.1.8 Data Integration

The vast amounts of data generated and managed by industries and research institutions are beginning to exceed current infrastructure capabilities. Improvements in how organizations operate involve various aspects of handling data, such as storage, management, maintenance, integration, and ensuring different systems work well together. Among these areas, focusing on data integration and interoperability can greatly enhance an organization’s overall performance. However, integrating and making different data systems work together is a complex challenge, especially when dealing with the diverse types of data that organizations use in big data settings. To effectively tackle these challenges, a thorough approach is essential (Kadadi et al., 2014).

5.1.9 Data Accuracy

Data accuracy is an essential part of data quality. It means that the information recorded for something is accurate. For a data value to be accurate, it needs to not only be the right value but also be presented in a clear and consistent way (Olson, 2003).

5.1.10 Data Timeliness

Offering a real-time context information service is challenging because of three main reasons: first, the information sources are always changing; second, users have different needs regarding how accurate the data should be and how quickly they want it; and third, the conditions of the system itself are always shifting (Han and Venkatasubramanian, 2007).

5.1.11 Role of XAI in Data Management

The emergence of AI has perturbed the field of healthcare in profound ways. These technologies offer spectacular means of diagnosing diseases, outcome prediction, and treatment design. XAI seeks to assist health practitioners in comprehending the decision-making and prediction processes of an AI system. There are two main categories of XAI methodologies: global approaches and local approaches. Global approaches are concerned with providing explanations for the general AI model reasoning processes, whereas local approaches deal with why a particular AI system rendered a specific response to a particular case, like the reasoning behind the diagnosis for a particular patient or the details surrounding an individual’s diagnostic images (Metta et al., 2024).

5.1.12 Role of XAI in Health Data Collection and Processing

A new trend in artificial intelligence is called explainable AI (XAI), which focuses on making AI models easier for people to understand. XAI explains how these models arrive at their decisions and predictions, which is particularly crucial in the healthcare field. By shedding light on how patient data is analyzed, XAI enhances clinical practices and encourages transparency, making it essential for improving healthcare solutions (Saraswat et al., 2022).

5.1.13 Advantages of Explainable Models

Explainable artificial intelligence (XAI) focuses on creating methods in machine learning that help people understand how these systems work. This understanding allows users to trust the technology more and create models that are easier to explain. When choosing the best way to develop an XAI application, it's important to have a solid grasp of the main concepts behind XAI and the programming tools that go with it (Dwivedi et al., 2023).

5.1.14 Reducing Algorithmic Bias

Algorithmic bias refers to the unfair treatment that algorithms can cause, particularly concerning protected characteristics like gender and race. Many researchers have attempted to define what fairness means and find ways to address bias, but there isn't a clear agreement on definitions and ways to measure fairness that fits all societies, times, and cultures. To keep the important aspects of the original data while removing bias-related information, we suggest a preprocessing method that relies on ideas from information theory. This method avoids conflicts in a dual optimization process by splitting the latent space into two separate areas (Kim and Cho, 2022).

The use of algorithm-based decision-making systems powered by artificial intelligence and machine learning is becoming more common in important areas like finance, healthcare, criminal justice, and hiring. These systems are meant to analyze data and make decisions automatically, but they have raised serious concerns about built-in biases that could lead to unfair treatment. These biases often come from factors such as past inequalities, unbalanced training data, and models that don't work well in all situations. For example, some resume screening tools have shown a bias against graduates from women's colleges, while certain healthcare algorithms have been found to unfairly estimate risks for different racial groups (Patel and Uddin, 2022).

5.1.15 Building Patient Trust and Acceptance

The rise of legal and ethical challenges surrounding AI applications, especially in the medical field, brings significant concerns since these decisions directly impact people's health and well-being. This situation creates difficulty in making informed choices for both patients and healthcare providers, as the reliability of AI can be questionable, leading to less accountability for mistakes. Consequently, the idea of what makes AI trustworthy remains vague. However, experts highlight three main areas essential for creating trustworthy AI: legitimacy, morality, and robustness. Legitimacy focuses on following laws and regulations, morality is about upholding values and ethical principles, and robustness deals with ensuring safety and security (Albahri et al., 2023).

5.2 PRIVACY AND SECURITY OF HEALTH DATA

This study analyzes data privacy regulations in the United States and Germany, particularly HIPAA, HITECH, BDSG, and PDSG. It investigates the implications of these regulations on healthcare delivery, research, and personalized treatment. The report also looks at the public health consequences, including how to comply with global regulations like GDPR and effectively address public health issues while upholding strict data protection guidelines. Aiming for a balance between regulation and healthcare innovation, the study offers strong policy analyses, critiques, and recommendations for both nations. The study emphasizes the significance of harmonized international data privacy standards in protecting patient information security and advancing public health.

Although their implementations differ, both Germany and the United States adopt elements of the Bismarck healthcare model (Adler-Milstein and Jha, 2017). Employers and employees often contribute to the cost of the insurance system used by the Bismarck model through payroll deductions (Myers, 2024). In the United States, 155 million Americans (Davis, 2022), According to the Bismarck model's tenets, around half of the population is insured by commercial insurance companies via their employers (Cwiek et al., 2023; Myers, 2024). Because of this common basis for providing healthcare, comparing the two countries is not only pertinent but also instructive, allowing us to examine the effects of data privacy regulations on healthcare in comparable healthcare systems.

Furthermore, Germany is in a unique situation when it comes to regulating data privacy. Germany was the birthplace of the world's first data privacy regulations in the years following World War II. These laws established a standard for data protection and are now used as a guide by nations worldwide. Germany is a perfect benchmark to evaluate and compare data privacy legislation in other countries because of its strong structure, which allows us to learn a lot about how data privacy regulation has changed over time. Therefore, this study honors the historical significance of Germany's contributions to the field of healthcare while also shedding light on the present condition of data privacy in this context (Myers, 2024).

In the United States, the data privacy concerning healthcare is under the purview of two acts: the Health Information Portability and Accountability Act (HIPAA) (Regulation, 2016) and the Health Information Technology for Economic and Clinical Health Act (HITECH) (Evans, 2018). HITECH supports HIPAA by emphasizing the importance of innovation in healthcare technology and the safeguarding of electronic health records. Undoubtedly, complex legislation and compliance requirements have dominated US healthcare for decades, and HIPAA is no exception. Gold and McLaughlin (2016) suggest that HIPAA has fundamentally shaped how health data is processed, exchanged, and protected within the American healthcare system.

In Germany, healthcare privacy is extensively covered by laws like the Federal Data Protection Act, which is known as BDSG (Abdelhadi, 2021) along with the Patient Data Protection Act, also termed as Patientendatenschutzgesetz (Myers, 2024). These legislations impose severe regulations on data processing and highlight the distinctive view of a European country towards the privacy of healthcare data.

The purpose of this study is to examine two nations' legal systems and comprehend how they affect public health and customized treatment. It seeks to identify the parallels and discrepancies between data privacy regulations and how they influence patient care and healthcare innovation.

The ethical use of genetic data, which is essential for the fair provision of tailored care, is the study's main focus. The study of genetics holds promise for transforming prognosis, diagnosis, and disease prevention (Saki, 2024). However, the possibility of abuse or illegal access jeopardizes personal freedom and rights. International data exchange is crucial, as seen by the convergence of genome research and public health. The scope and depth of datasets accessible for study may be restricted in the absence of stringent laws due to data privacy and security issues (Olorunsogo et al., 2024). Developing public health policy that regulates genomic and personalized medicine research begins with addressing these issues. Health equity is promoted by actions to strengthen genetic information security and privacy, which enables more thorough and representative study results.

5.2.1 XAI and Privacy

Prior to the digital age, in-person consultations were the main method used to gather patient health data, which was then physically entered onto paper (Khatiwada et al., 2024). Following that, these records—which included imaging tests, lab test results, clinical observations, and doctor's notes—were physically stored at medical institutions. The procedure was laborious and frequently required faxing or mailing, which might cause delays or result in the loss of important data. A paradigm shift toward electronic health records (EHRs) was brought about by technological advancements in healthcare, which made it easier to store, retrieve, and share patient data. Another significant step toward the introduction of patient-generated health data (PGHD) is this discovery (Khatiwada et al., 2024).

Patients now have unparalleled access to a wealth of health data thanks to the digital age, which has increased demand for platforms and technologies that allow tracking of individual health indicators. Wearable technology and home monitoring systems have responded to the need for improved healthcare outcomes by offering useful data outside of conventional clinical settings (Liu et al., 2016).

Patients may now more easily document their everyday experiences, including the development of symptoms and the usage of drugs, thanks to the increasing use of digital platforms. The implications of this shift go beyond the realm of routine data collection. Researchers, medical experts, and industrial stakeholders might all have diverse perspectives on PGHD. When the phrases "health data," "patient data," or "generated data" are used, they should be interpreted as particularly referring to patient-generated health data (PGHD), as it is commonly used to describe health data created by patients (Khatiwada et al., 2024; Winter and Davidson, 2022).

Over the past several years, explainable AI (XAI) has expanded dramatically and emerged as a vibrant area of study within the broader subject of artificial intelligence (AI). With study themes spanning areas beyond computer science, it has developed into a multidisciplinary, interdisciplinary, and transdisciplinary field (Minh et al., 2022). The expansion of XAI can be linked to the growing usage of AI, especially in machine learning and deep learning methods that are applied in vital fields like healthcare and finance. In response to this need, XAI was created with the goal of developing frameworks for describing AI systems and their results (Adadi and Berrada, 2018).

But there are a lot of issues and topics that need further thought, investigation, and research. Explainability, along with respect for human autonomy, damage reduction, and fairness, is regarded as one of the four ethical criteria for trustworthy AI. A thorough evaluation of XAI's overall influence on the development of trustworthy AI systems is hampered by the lack of clarity surrounding its precise relationship to other prerequisites for reliable AI. Recent research has looked at the link between explainability and robustness, the relationship between explainability and trustworthiness, and certain XAI myths and drawbacks (Longo et al., 2024).

The community is beginning to critically examine the path thus far and the justifications offered in the literature to support it as XAI research develops. "Explainable AI: Beware of Inmates Running the Asylum," for instance, demonstrates how explainability research frequently overlooks information from fields other than computer science (Millers et al., 2017). According to a discussion of the connection between explainability and transparency, explanations ought to be customized for the model's target audience, which may include developers, designers, regulators, or members of the general public. This has increased the complexity of XAI and rekindled the need to modify explanations according to the audience and take domain-specific expertise into account while creating them (Felzmann et al., 2020).

To provide useful explanations for all parties impacted by and involved with AI systems, interdisciplinary cooperation is essential. On the other hand, empirical research on the efficacy of explanations is far too limited. XAI frequently puts comprehensibility ahead of thorough and accurate explanations, which might lead to explanations that don't match how the AI system really produced a prediction (Longo et al., 2024).

The community urgently needs a global vision and discussion about how to move forward in the future development of XAI (Longo et al., 2024). In order to meet this requirement, this research publication brings together a diverse group of specialists to jointly identify and address unresolved issues in XAI research. The objective is to provide a proposal that is amenable to debate and provides fresh viewpoints and ideas for creating and refining techniques as well as utilizing current techniques in new fields (Antons et al., 2023; Longo et al., 2024). An international privacy guideline called "privacy by design" was approved in 2010 to safeguard personal information kept in organizations. It seeks to swiftly and effectively identify and address data breaches. With a focus on data reduction and pseudonymization, the GDPR addresses this approach as a legal requirement for data controllers and processors. In order to ensure GDPR compliance and safeguard data subjects, these regulations are taken into account early on in the development of IT systems. Privacy by design is predicated on seven principles: proactive rather than reactive; preventative rather than corrective; privacy by default; privacy included into the design; end-to-end security—complete lifecycle protection; full functionality—positive-sum, not zero-sum; openness and visibility—maintain it open; and respect for user privacy—maintain it user-centric (Alshammari, 2019). Since the GDPR was implemented in 2016, privacy by design has been widely accepted, with the European Commission supporting this approach to promote data security. Since developers and engineers are ultimately in charge of making goods, it is their duty to promote privacy by design while adhering to GDPR (Tamò-Larrieux et al., 2018).

To sum up, privacy by design is a proactive strategy for safeguarding user privacy, minimizing data, and preserving personal information. It is included in the user interface and design, preventing erroneous divisions between security and privacy.

5.3 THREATS AND SOLUTIONS

5.3.1 Cybersecurity Risks in Healthcare

The healthcare industry is one of the most targeted sectors by cybercriminals due to the high value of medical data. Personal health information (PHI) contains sensitive details such as names, addresses, medical histories, and financial records, making it a lucrative target for hackers. Unlike financial data, which can be quickly devalued by canceling credit cards, PHI retains its value for longer periods, allowing cybercriminals to use it for fraudulent activities, including identity theft and insurance fraud. The increasing digitization of healthcare records has amplified these risks, making cybersecurity a critical concern for healthcare organizations worldwide. One of the most pressing cybersecurity threats in healthcare is data breaches. Such incidents happen when people who are not permitted access to patient records get into them, often resulting in the leakage or unauthorized access of private medical information. Leaked healthcare information can be sold on the dark web or used to perpetrate deceptive schemes. Sometimes, attackers exploit such sensitive information to submit fraudulent health insurance claims or unlawfully acquire prescription medications. An entire industry painstakingly builds its reputation over decades, only to face colossal financial and reputational damages from data breaches that can apparently affect thousands, if not millions, of patients' private credentials (Wall Street Journal, 2024).

Another growing concern is ransomware attacks, in which cybercriminals encrypt healthcare data and demand a ransom to restore access. These attacks can paralyze hospital operations, preventing medical staff from accessing critical patient information. In severe cases, hospitals have been forced to cancel surgeries, delay treatments, and divert patients to other facilities. The financial impact of ransomware attacks can be devastating, as healthcare providers may be pressured to pay the ransom to restore services quickly. However, there is no guarantee that attackers will unlock the data even after payment, leaving organizations vulnerable to further exploitation. Phishing attacks are also a major cybersecurity risk in the healthcare sector. Cybercriminals often use deceptive emails and messages to trick employees into revealing login credentials or downloading malware (*The Guardian*, 2024). These attacks exploit human error, making them particularly dangerous in fast-paced healthcare environments. Once inside a system, attackers can move laterally, gaining access to sensitive databases and infrastructure. Phishing attacks are responsible for a significant portion of healthcare breaches, highlighting the need for continuous employee training on cybersecurity best practices. Internet of Medical Things (IoMT) vulnerabilities add another layer of cybersecurity risk (Reuters, 2025). Many healthcare organizations rely on interconnected medical devices such as pacemakers, insulin pumps, and remote monitoring systems. While these devices enhance patient care, they often lack robust security measures, making them easy targets for hackers. A compromised medical device could be manipulated to cause physical harm to patients or serve as an entry point for attackers to access an entire hospital network. As the use of IoMT expands, securing these devices is becoming increasingly important. Weak access controls and inadequate authentication mechanisms further expose healthcare organizations to cyber threats. Many hospitals and clinics still use outdated security practices, such as shared login credentials and weak passwords, which make it easier for attackers to gain unauthorized access. Implementing multifactor authentication (MFA) and strict role-based access controls can significantly reduce the risk of unauthorized data exposure. However, many organizations struggle to implement these security measures due to legacy systems and budget constraints (Reuters, 2024).

Supply chain attacks also pose a growing risk in the healthcare industry. Many healthcare providers rely on third-party vendors for services such as cloud storage, electronic health record (EHR) management, and medical device manufacturing. If a vendor's system is compromised, attackers can use it as a gateway to infiltrate healthcare networks. Supply chain vulnerabilities highlight the need for rigorous vendor risk assessments and cybersecurity compliance standards to protect patient data. Regulatory and compliance challenges further complicate the cybersecurity landscape in healthcare. Organizations must comply with regulations such as the Health Insurance Portability and Accountability Act (HIPAA) in the United States, the General Data Protection Regulation (GDPR) in Europe, and other data protection laws worldwide. However, achieving full compliance can be challenging, especially for smaller healthcare providers with limited resources. Non-compliance not only increases the risk of cyberattacks but also results in hefty fines and legal consequences. As cyber threats continue to evolve, healthcare organizations must adopt a proactive approach to cybersecurity. This includes investing in advanced security technologies such as artificial intelligence (AI)-driven threat detection, implementing comprehensive employee training programs, and regularly updating security protocols. By strengthening cybersecurity defenses, healthcare providers can protect patient data, maintain trust, and ensure uninterrupted medical services in an increasingly digital world (The Guardian, 2024).

5.3.2 Proposed Solutions

In the evolving landscape of healthcare, safeguarding patient data is paramount. Two innovative solutions have emerged to address cybersecurity challenges: blockchain technology and explainable artificial intelligence (XAI). These technologies offer promising avenues for enhancing data security and transparency in healthcare systems.

5.3.3 Blockchain for Data Security

The implementation of blockchain technology brings a new dimension to a decentralized, globally distributed, and immutable ledger system, which further enhances the integrity and security that health data entails. As stated by Deloitte (2016), the patient's data is encrypted and shared across a network, making it impossible for unauthorized personnel to gain access to the data. It guarantees that the medical records are stored on the blockchain in a manner that enables them to be accessed only by the parties given explicit permission, which enhances the privacy of the patient alongside the security of the data. This protocol provides a secure login alongside defined methodologies for key sharing and data sharing between authorized representatives, which gives more security to the medical records. Alzubi et al. (2023) propose the immediate application of this protocol on sensitive medical data to offer protection in real time. In addition, the blockchain's quality of transparency bolsters users' confidence alongside its unchangeability, allowing smooth data sharing across healthcare providers. This is significant for Health Information Exchanges and aids in the advancement of electronic medical records into more advanced, self-contained, and secure technologies. Blockchain technology improves the self-governed, confidential, and cross-compatible aspects of health data by focusing on patients as the core of the healthcare ecosystem.

5.3.4 Explainable Artificial Intelligence (XAI) for Real-Time Threat Detection and Monitoring

Explainable artificial intelligence (XAI) enhances transparency in AI-driven systems by providing clear explanations of decision-making processes. In healthcare, XAI can be utilized to monitor network activities and detect anomalies indicative of cyber threats in real time. By understanding the rationale behind AI decisions, healthcare providers can trust and effectively respond to potential security incidents (Arrieta et al., 2020). A survey by Tjoa and Guan (2020) highlights the application of XAI techniques in healthcare, particularly in medical imaging. The study categorizes various XAI methods and emphasizes their role in increasing interpretability in medical imaging topics. This interpretability is crucial for clinicians to understand and trust AI-driven diagnostic tools, thereby facilitating their integration into clinical practice. Furthermore, XAI can be applied to intrusion detection systems (IDS) in healthcare. By integrating XAI into IDS, healthcare organizations can enhance transparency, trust, and accountability in their cybersecurity measures.

This integration allows for the real-time detection of cyber threats, enabling prompt and effective responses to potential security incidents.

5.3.5 Ethical Challenges

Implementing advanced technologies in healthcare necessitates a careful approach to ethical considerations, particularly in handling patient data and ensuring algorithmic transparency. Key areas of focus include maintaining patient confidentiality, obtaining informed consent for data usage, and preventing algorithmic biases. Healthcare providers must establish ethical guidelines and governance frameworks to uphold trust and accountability in AI-driven systems.

5.3.6 Patient Confidentiality

Protecting patient confidentiality is paramount in healthcare. The integration of AI systems often requires extensive data collection, raising concerns about how patient information is stored, accessed, and shared. Ensuring that data is anonymized and securely stored is essential to prevent unauthorized access and potential breaches. According to a study published in BMC Medical Ethics, key ethical considerations for AI in healthcare include the privacy of patient data and the need for robust data protection measures (Hasan et al., 2024).

5.3.7 Informed Consent

Informed consent for data usage is one of the ethical challenges that require the utmost attention. The development of an AI system certainly uses data, and patients must know how their information is utilized. Trust is built when there is clear communication about how data is used, which helps patients take control over their information. The CDC underlines that the consent must be informed, which means, as a patient, you must be educated about how your information is going to be applied and for what reasons in health AI systems (CDC, 2024).

5.3.8 Preventing Algorithmic Bias

Algorithmic bias in AI systems can lead to unequal treatment and exacerbate existing health disparities. Biases often stem from non-representative training data, resulting in AI models that perform inadequately for certain populations. Addressing this issue requires careful dataset curation and ongoing monitoring to ensure fairness and equity in AI-driven healthcare solutions. A review in *Frontiers in Surgery* discusses the ethical challenges posed by AI, including the risk of bias and discrimination, emphasizing the need for vigilant oversight (Naik et al., 2022).

5.3.9 Establishing Ethical Guidelines and Governance Frameworks

To navigate these ethical challenges, healthcare organizations should develop comprehensive guidelines and governance frameworks. These frameworks should outline best practices for data handling, algorithm development, and system deployment, ensuring that ethical considerations are integrated at every stage. The HITRUST Alliance underscores the importance of such frameworks, highlighting key areas like safety, liability, patient privacy, and data ownership as critical components of ethical AI implementation in healthcare (HITRUST Alliance, 2024).

5.3.10 Integrating Blockchain and Explainable AI (XAI)

Combining blockchain with XAI allows healthcare organizations to improve the security, transparency, and ethical governance of sensitive patient information. The decentralized blockchain ledger upholds data accuracy and protection while XAI enables responsible and trustworthy access to processes made by AI. Applied Sciences describes the ways in which blockchain offers security, reliability, privacy, and interoperability, fundamentally transforming the healthcare system (Alabdulatif et al., 2022).

5.4 REAL-WORLD APPLICATIONS AND CASE STUDIES

5.4.1 Applications of XAI Methods

Numerous industries, including banking, education, agriculture, environmental research, and medicine and healthcare, have made extensive use of XAI techniques. Some of the numerous uses of XAI techniques are covered in this section. Providing case studies and examples to stakeholders is the aim.

5.4.2 Medicine, Healthcare, and Bioinformatics

Clinical Decision Support Systems and other AI-based systems are essential for medical decision-making, patient communication, and therapy selection. However, since erroneous diagnoses can have a serious effect on patients, faith in AI-supported medical judgments is essential. It can be useful to measure trust and dependence by comprehending AI-supported judgments. In high-stakes situations like electronic medical records, COVID-19 identification, chronic renal illness, and fungal or bloodstream infections, XAI techniques like LIME, SHAP, and Anchors have been used. Although explainability is a complicated topic with cultural, ethical, legal, and medical factors, AI-based systems may be able to diagnose problems more accurately than human specialists. Linking XAI to the standards for reliable AI in this field is crucial. According to the EU AI Act, a thorough examination of the reliability standards for a real-world case study in AI for healthcare promotes adherence to regulations in high-risk situations.

5.4.3 Finance

Banks and financial organizations are using AI to increase service security, save costs, automate procedures, and obtain a competitive edge. Artificial intelligence (AI) algorithms are used to diagnose investment portfolios for optimization, identify fraud, and forecast credit risk. However, for legal reasons, this frequently calls for explainability and openness. This is especially crucial in the consumer banking industry, where banks are required to adhere to stringent laws such as the USA Fair Housing Act (FHA) and the USA Equal Credit Opportunity Act (ECOA) in order to reveal unfavorable action codes and give concise justifications for their choices. The General Data Protection Regulation (GDPR) law in Europe has similar regulations and enforcement.

The use of AI algorithms makes it more challenging for banks to offer reliable and consistent justifications. Banks may face regulatory fines and lose the trust of their customers as a result of this explainability issue. The requirement to guarantee the resilience and stability of AI systems—which may be exposed to harsh market conditions and unforeseen circumstances—drives the need for XAI in investment banking.

5.4.4 Environmental Science and Agriculture

The intelligent study, modeling, and management of agricultural and forest ecosystems—which are essential to protecting our planet for coming generations—have seen a rise in the use of AI. For example, drones may be used to gather data and machine learning techniques can be used to estimate the amount of carbon stored in forests. Forest carbon stock is a crucial measure for climate study and management. Because it offers vital information on forest attributes including tree species, size, and density, forest inventories are also essential to forest engineering.

However, high-dimensional and heterogeneous data are frequently collected using sensor-based technologies, which result in models that are not very robust. The reliability of such models is undermined by the fact that even small changes in the input data can have a substantial impact on the model's output. Since AI techniques for creating forest inventory models are susceptible to a number of sources of uncertainty, such as measurement error, geographic variability, and model misspecification, it is difficult to build techniques for quantifying and propagating uncertainty in realistic settings. As a result, it is crucial to evaluate and improve the resilience of AI techniques for the models and conclusions they generate.

5.4.5 Education

The Artificial Intelligence in Education (AIED) area attempts to develop educational technologies powered by AI to assist teachers, learners, and educational bodies in performing their functions (Chen et al., 2025). The objective of AIED is to develop models and adaptive systems that identify the capabilities and shortcomings of the students so that they may be provided with the appropriate material and instruction designed to fulfill their learning needs. These resources can enhance metacognitive functions including planning, introspection, and self-monitoring (Sufyan Ghaleb and Alshiha, 2023).

AIED technologies can reduce dropout rates by serving as intelligent teaching assistants for teachers, helping with classroom management, grading tests, and responding to student inquiries. Using Large Language Models (LLMs) to create new textual material in response to human input prompts is the most current use of AIED (Almusaed et al., 2023). The control of AI-based technologies, especially educational recommender systems, which are being used more and more to automate and customize learning activities, has drawn criticism. Fairness, accountability, explainability, ethics, and the effect on students' agency and self-regulated learning are among the issues raised by these technologies (Srinivasa et al., 2022).

REFERENCES

Abdelhadi, M. A. (2021). The right to privacy in the age of pandemics "a study in German and European law". 60–1 ,(1)7 ,مجلة الدراسات القانونية والاقتصادية.

Adadi, A., and Berrada, M. (2018). Peeking inside the black-box: A survey on Explainable Artificial Intelligence (XAI). *IEEE Access*, 6, 52138–52160.

Adler-Milstein, J., and Jha, A. K. (2017). HITECH Act drove large gains in hospital electronic health record adoption. *Health Affairs*, 36(8), 1416–1422.

Alabdulatif, A., Khalil, I., and Saidur Rahman, M. (2022). Security of blockchain and AI-empowered smart healthcare: Application-based analysis. *Applied Sciences*, *12*(21), 11039.

Albahri, A. S., Duhaim, A. M., Fadhel, M. A., Alnoor, A., Baqer, N. S., Alzubaidi, L., Albahri, O. S., Alamoodi, A. H., Bai, J., and Salhi, A. (2023). A systematic review of trustworthy and explainable artificial intelligence in healthcare: Assessment of quality, bias risk, and data fusion. *Information Fusion*, 96, 156–191.

Almusaed, A., Almssad, A., Yitmen, I., and Homod, R. Z. (2023). Enhancing student engagement: Harnessing "AIED"'s power in hybrid education—A review analysis. *Education Sciences*, 13(7), 632.

Alshammari, M. (2019). *A principled approach for engineering privacy by design*. University of Oxford.

Alzubi, J. A., Alzubi, O. A., and Alzubi, A. A. (2023). Securing patient data in the healthcare industry: A blockchain-driven approach. *Journal of Healthcare Engineering*, 1–12. https://doi.org/10.1155/2023/11081437

Antons, D., Breidbach, C. F., Joshi, A. M., and Salge, T. O. (2023). Computational literature reviews: Method, algorithms, and roadmap. *Organizational Research Methods*, 26(1), 107–138.

Arrieta, A. B., Díaz-Rodríguez, N., Del Ser, J., Bennetot, A., Tabik, S., Barbado, A., ... Herrera, F. (2020). Explainable Artificial Intelligence (XAI): Concepts, taxonomies, opportunities and challenges toward responsible AI. *Information Fusion*, 58, 82–115. https://doi.org/10.1016/j.inffus.2019.12.012

Centers for Disease Control and Prevention (CDC). (2024). *Importance of informed consent in AI applications for healthcare*. https://www.cdc.gov/pcd/issues/2024/24_0245.htm

Chen, J., Chen, Y., Du, X., Li, C., Lu, J., Zhao, S., and Zhou, X. (2013). Big data challenge: A data management perspective. *Frontiers of Computer Science*, 7, 157–164.

Chen, X., Li, X., Zou, D., Xie, H., and Wang, F. L. (2025). Metacognition research in education: Topic modeling and bibliometrics. *Educational Technology Research and Development*, 1–29. https://link.springer.com/journal/11423/online-first?filterOpenAccess=false&page=2

Cilliers, L. (2020). Wearable devices in healthcare: Privacy and information security issues. *Health Information Management Journal*, 49(2–3), 150–156.

Cowie, M. R., Blomster, J. I., Curtis, L. H., Duclaux, S., Ford, I., Fritz, F., Goldman, S., Janmohamed, S., Kreuzer, J., and Leenay, M. (2017). Electronic health records to facilitate clinical research. *Clinical Research in Cardiology*, 106, 1–9.

Cwiek, M., Kikano, G., Brown, J., Maher, V., Roth, B., and Zaman, F. (2023). *Electronic health records: The wonders and the worries*. Editors N. Delener and Christina Schweikert. 24th Annual International Conference. Global Business and Technology Association 22 Cobblers Lane I Dix Hills, New York 11746I U.S.A. https://www.researchgate.net/profile/Azwihangwisi-Mphidi/publication/384355329_2023_GBATA_READINGS_BOOK_THEME_EMBRACING_THE_POSITIVE_IMPACT_OF_DISRUPTION_IN_THE_FIELD_OF_FUTURISM_GBATA-2023-ReadingsBook_pages_445_to_454_Title_of_the_Paper_Corporate_Fraud_at_the_Small_Enterprise_/links/66f54cf7869f1104c6b53a62/2023-GBATA-READINGS-BOOK-THEME-EMBRACING-THE-POSITIVE-IMPACT-OF-DISRUPTION-IN-THE-FIELD-OF-FUTURISM-GBATA-2023-ReadingsBook-pages-445-to-454-Title-of-the-Paper-Corporate-Fraud-at-the-Small-Enterpris.pdf#page=134.

Davis, J. R. (2022). *Healthcare entities and data breach threat indicators and deterrence: A quantitative study*. Northcentral University.

Deloitte. (2016). *Blockchain: Opportunities for health care*. Deloitte Insights. https://www2.deloitte.com/us/en/pages/public-sector/articles/blockchain-opportunities-for-health-care.html

Dwivedi, R., Dave, D., Naik, H., Singhal, S., Omer, R., Patel, P., Qian, B., Wen, Z., Shah, T., and Morgan, G. (2023). Explainable AI (XAI): Core ideas, techniques, and solutions. *ACM Computing Surveys*, 55(9), 1–33.

Evans, B. J. (2018). HIPAA's individual right of access to genomic data: Reconciling safety and civil rights. *The American Journal of Human Genetics*, 102(1), 5–10.

Felzmann, H., Fosch-Villaronga, E., Lutz, C., and Tamò-Larrieux, A. (2020). Towards transparency by design for artificial intelligence. *Science and Engineering Ethics*, 26(6), 3333–3361.

Gold, M., and McLaughlin, C. (2016). Assessing HITECH implementation and lessons: 5 years later. *The Milbank Quarterly*, 94(3), 654–687.

Han, Q., and Venkatasubramanian, N. (2007). Timeliness-accuracy balanced collection of dynamic context data. *IEEE Transactions on Parallel and Distributed Systems*, 18(2), 158–171.

Hasan, H. E., Jaber, D., Khabour, O. F., and Alzoubi, K. H. (2024). Ethical considerations and concerns in the implementation of AI in pharmacy practice: A cross-sectional study. *BMC Medical Ethics*, 25(1), 55.

Häyrinen, K., Saranto, K., and Nykänen, P. (2008). Definition, structure, content, use and impacts of electronic health records: A review of the research literature. *International Journal of Medical Informatics*, 77(5), 291–304.

HITRUST Alliance. (2024). *The ethics of AI in healthcare: Addressing safety, liability, and patient privacy*. https://hitrustalliance.net/blog/the-ethics-of-ai-in-healthcare

Holzinger, A., Haibe-Kains, B., and Jurisica, I. (2019). Why imaging data alone is not enough: AI-based integration of imaging, omics, and clinical data. *European Journal of Nuclear Medicine and Molecular Imaging*, 46(13), 2722–2730.

Kadadi, A., Agrawal, R., Nyamful, C., and Atiq, R. (2014). *Challenges of data integration and interoperability in big data.* 2014 IEEE International Conference on Big Data (big data).

Katal, A., Wazid, M., and Goudar, R. H. (2013). *Big data: Issues, challenges, tools and good practices.* 2013 Sixth International Conference on Contemporary Computing (IC3),

Khatiwada, P., Yang, B., Lin, J.-C., and Blobel, B. (2024). Patient-generated health data (PGHD): Understanding, requirements, challenges, and existing techniques for data security and privacy. *Journal of Personalized Medicine*, 14(3), 282.

Kho, A. N., Rasmussen, L. V., Connolly, J. J., Peissig, P. L., Starren, J., Hakonarson, H., and Hayes, M. G. (2013). Practical challenges in integrating genomic data into the electronic health record. *Genetics in Medicine*, 15(10), 772–778.

Kim, J.-Y., and Cho, S.-B. (2022). An information theoretic approach to reducing algorithmic bias for machine learning. *Neurocomputing*, 500, 26–38.

Lavallee, D. C., Chenok, K. E., Love, R. M., Petersen, C., Holve, E., Segal, C. D., and Franklin, P. D. (2016). Incorporating patient-reported outcomes into health care to engage patients and enhance care. *Health Affairs*, 35(4), 575–582.

Liu, L., Stroulia, E., Nikolaidis, I., Miguel-Cruz, A., and Rincon, A. R. (2016). Smart homes and home health monitoring technologies for older adults: A systematic review. *International Journal of Medical Informatics*, 91, 44–59.

Longo, L., Brcic, M., Cabitza, F., Choi, J., Confalonieri, R., Del Ser, J., . . . Holzinger, A. (2024). Explainable Artificial Intelligence (XAI) 2.0: A manifesto of open challenges and interdisciplinary research directions. *Information Fusion*, 106, 102301.

Metta, C., Beretta, A., Pellungrini, R., Rinzivillo, S., and Giannotti, F. (2024). Towards transparent healthcare: Advancing local explanation methods in explainable artificial intelligence. *Bioengineering*, 11(4), 369.

Millers, T., Howe, P., and Sonnenberg, L. (2017). Explainable AI: Beware of inmates running the asylum. *ArXiv Report.*

Minh, D., Wang, H. X., Li, Y. F., and Nguyen, T. N. (2022). Explainable artificial intelligence: A comprehensive review. *Artificial Intelligence Review*, 55(5), 3503–3568. https://doi.org/10.1007/s10462-021-10088-y.

Myers, M. C. (2024). *Data privacy laws in the united states and Germany: Implications for genomics research and personalized medicine.* Master Essay, University of Pittsburgh.

Naik, N., Hameed, B. Z., Shetty, D. K., Swain, D., Shah, M., Paul, R., ... Somani, B. K. (2022). Legal and ethical consideration in artificial intelligence in healthcare: Who takes responsibility?. *Frontiers in Surgery*, 9, 862322.

Olorunsogo, T. O., Balogun, O. D., Ayo-Farai, O., Ogundairo, O., Maduka, C. P., Okongwu, C. C., and Onwumere, C. (2024). Bioinformatics and personalized medicine in the US: A comprehensive review: Scrutinizing the advancements in genomics and their potential to revolutionize healthcare delivery. *World Journal of Advanced Research and Reviews*, 21(1), 335–351.

Olson, J. E. (2003). *Data quality: The accuracy dimension.* Elsevier.

Patel, P., and Uddin, M. N. (2022). AI for algorithmic auditing: Mitigating bias and improving fairness in big data systems. *International Journal of Social Analytics*, 7(12), 39–48.

Regulation, P. (2016). Regulation (EU) 2016/679 of the European parliament and of the council. *Regulation* (EU), 679, 1–209.

Reuters. (2024, December 27). *Biden administration proposes new cybersecurity rules to limit impact on healthcare.* https://www.reuters.com/technology/cybersecurity/biden-administration-proposes-new-cybersecurity-rules-limit-impact-healthcare-2024-12-27

Reuters. (2025, January 30). *U.S. FDA identifies cybersecurity risks in certain patient monitors.* https://www.reuters.com/business/healthcare-pharmaceuticals/us-fda-identifies-cybersecurity-risks-certain-patient-monitors-2025-01-30

Saki, S. (2024). Advancements in genomic research: Paving the way for future personalized medicine. *International Journal of BioMed Insights*, 1(1), 1–15.

Saraswat, D., Bhattacharya, P., Verma, A., Prasad, V. K., Tanwar, S., Sharma, G., Bokoro, P. N., and Sharma, R. (2022). Explainable AI for healthcare 5.0: Opportunities and challenges. *IEEE Access*, 10, 84486–84517.

Srinivasa, K., Kurni, M., and Saritha, K. (2022). *Harnessing the power of AI to education learning, teaching, and assessment methods for contemporary learners: Pedagogy for the digital generation* (pp. 311–342). Springer.

Sufyan Ghaleb, M. M., and Alshiha, A. A. (2023). Empowering self-management: unveiling the impact of artificial intelligence in learning on student self-efficacy and self-monitoring. *Eurasian Journal of Educational Research (EJER),* 107, 68.

Tamò-Larrieux, A., Tamò-Larrieux, S., and Seyfried, M. (2018). *Designing for privacy and its legal framework.* Springer.

The Guardian. (2024, November 29). *Alder hey children's hospital explores data breach after ransomware claims.* https://www.theguardian.com/technology/2024/nov/29/alder-hey-childrens-hospital-explores-data-breach-after-ransomware-claims

Tjoa, E., and Guan, C. (2020). A survey on Explainable Artificial Intelligence (XAI): Toward medical XAI. *IEEE Transactions on Neural Networks and Learning Systems*, 32(11), 4793–4813. https://doi.org/10.1109/TNNLS.2020.3027314

Wall Street Journal. (2024, April 12). *UnitedHealth estimates change healthcare hack impacted about 190 million people.* https://www.wsj.com/articles/unitedhealth-estimates-change-healthcare-hack-impacted-about-190-million-people-9564533c

Winter, J. S., and Davidson, E. (2022). Harmonizing regulatory regimes for the governance of patient-generated health data. *Telecommunications Policy*, 46(5), 102285.

6 Decision Support Systems in Healthcare

Applications, Benefits, Challenges, and Future Trends

R. S. M. Lakshmi Patibandla

6.1 INTRODUCTION

Decision Support Systems (DSSs) are one of the technologies of the modern healthcare setting, aimed at enhancing patient outcomes, maximizing utilization of the resources, and facilitating clinical decision-making. DSSs utilize gigantic databases, algorithms, and artificial intelligence methodologies in order to produce useful information for clinicians. Some of the basic concepts of DSSs, fundamental components, day-to-day uses, benefits, and intrinsic drawbacks in the clinical environment are included in this chapter.

6.1.1 Principles of Decision Support Systems (DSSs)

Decision Support Systems (DSSs) are applicable in medicine, leveraging the ability of computers to process large volumes of medical information and provide clinicians with useful information to make decisions. DSSs are middle-level systems that bridge raw medical information and clinical knowledge, transforming unstructured information into context-specific recommendations. DSSs range from simple rule-based alert systems to advanced artificial intelligence-based analytics, which forecast patient outcomes and provide best practice recommendations (Divya et al., 2025). By incorporating machine learning paradigms, statistical algorithms, and expert knowledge bases, DSSs provide actionable information that minimizes diagnostic errors, enhances therapeutic efficacy, and enhances the overall quality of patient care.

The foundation of DSSs in medicine lies in human–computer interaction models, analytical techniques, and information management. Firm patient medical history, genomic information, imaging, and laboratory results are the foundations of effective DSS to make timely and accurate suggestions. DSSs combine real-time monitoring data, clinical guidelines, and electronic health records (EHRs) to support medical

DOI: 10.1201/9781003605416-6

staff in making evidence-based treatment decisions. DSSs also enhance operational efficiency by streamlining hospital processes, resource allocation, and supply chain management methods. The continuous technological developments in artificial intelligence, cloud computing technology, and Big Data analytics are also further driving the development of DSSs, which are becoming more adaptive, predictive, and personalized for clinicians and patients.

6.1.2 Components of DSSs

A standard healthcare Decision Support System (DSS) consists of a Data Management System (DMS) as a sophisticated platform carefully optimized to efficiently collect, store, categorize, and process large-scale healthcare information. These include patient records, medical images, laboratory tests, treatment histories, prescriptions, and other vital health-related information. The system retains the information in an organized fashion, easily retrievable, and securely stored, thereby making interoperability between different healthcare departments easy. By implementing efficient data processing and retrieval procedures, a DMS enables improved decision-making among healthcare professionals, clinical research studies, and improved patient care through the availability of timely, accurate, and updated information. Additionally, such systems typically include efficient security procedures like encryption, access controls, and audit trails to secure sensitive patient information and ensure compliance with regulatory mandates like Health Insurance Portability and Accountability Act (HIPAA) and General Data Protection Regulation (GDPR).

A Model Management System (MMS) is a tailor-made system for predictive model development, management, and use of sophisticated statistical analysis to extract meaning from complex health-related data. The system enables healthcare practitioners and researchers to utilize machine learning algorithms, statistical processes, and artificial intelligence (AI) for pattern, trend, and correlation identification in medical data. The MMS covers the entire predictive modeling life cycle from data preprocessing to feature selection, model training, validation, deployment, and continuous performance monitoring. Its applications include disease outbreak forecasting, patient outcome prediction, high-risk individual identification, treatment protocol optimization, and clinical decision-making process optimization. An MMS also maintains the long-term accuracy and reliability of the models by monitoring parameters such as accuracy, precision, recall, and receiver operating characteristic (ROC) curves continuously.

To ensure transparency and ethical healthcare AI practice, an MMS is also equipped with explainability tools, bias detection mechanisms, and regulatory compliance measures such as HIPAA and GDPR. With seamless interoperability with electronic health records (EHRs) and other healthcare IT systems, the Model Management System facilitates data-driven healthcare decision-making, enhances patient experience, and drives medical research efforts. A Knowledge-Based System (KBS) is a very advanced Decision Support System that indexes, organizes, and applies clinical guidelines, best practice medical procedures, and expert knowledge to improve the process of decision-making in the healthcare industry. A KBS is an electronic repository of medical knowledge (Ben Khalfallah et al., 2025), which integrates systematic knowledge consisting of disease management protocols, treatment guidelines, diagnostic criteria, and drug interaction information (Figure 6.1).

With the help of rule-based reasoning, machine learning, and artificial intelligence, a Knowledge-Based System (KBS) helps healthcare professionals to diagnose diseases, suggest treatments, and predict the patient's prognosis. Besides this, KBSs can be designed to interface with electronic health records (EHRs) in such a way that provide context-relevant and timely suggestions taking into account the unique features of each patient. Further, a KBS enhances clinical workflows by minimizing errors, streamlining care protocols, and informing health professionals of the most recent evidence-based information. In an attempt to keep pace with accuracy and relevance, these systems are regularly updated with new information in medical research, regulatory guidelines, and expert opinions, thus ultimately driving improvements in patient safety, treatment efficacy, and overall effectiveness of healthcare processes.

The user interface (UI) of a health system is the main interface for healthcare workers with the base data analysis, management, and Decision Support Systems. Designed to maximize efficiency and user satisfaction, the UI provides easy-to-use interactive dashboards integrating relevant patient information, diagnosis reports, treatment guidelines, and predictive analysis into an integrated visual form. Dashboards enable healthcare workers to quickly analyze the patient's health condition, track the disease progression, and compare the outcomes of different treatments. Apart from the dashboards, the user interface includes real-time alerts and notifications designed to improve patient safety and simplify clinical workflows. Alerts can also be presented as notifications for abnormal laboratory results, drug interaction warnings, patient deterioration risk warnings, and medication reminders. The user interface should be dynamic and role-based access control should be offered so that information relevant to various stakeholders, such as physicians, nurses, and administrative staff, can be viewed. To ensure maximum utilization, the UI utilizes responsive design, voice-controlled recognition, and touch-sensitive interfaces to be

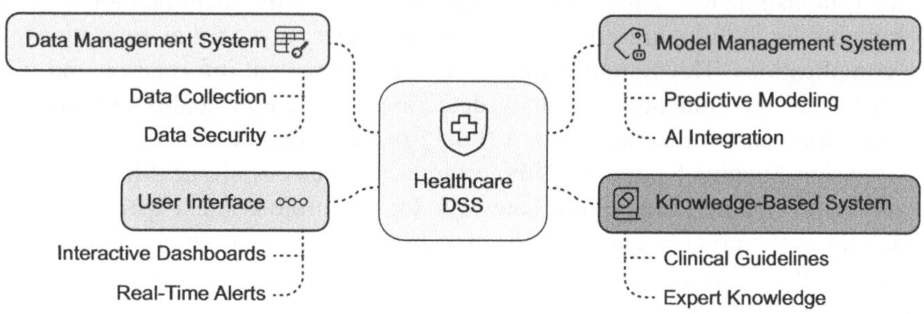

FIGURE 6.1 Components of healthcare DSSs.

utilized on several platforms, i.e., desktops, tablets, and mobile applications. The accessibility features, i.e., user-controllable display options, assistive technology, and language options, are also given importance to support a broad range of user requirements. By adopting function and user-centered design, the UI maximizes clinical decision-making tasks, minimizes cognitive burden, and maximizes overall productivity in patient treatment (Manta et al., 2024).

6.2 TYPES OF DECISION SUPPORT SYSTEMS (DSSS)

Decision Support Systems (DSSs) in the healthcare sector can be classified into various types based on their functionality in the context of operations and automation levels.

6.2.1 Clinical Decision Support Systems (CDSSs)

These enable healthcare professionals to perform diagnosis, treatment choice, and risk determination procedures. The Clinical Decision Support System (CDSS) is a new healthcare technology that has been carefully developed to assist healthcare professionals in making accurate, evidence-based decisions for patient diagnosis, choice of treatment, and risk determination. CDSSs combine medical knowledge with patient-specific data and predictive analyses to optimize the clinical processes and capability of health practitioners in an evidence-based decision-making process. This refers further to the provision of decision support in diagnostics whereby the system analyzes the symptoms of a patient, lab results, imaging studies, and history to provide suggestions on possible diagnoses. Based on rule-based reasoning, machine learning models, and pattern recognition techniques, the CDSS helps diagnose rare diseases, reduces diagnostic mistakes, and enhances diagnostic accuracy. Another significant task for the CDSS is providing clinical data for personalized treatment selection based on clinical guidelines or interactions between drugs, genetics, or individual patient data. This infrastructure uses large medical databases, with real-time tracking of patient data, to help clinicians select the best treatment regimens, medications, and intervention strategies.

Clinical Decision Support Systems (CDSSs) play a vital role in risk assessment and the establishment of early warning systems through the identification of high-risk patients for developing conditions such as sepsis, myocardial infarctions, or drug complications. The system continues to monitor patient information and initiates alerts and recommendations upon detection of potential health hazards, thus allowing clinicians to take action in a timely manner. Besides, modern computerized Decision Support Systems combine forces with electronic healthcare records and other information technology gateways for real-time context-specific recommendations at the point of care. CDSSs significantly contribute to better healthcare outcomes and operational efficiency by improving clinical efficiency, reducing the variability of treatment decisions, and ensuring patient safety.

6.2.2 Operational and Administrative DSSs

These systems help in optimizing hospital operations, staff scheduling, and resource allocating. It is a very specialized Decision Support System, operational and administrative, which focuses on improving service effectiveness, refining administrative tasks, and appropriating resources to improve healthcare facilities. Using data analytics, artificial intelligence techniques, and real-time monitoring, the system allows healthcare administrators to make the best possible decisions regarding staff scheduling, resource distribution, and the overall governance of the grain. With scheduling of staff being the core process, this involves demand for patient, shift pattern, and workforce availability to create schedules for physicians, nurses, and allied staff (Figure 6.2).

Balancing a workload means minimizing overtime while optimizing overall satisfaction on the part of the employees, thereby reducing extreme cases of either

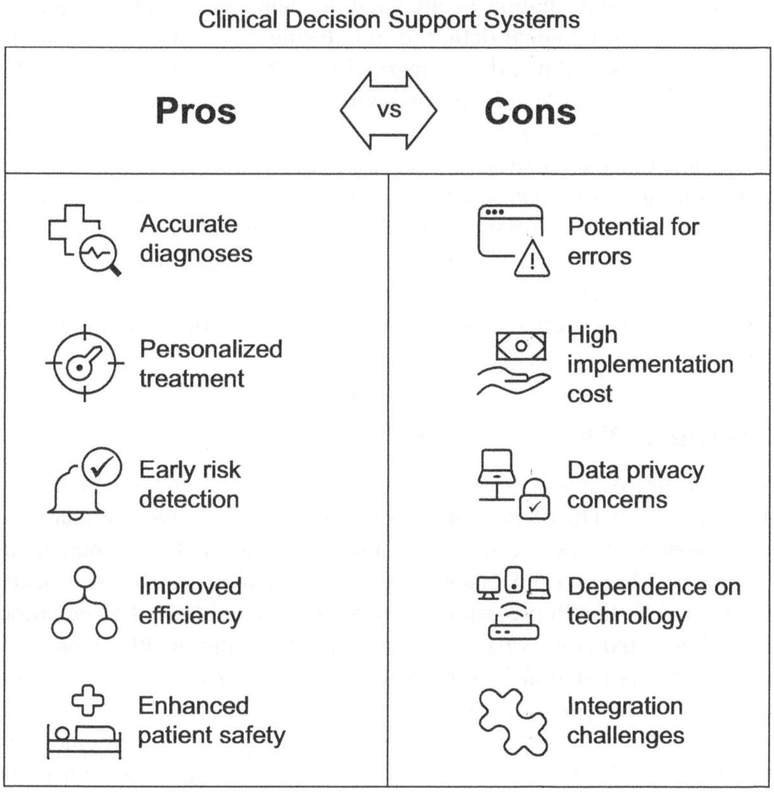

FIGURE 6.2 Clinical Decision Support Systems.

burnout or a decrease in employee performance, thus overall enhancing the quality of care. An equally important aspect concerns resource allocation and hospital asset management, such as ICU beds, surgical theaters, medical equipment, and drug inventory. The DSS continuously monitors resource use, predicts demand, and allocates resources to prevent shortages and waste while optimally responding to patient flow. For instance, during emergencies, the system enables the aberrant redistribution of beds and staff, directing them in real time to critical areas in this sense to provide immediate care to the patients.

Also, it is the optimization of facilities that enables hospital administrators to detect bottlenecks in admitting, discharging, and transferring patients. Using data from the past combined with real-time data offers some concrete approaches to decrease wait times, advance patient throughput, and better utilization of hospital resources. Current Operational and Administrative DSS solutions are designed to seamlessly integrate into EHRs, financial management systems, and predictive analytics applications, enabling data-driven decision-making (Jammal et al., 2025).

Additionally, facilitate public health planning and policy formulation through the analysis of epidemiological data, the monitoring of disease outbreaks, and the evaluation of the effects of healthcare regulations. These insights can be utilized by governmental entities and healthcare policymakers to enact evidence-based health policies, allocate resources for preventive care initiatives, and prepare for potential public health emergencies such as pandemics. Furthermore, the practice of competitive benchmarking and market analysis permits hospital executives to assess their institution's performance in relation to industry benchmarks and competitors. This evaluation is crucial for informed strategic decision-making. Through the automation of repetitive administrative tasks and amplified capability in managing resources, such systems lead to cost-effectiveness, operational reliability, and a higher level of patient care.

6.2.3 Strategic DSSs

Support healthcare executives and policymakers in making long-term, informed decisions. A Strategic Decision Support System (DSS) is a powerful analytical tool designed to support healthcare executives, administrators, and policymakers in making well-informed, long-term decisions that determine the course of healthcare organizations and public health programs. Through the integration of large amounts of information harvested from varied sources like electronic health records (EHRs), payment systems, population health trends, and predictive analytics, a Strategic Decision Support System (DSS) offers informed suggestions that form the basis of policy development, resource allocation, and strategic organizational decision-making. It is one of the strengths of the system that it facilitates long-term planning for resources, which allows hospital managers and policymakers to project future demands in terms of healthcare services, infrastructure, and manpower issues. With historical trend analysis, population statistics, and disease prevalence, Strategic DSS can help with new healthcare facility opening strategies, resource financial plans, and prioritization of medical specialties. Budget and finance analysis is also required in this regard, helping executives simplify financial expenditure, monitor income streams, and determine areas where cost savings can be achieved. Through analysis of various funding plans, reimbursement plans, and operational costs, the system provides long-term financial stability of healthcare facilities while at the same time providing high levels of patient care.

Strategic Decision Support Systems facilitate decision-making regarding mergers, acquisitions, service growth, and the integration of new healthcare technologies. Through machine learning, predictive modeling, and data visualization, a Strategic DSS transforms complex healthcare data into actionable intelligence, enabling leaders to make proactive, data-driven decisions that drive improved healthcare delivery, patient outcomes, and operational effectiveness in the IDSS use in Health Care: As a tool, the Decision Support System has been integrated in many healthcare settings for differing reasons.

6.2.4 Clinical Decision Support Systems (CDSSs) with Diagnostic Support

AI diagnostic assistance systems increase the speed and rate of accuracy. Contemporary healthcare AI-support diagnostic systems are transforming healthcare by amplifying precision, efficiency, and the speed at which diseases are diagnosed and medical decisions are made. These systems make use of advanced technologies such as effective machine learning (ML), deep learning (DL), Natural Language Processing (NLP), and computer vision to analyze Big Data within the medical field, recognize complex patterns, and offer real-time diagnostic decisions to health workers. One core use of AI in diagnostic imaging is for the examination of medical images. Powered by AI algorithms, radiographs, MRIs, CT scans, and ultrasounds are rapidly assessed for anomalies like tumors, fractures, or organ damage. Since these pieces of equipment are trained on large data, they make fewer human mistakes when learning, help radiologists prioritize urgent cases, and standardize healthcare sectors. AI is revolutionizing clinical pathology and laboratory diagnostics by examining blood samples, genetic data, and microbiological specimens to identify infections, genetic abnormalities, and metabolic disorders. Advanced AI-driven pathology tools can now detect malignant cells in biopsy samples with accuracy comparable to or even greater than that of experienced pathologists. This advancement enables quicker diagnoses and more precise treatment strategies. AI is transforming healthcare by making diagnoses faster, more precise, and more efficient. By analyzing electronic health records (EHRs) and vast medical databases, AI can assess a patient's medical history, symptoms, test results, and past diagnoses. This advanced technology helps doctors recognize rare conditions that might otherwise go undetected by identifying patterns in patient data and global healthcare trends. In both primary care and telemedicine, AI-driven chatbots and virtual assistants are improving healthcare accessibility. These intelligent tools analyze patient-reported symptoms and medical backgrounds, offering initial diagnostic insights and directing individuals to appropriate medical services or urgent care when necessary. This technology is particularly beneficial for people in remote or underserved regions, as AI-powered consultations provide real-time medical assistance and help close gaps in healthcare access. AI improves diagnostic accuracy when combined with Clinical Decision Support Systems (CDSSs). These innovative technologies use predictive modeling, risk assessment, and precision medicine to help doctors make better decisions. In cardiology, AI can evaluate ECG data to determine the risk of heart disease, while in oncology, it may examine genetic markers to offer individualized cancer treatment plans. By increasing diagnosis accuracy, cutting wait times, and enabling data-driven medical decision-making, artificial intelligence is revolutionizing healthcare. Along with faster treatments and improved patient outcomes, these advancements contribute to the creation of a healthcare system that is more effective and accessible for all (Hussain et al., 2024).

6.3 MEDICATION MANAGEMENT

Modern medication delivery is being revolutionized by artificial intelligence, leading to significant gains in both accuracy and patient well-being. Intelligent systems are now central to ensuring medications are used safely and effectively, dramatically reducing the likelihood of errors. Utilizing AI, machine learning, and sophisticated clinical decision support, these platforms empower medical professionals throughout the prescribing, dispensing, and monitoring stages.

Through integration with electronic health records, extensive drug databases, and current clinical guidelines, they deliver real-time warnings, informed suggestions, and data-backed insights to enhance treatment and mitigate potential harm. A core feature of these systems is their ability to rigorously scrutinize prescriptions, proactively identifying and averting hazardous drug combinations.

By comparing a patient's medication inventory with databases of known drug interactions, the system alerts doctors to potentially harmful combinations that could result in serious side effects, decreased treatment efficacy, or even death. For instance, medication management systems can quickly identify that some anticoagulants can raise the risk of serious bleeding when used with specific antibiotics. These technologies also help reduce dosing errors by verifying the accuracy of prescriptions based on patient-specific factors including age, weight, liver health, and renal function. Automated dose-verification algorithms ensure that prescribed pharmaceuticals stay within the safe therapeutic range, reducing the chance of overdosing or underdosing (Figure 6.3).

These methods provide weight-adjusted dose estimates, which are vital in order to protect both younger and older patients from the possibly detrimental effects of medicines. Another important component is a warning tool for allergies and contraindications that checks a patient's medical record for known allergies or pre-existing conditions that may render certain medicine unsafe. For example, an antibiotic in the penicillin world would instantly alert the practitioner if the practitioner attempted to prescribe it for a penicillin-allergic patient. Medication management systems dramatically reduce the risk of human error in hospitals and pharmacies by enabling automated dispensing and barcode scanning.

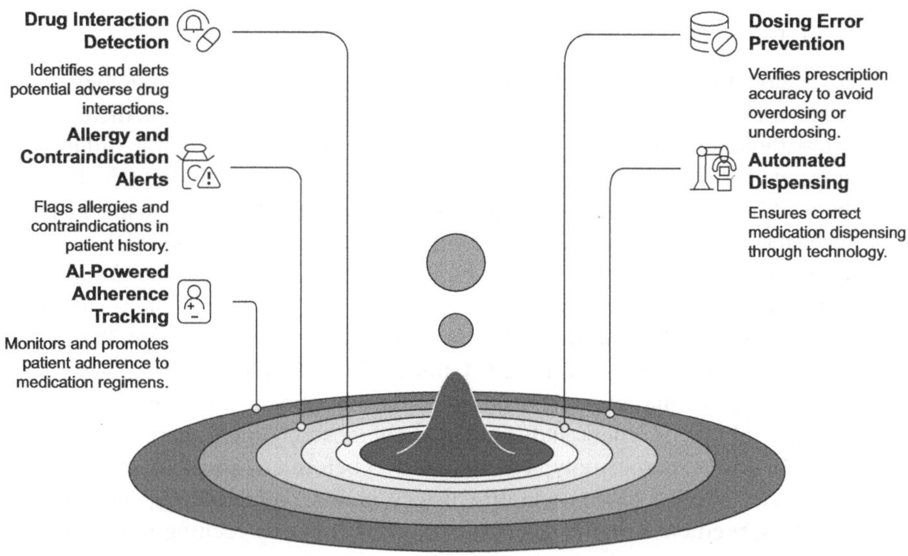

FIGURE 6.3 Medication management outcomes.

Pharmacists and nurses employ these systems to confirm that the right drug, dose, and route of administration are assigned to the correct patient, thereby ensuring compliance with the "five rights" of medication safety: right patient, right drug, right dose, right route, and right time. Moreover, AI-enhanced adherence-monitoring applications help guarantee that patients adhere to their medications correctly by sending reminders, tracking each patient's refill of prescription medication, and analyzing patterns in patient compliance with their medications. This is particularly important in the management of chronic conditions such as diabetes, hypertension, and cardiovascular disorders, where missed doses may compromise patient health. As medication management systems eliminate prescription errors, augment pharmaceutical safety, and guarantee compliance with clinical best practices, they greatly enhance patient outcomes by decreasing hospital readmissions and promoting efficiency in health service delivery (Houssem et al., 2023a).

6.4 PREDICTIVE ANALYTICS

They also help in evaluating the risks of certain conditions like cancer and diabetes. Predictive analytics analyzes risk factors leading to diseases such as cancer, diabetes, cardiovascular diseases, and neurodegenerative conditions within the early α-phase of their onset in healthcare using ML, AI, statistical methodologies, and extensive data. Predictive analytics provides medical professionals with insights through the study of vast data sets, including EHRs, genomic data, imaging diagnostics, fitting into lifestyles, and other medical histories about the detection, prevention, diagnosis, and management of disease progression before it becomes difficult to handle.

6.4.1 Detection of Cancer Early in Time

Predictive modeling is one of the main Global Foundries (GF) technology tools employed for the early identification of cancer by a combination of medical imaging, histopathological findings, genetic tendencies, and lifestyle factor influences. AI-enhanced vision recognition creates a combined picture set of radiological scans. AI-enhanced imaging tools trained with huge collections of radiological scans can detect even the slightest abnormalities in mammograms, CT scans, and MRIs, usually well before they can be detected through human observation, such as mammography is an instrumental AI tool providing insight into the identification of microcalcifications and tumor patterns that are early-stage indicators of breast cancer. Predictive algorithms can also analyze low-dose CT imaging for the identification of nodules that may advance to malignancy, enabling earlier treatment intervention that can improve survival rates. Genetic indicators and colonoscopy images are analyzed by AI to identify pre-cancerous polyps to be removed before any progression. By identifying high-risk patients based on family history, genetic vulnerability, and environmental factors, predictive analytics enables tailored cancer screening programs and targeted interventions to reduce mortality.

6.4.2 Diabetes Prediction and Prevention-Predictive

Analytics Technology AI is of catalytic importance in identifying high-risk patients, preventing complications, and refining treatment strategies in diabetes management. Through patient data—microscopic levels, such as HbA1c trends, body mass index, feeding habits, activity levels, and genetic predispositions—AI frameworks can predict the probability of developing hyperglycemic conditions long before it could even be identified.

6.4.2.1 Diabetes Management

Early on, we can use smart computer systems to spot trends in how blood sugar levels change and how the body responds to insulin. This helps doctors implement preventive steps to prevent problems, like suggesting changes in diet and exercise habits or prescribing medication. Predictive tools make it possible to establish whether an individual might be susceptible to organ damage, retinal issues, or kidney problems due to diabetes. Such facilities let us act beforehand before the emergence of such ailments and phenomena of any nature. For the mothers, there are special apps employing artificial intelligence technologies to monitor metabolic changes to pick up on variations in gestational diabetes. This also helps ensure both the mother's and baby's well-being.

6.4.3 Predicting and Preventing Other Diseases

Another domain that these predictive tools extend into, apart from the previously mentioned conditions, is the early identification of heart diseases, strokes, septicemia, and brain-related conditions like Alzheimer's and Parkinson's diseases. They enable proactive healthcare by treating these conditions before they really begin to show.

6.4.3.1 Diagnosing Heart Problems

The artificial intelligence-based study of ECG readings combined with wearable monitoring can detect predispositions to heart attack and stroke very early by identifying arrhythmia, hypertension, and arterial blockage. Advanced predictive models running on vital signs, lab tests, and bedside clinical histories in intensive care units can predict whether sepsis may develop, which allows early intervention can drastically decrease mortality rates. Neurological conditions such as artificial intelligence-enabled speech and movement analyses can detect early subtle cues of Alzheimer's and Parkinsonism and could prompt cognitive rehabilitation therapy and lifestyle changes. Predictive analytics in preventive healthcare includes real-time scanning, wearables, genomic analysis, and deep learning algorithms, thus offering early disease detection and risk stratification, leading to customized treatments, lower care costs, and improved patient outcomes (Houssem et al., 2023b).

6.4.3.2 Treatment Planning

Personalized treatment recommendations based on patient history, the Modern-Day Care, is extremely important. Advanced techniques like artificial intelligence, machine learning, predictive analysis, and clinical decision-aid systems are used for personalized treatment offerings addressed toward separate patients. Such sophisticated systems will take a detailed look at a patient's medical history, genetic make-up, lifestyle variables, disease progression, and responses to previous treatments for suggesting the best treatments while at the same time minimizing risk and adverse effects.

6.4.4 Personalized Medicine and Precision Treatment

This major breakthrough in treatment planning is toward personalized medicine through AI-based tools. These tools analyze genetic and biomarker information to provide recommendations on targeted therapeutic interventions. For example, by securing AI-facilitated molecular profiling, oncology assists in identifying the most efficient chemotherapy, immunotherapy, or targeted treatment according to a patient's unique cancer mutations. In cardiology, interventions have been becoming finely tuned, guided by ECG assessments, cholesterol levels, and genetic predispositions, in further refinement of pharmacological treatment of hypertension and cardiovascular diseases. In diabetes management, AI systems can decipher the recommended routes for the delivery of insulin and dietary management, using continuous glucose m(CGM), insulin responses, and lifestyle practices data.

6.4.5 AI-Driven Drug and Therapy Selection

AI-assisted treatment planning tools recommend optimal medications and dosages, as well as combinations that allow various treatments based on the large datasets of clinical trials, real-world patient outcomes, and medical research. Besides being able to avert negative drug interactions and contraindications, such systems can detect a recognized combination of drugs with an individual contraindication, drug–drug interaction, and patient-specific risk factors. In pharmacogenomics, AI examines genetic variations with potential influence on pharmacokinetics to avoid administration of drugs not compatible with the patient's genetic profile. In autoimmune diseases, an AI assessment allows the choice of biologic therapies based on the immunological response characteristics of the patient, thus allowing adequate treatment of rheumatoid arthritis and multiple sclerosis.

6.4.6 Real-Time Monitoring and Adaptive Treatment Adjustments

AI-assisted treatment planning tools use real-world datasets from clinical trials, medical research, and patient outcomes to find the optimal drug, its dosage, and the combination for different kinds of therapies. Such systems also avert negative drug–drug interactions and indications by looking into drug and individual drug interaction. Pharmacogenomics works on genetic changes that hamper a drug's pharmacokinetics so that patients receive drugs that will not cause an adverse effect. Autoimmune diseases, AI assessments allow the selection of biologic therapies according to the immune response characteristics of the patient.

Artificial intelligence is continuing in evaluating health metrics through wearables, mobile applications, and IoT-connected devices, thus providing real-time monitoring of treatment efficacy and modifying plans accordingly. For chronic illness, AI assesses patient responses and dynamically prescribes pharmaceutical or lifestyle changes. Due to the unfolding advances in AI in rehabilitation protocols for post-surgical recovery, the monitoring of patient mobility, pain levels, and amount of recovery has allowed the further refinement of physical therapy recommendations. In accordance with electronic health records (EHRs) and Clinical Decision Support Systems (CDSS), treatment planning tools normally complement EHRs to supply context-sensitive, real-time suggestions based on a patient's complete medical history, subsequent lab test results, imaging evaluations, and their previous responses to treatments. The CDSS platforms support doctors in decision-making by presenting evidence-based therapeutic alternatives that conform to clinical guidelines and best practice. By tapping Big Data, AI, and predictive analytics, contemporary treatment planning systems bridge the trial-and-error nature of medical treatment, improve patient outcomes with lowered risks and a push for precision medicine, ensuring safer, effective, and exquisite individualized healthcare (Liyun et al., 2023).

6.5 OPERATIONAL AND ADMINISTRATIVE DECISION SUPPORT SYSTEMS (DSSS)

6.5.1 Hospital Resource Management

This helps in improving bed allocation, medical equipment utilization, and workforce resource planning. Management of hospital resources constitutes, therefore, one of the most decisive operational domains for guaranteeing that healthcare institutions function efficiently through the optimization of hospital beds, medical equipment, and human resources. As patient inflow, variability of healthcare needs, and the exigency for cost-effective operations are escalating, hospitals have begun embracing data-centric Decision Support Systems, artificial intelligence (AI), and predictive analytics to enhance resource distribution, patient care, and operational profit impediment.

6.5.1.1 Bed Allocation and Capacity Management

The proficient allocation of hospital beds is paramount for diminishing patient wait times, averting overcrowding, and facilitating timely admissions and discharges. AI-augmented bed management systems monitor real-time bed occupancy, patient acuity assessments, and discharge timelines to maximize bed accessibility (Antoniadi et al., 2021).

6.5.1.2 Dynamic Bed Assignment

Appropriate hospital bed assignment is central to shortening patient waiting time, controlling the patient queuing system, and allowing timely admitting and discharging of patients. AI-augmented bed management systems offer the real-time statuses of occupancy, patient acuity assessment, and discharge timeline for bed accessibility maximization.

AI continuously assesses admission trends, patients' medical status, and expected length of stays as new data are entered into the system, and allocates beds, on the basis of clinical urgency. In predictive modeling of patient flow, machine learning algorithms analyze frequencies of hospital admits, surges of Emergency Department (ED) visits, and ICU demand, allowing steps beforehand to change bed counts. In automated discharge planning, AI systems optimize nurse flow with lab tests and prescriptions to expedite the discharge and minimize bed turnaround time.

6.5.1.3 Medical Equipment Utilization

Hospitals have under their supervision thousands of expensive and critical medical devices, such as MRI machines, ventilators, surgical instruments, and infusion devices. They require efficient management and maintenance. IoT devices and AI-based tracking systems accomplish better utilization of the equipment in these specific ways:

6.5.1.4 Real-Time Asset Tracking

Radio frequency identification (RFID) and IoT sensors monitor the location as well as the availability of critical medical equipment, thus reducing delays in patient care. AI studies the usage trends and wear-and-tear data in scheduling routine maintenance such that service does not harm or suspend any critical medical activities. Scheduling MRI scans, CT imaging, and operating room bookings enhanced by AI stimulates both patient throughput and equipment utilization.

6.5.2 Workforce Planning and Scheduling

It includes managing health workers such as physicians, nurses, technicians, and administrative staff to ensure a proper functioning hospital and avoid employee burnout. AI-enabled workforce management systems will give hospitals the ability to optimize department-level complete staffing for.

6.5.2.1 Automated Staff Scheduling

It allows for combination and shift generation according to preferences, patient loads, skill competencies, and labor laws, all efficiently generated by algorithms.

6.5.2.2 Predictive Demand Modeling

Machine learning to forecast peak hours of operations, seasonal flu spikes, and surges in emergencies allows hospitals to allocate personnel ahead of time.

6.5.2.3 Workload Distribution

AI monitors the nurses-to-patient ratio and physicians work to ensure equal distribution of workloads to minimize burnout and improve quality of patient care.

6.6 SUPPLY CHAIN AND INVENTORY MANAGEMENT

It is sure that the hospital runs smoothly by observing the equality. This means that it can be concentrated in the supply series that there are sure to be important things, such as treatment, individual security instruments, and other necessary things that are always available in need. Artificial intelligence can correct this supply series (Lyu and Zhang, 2019).

6.6.1 The Pre-inference of Future Needs

The historical data and the patients are used to infer that the equality of medicines and others can be inferred. In investment controls, fill the objects on the basis of the current stock level, protecting the hospital's well-connected supply, and avoid the absence of excessive accumulation.

6.6.2 Upgradation Expenditure

AII purchasing policies are acquired, so that less expenditure and more skills of budget can be used (Haque et al., 2018).

6.6.3 Emergency Response and Surge Capacity Planning

Epidemic, collective accidental events, or natural disasters, and the artificial intelligence (AI)-religious-Aspata-Recurrent Management system are included in the context of crisis.

6.6.4 Real-Time Capacity Observation

This work capacity is accessible to the deep-sized deepness of the depths, vegetables, and united by the available deepness, which makes the skillful allocation of resources in the resources of the peaks. Elgoridam is re-appointed to the high-managed fields of health service employees, which is ensuring a quick and effective reaction to emergency. In cooperation with the regional health service nets, hospitals can make the patient analysis of the patient resources and resources, the internet decision, and self-ordinary determination. Hospital resources management system increases, values reduce values, enhance the results of patients and include progressive progress that health services are easy to conduct regularly, unexpected, essential, and long-term planning. Finally, health services and resources are strongly enriched.

Modern epidemiological surveillance systems integrate mobile applications, artificial intelligence (AI) technologies, and Bluetooth functionality to monitor potential disease exposure and notify individuals who may have been affected. For instance, digital contact tracing solutions such as the Apple/Google Exposure Notification System provide anonymous alerts to individuals who have been in proximity to confirmed cases. AI-powered risk assessment tools enable public health authorities to analyze mobility data and transmission patterns, facilitating the design of localized lockdowns, quarantine protocols, and vaccination strategies. Moreover, AI-enabled telemedicine platforms allow remote monitoring of patients in home isolation, supporting timely medical interventions and reducing the burden on healthcare facilities.

6.7 SUPPLY CHAIN MANAGEMENT

The inner supply series of health service areas (SCM) is an important process that the medical materials, drugs, surgeries, personal securities and medical materials, hospitals, medicines, and drugs work in time of expenditure influence. The supply series reduces the removal, prevents lack, reduces expenditure, ensures the availability of necessary medical resources when they are needed. Architecture (AI), machine learning (ML), the Internet of Things (IoT), and blockchain technology, investigating inventory tracking, Authority Professional Profession, and Speak Supply Resistance are empowered.

6.7.1 Demand Forecasting and Inventory Optimization

To avert shortages and the accumulation of excessive inventory, contemporary supply chain management systems leverage predictive analytics to anticipate demand patterns predicated on historical data, patient admission rates, seasonal illness trends, and emergency situations.

6.7.1.1 Authorized Inventory Tracking and Just-in-Time (JIT) Inventory Management

Authorized inventory tracking utilizes advanced technologies, including the Internet of Things (IoT) and Radio Frequency Identification (RFID), to monitor real-time stock levels within healthcare facilities. This accurate and timely tracking enables procurement teams to optimize their supply chain management practices effectively, ensuring critical resources are continuously available without excess inventory. Additionally, the implementation of Just-In-Time (JIT) inventory management further enhances operational efficiency by reducing unnecessary inventory holding costs. JIT ensures that medical supplies and pharmaceuticals are delivered precisely when needed, minimizing storage expenses, decreasing waste, and allowing healthcare facilities to allocate resources more strategically. This integrated approach to inventory management, supported by IoT and RFID systems, helps healthcare institutions achieve cost-effective, efficient, and reliable supply chain management practices. (Faust and Acharya, 2021).

6.7.2 Efficient Procurement and Supplier Coordination

Healthcare supply chains depend on robust supplier relationships and streamlined procurement processes to ensure that medical facilities are provided with high-quality supplies in a timely manner.

6.7.2.1 Automated Procurement Systems

AI-enabled systems align issuer availability with sanatorium necessities, thereby reducing guide hard work and expediting the ordering system.

6.7.2.2 Multiprovider Approach

This method diversifies sourcing options to decrease reliance on an unmarried provider, for this reason stopping disruptions throughout global delivery chain crises (e.g., within the course of pandemics).

6.7.2.3 Vendor Performance Monitoring

AI continuously video display units provider reliability, delivery performance, and product fine, ensuring that hospitals engage with the most straightforward suppliers.

6.7.3 Logistics and Distribution Optimization

After the purchase of medical supply, effective logistics management guarantees timely delivery of these resources to hospitals, pharmacies, and clinics, while at the same time transport reduces costs and delays.

6.7.3.1 AI-POIL Route Optimization

Logistics system appoints AI to detect the fastest and economically viable transport paths, which increases delivery efficiency.

6.7.3.2 Cold Chain Control for Drugs

Vaccines, insulin, and biology require temperature-regulated storage and transport; IoT competition; tracking devices facilitate real-time monitoring of temperature variations.

6.7.3.3 Stock Automation

Robotic systems and AI-enhanced warehouse management software reduce human errors, accelerate order fulfillment processes, and increase the flexibility of supply chains.

6.7.4 Waste Management

Covering medical waste, expired medicines, and uncontrolled services is quite a challenge in health services. Advanced supply chain management functions contribute to a reduction in waste and ensure subsequent availability of important resources (Jin et al., 2020).

6.7.4.1 Exit Tracking System

AI-operated tracking mechanisms (first ending, first out—FEFO function) Avoid drug waste by preferring the use of medications that come into contact.

6.7.4.2 Automatic Low Warehouse Notification

Health services receive immediate information to fill out the required supply before reduction.

6.7.4.3 Revolution of Surplus Stock

AI identifies surplus portfolios in a function and rebuilds it for places that reduce it.

6.7.5 Emergency Preparedness and Supply Chain Resilience

In the times of crises such as pandemics, natural disasters, or major damage such as crisis, health services require rapid access to important supply to important supply including fan, personal safety equipment (PPE), and life-saving medicines. Emergency preparation through AI enhanced supply series administration.

Crisis demand modeling, which is a predicted analysis, considers dedicated supply requirements for historical public healthcare and increases in positive entrance. Automatic emergency measurement: guarantees that the important supplies are premixed for disaster response, leading to the defect at the last minute. Collaboration with regional and national supply chains: AI-driven structures facilitate coordination with public agencies, non-governmental organizations (NGO), and international suppliers to speed up resource sharing during emergencies (Pappada et al., 2020).

6.7.6 Blockchain for Transparency and Security

Blockchain technology is adopted to secure gradually and adapt to the health system's supply chain by ensuring this.

6.7.6.1 Authenticity Confirmation of Medical Products

Blockchain technology stops false drugs from infiltrating the supply chain by documenting each transaction on an irreversible account book. End-to-end traceability: original, storage status, and medical supply distribution roads guarantee widespread visibility. Compliance: by presenting tamper-proof items over all transactions, the rules of the healthcare system (e.g., FDA, such as medical equipment regulations in the EU) are streamlined. AI, IoT, Predictive Analytics, Blockchain and Automatic Logistics, Contemporary Healthcare Supply Chain Management System are used in right places and in correct amounts, securing medical supply and efficient distribution of medicines to the right amounts. This progression leads to a reduction in costs, increased patient safety, supply, and permanent health system's flexibility, resulting in the patient results being improved and adapted to hospital operations.

6.7.7 Public Health Decision Support

6.7.7.1 Epidemiological Surveillance

Monitoring epidemiology constitutes an indispensable function in public health, including the outbreak of the disease, new health hazards and real-time observation, data interpretation, and future analysis to eliminate public health patterns. By using extensive datasets, artificial intelligence (AI), machine learning (ML), Geographical Information System (GIS), and Internet of Things (IoT), a unit capable of IoT, modern surveillance frameworks are well-equipped to identify outbreaks in an initial stage and to identify outbreaks in direct public health services (Kannan, 2022).

6.7.7.2 Detection

Epidemiological monitoring systems operate by continuously aggregating and analyzing health data collected from hospitals, clinics, laboratories, and public health organizations to identify patterns or increases in disease incidence. AI-enabled systems detect potential outbreaks through surveillance monitoring.

6.7.7.2.1 Electronic Health Records (EHRS)

AI checks the information to an anonymous patient for groups of functioning analogy symptoms that may indicate a possible outbreak. Social media and news reports: AI-competent equipment checks dynamics of social media, news publications, and online search examination to understand the first indicators of disease spread.

6.7.7.2.2 Waste Water Analysis

Monitoring of viral concentrations (e.g., COVID-19, Polio virus) in wastewater tests produces advance alerts before the emergence of widespread clinical cases.

6.7.7.2.3 Portable Health Equipment

IoT-integrated wear, such as smartwatch, body temperature, heartbeat, and compilation of oxygen-saturation data may indicate early signs of population level infection.

6.7.8 Geographic Tracking and Mapping of Disease Spread

Sophisticated Geographical Information System (GIS) emphasizes public health authorities to imagine and predict the spread of diseases by using the method of outbreak of real-time mapping.

6.7.8.1 Heatmaps of Infections

Geographic Information Systems (GIS) in the Epidemic Risk Assessment (ERA) framework highlights high-risk areas, sources of contamination, and transmission pathways. These visualizations support the development and implementation of targeted disease control strategies.

6.7.8.2 Population Motion Analysis

AI amalgamates mobile phone geolocation records and excursion logs to hint at the propagation of diseases during numerous regions. Climate and environmental elements: AI algorithms set up correlations among meteorological conditions, air superb, and pollutant metrics with the superiority of ailments (e.g., examining how vector-borne illnesses include malaria and dengue in response to fluctuations in temperature).

6.7.9 Predictive Analytics for Disease Trends and Risk Assessment

Through the evaluation of historic fitness facts, system learning algorithms forecast the opportunity of ailment outbreaks, seasonal versions, and impending public fitness emergencies.

6.7.9.1 Influenza Forecasting

AI monitors trends in flu seasons to anticipate height contamination durations and decorate vaccine distribution techniques.

6.7.9.2 Pandemic Preparedness

AI-facilitated fashions compare international sickness surveillance information (e.g., CDC, WHO, country-wide fitness institutions) to foresee the ability of pandemics and biothreats.

6.7.9.3 Non-Communicable Disorder (NCD) Tracking

Predictive fashions evaluate trends in diabetes, cardiovascular disorder, and cancer, helping policymakers in the allocation of assets for preventive healthcare projects.

6.8 AUTOMATED CONTACT TRACING AND PUBLIC HEALTH INTERVENTIONS

Modern epidemiological surveillance systems integrate mobile applications, artificial intelligence (AI) technologies, and Bluetooth functionality to monitor potential disease exposure and notify individuals who may have been affected. For instance, digital contact tracing solutions such as the Apple/Google Exposure Notification System provide anonymous alerts to individuals who have been in proximity to confirmed cases. AI-powered risk assessment tools enable public health authorities to analyze mobility data and transmission patterns, facilitating the design of localized lockdowns, quarantine protocols, and vaccination strategies. Moreover, AI-enabled telemedicine platforms allow remote monitoring of patients in home isolation, supporting timely medical interventions and reducing the burden on healthcare facilities (Shafi et al., 2021).

6.8.1 Integration with Global Health Networks and Policymaking

Surveillance structures, in collaboration with the World Health Organization (WHO), Disease Control and Prevention Center (CDC), and the European Center Disease Prevention and Control (ECDC), facilitate the relationship between nationwide and nationwide training institutions and groups around the world, which allows coordination of real-time activities.

6.8.1.1 Standardized Statistics Sharing

The utilization of artificial intelligence (AI) automates the processes of reporting and harmonizing epidemiological records throughout diverse areas. Vaccine distribution making plans: Predictive analytics decorate the optimization of vaccine deployment by way of evaluating populace immunity tiers, bloodless chain logistics, and demographics taken into consideration to be at high chance. Public health policy method: Insights derived from records—pushed methodologies assist governments in setting up quarantine measures, imposing tour regulations, and facilitating resource allocation in response to outbreaks (Hamedan et al., 2020).

6.8.2 AI and Blockchain for Data Security and Transparency

To guarantee the privacy and accuracy of data, the modern monitoring system covers blockchain technology with safe AI models. Tampering-proof record: Implementation of blockchain technology ensures that disease reports and laboratory results maintain their authenticity and remain untouched. Unknown patient tracking: AI systems analyze data without violating privacy rights, ensuring the following rules such as HIPAA and GDPR. Belief in public health data: Transparent structure for sharing data that has been worked in the Health Council to combat misinformation and promote public trust. The area for monitoring epidemiology undergoes significant development through the integration of AI, Big Data Analytics, Internet of Things (IoT), and Geographical Information System (GIS) and provides overall facilities for detecting outbreaks, tracing real-time diseases, forecast modeling, and global coordination. These technological advances significantly increase public health preparation, enable time intervention and eventually preserve life by preventing and reducing the results of infectious diseases and chronic health hazards globally.

6.8.2.1 Policymaking and Population Health Management

To guide future models, politics and population health management, predictive analysis, artificial intelligence (AI), and health policy using Big Data create evidence-based health policy with a view of improving the overall public health services. Through the investigation of extensive health records, demographic data, disease trends, and environmental factors, the future equates the chair-models—the insight required to take resource allocation to decision-makers, access to healthcare and long-term health strategies to make informed decisions (Ylenia et al., 2021).

6.8.3 Data-Driven Healthcare Policy Formulation

Predictive models analyze historical and health data in real time, which understand the pattern, evaluate risks, and suggest policy interventions. Important applications include the following.

6.8.3.1 Exam Forecast

AI prohibits outbreaks of function, seasonal diseases, and new health hazards, so that governments can implement active control strategies.

6.8.3.2 Prevention of Chronic Illness

Future staging models examine diabetes, heart disease, and obesity-related trends and support decision-makers in producing targeted health campaigns and preventive care initiatives.

6.8.3.3 Health Access and Equity Analysis

AI technologies assess inequalities in health services access between different demographics, thus informing guidelines aimed at increasing health services in the countryside, improving health services in the countryside, making telemedicine access to expand access to telecommunications and reducing socio-economic health.

6.8.4 Resource Distribution and Health Infrastructure Scheme

Government bodies and health organizations analyze the future to limit the distribution of resources and expect future healthcare requirements.

6.8.4.1 Hospital Capacity Scheme

AI estimated the demand for patient entrance rate, intensive care unit, and emergency room and ensured that hospitals are adequately prepared for seasonal influence, epidemic or natural disasters.

6.8.4.2 Vaccine Distribution Adjustment

Machine learning models predict vaccination, population level, and cold chain logistics, which leads to an effective roll-out of vaccine.

6.8.4.3 Medical Work Planning

Artificial intelligence (AI) performs intensive analysis of demographic infection and the spread of illness to detect future healthcare requirements, which reduces potential deficiency of medical doctors, nursing professionals, and special suppliers.

6.8.5 The Population's Health Evaluation and Intervention Strategies

Predictive analyses strengthen government institutions to understand demographic groups with high risk and perform targeted health intervention.

6.8.5.1 Social Determiners of Health (SDOH) Analysis

AI synthesizes data to predict health results related to income inequalities, housing status, education, and availability of nutritious food.

6.8.5.2 Prevention of Mental Health and Drug Intake

AI monitors trends in opioid addiction, identifies the risk indicators of suicide, and detects mental health emergencies, which help with the allocation of resources for rehabilitation facilities, mental health services, and public consciousness initiatives.

6.8.5.3 Mother and Child Health Program

Prognosis models check birth results, access to care before delivery, and infant mortality figures to increase the framework for health policies.

6.8.6 Crisis Management and Emergency Preparedness

AI-driven policy frameworks increase public fitness emergency preparedness with the aid of forecasting disease outbreaks, natural calamities, and vulnerabilities inside healthcare systems.

6.8.6.1 Pandemic Reaction Making Plans

AI fashions numerous virus transmission eventualities, aiding governmental bodies inside the implementation of quarantine protocols, travel restrictions, and mass trying out projects.

6.8.6.2 Disaster Response Coordination

Predictive models refine ambulance dispatch, clinic surge capacity, and clinical supply inventories in practice for natural screw ups inclusive of hurricanes or earthquakes.

6.8.6.3 Biothreat and Biosecurity Monitoring

AI evaluates capacity bioterrorism threats and laboratory protection measures, steering national safety coverage development (Fernandes et al., 2020).

6.8.7 AI and Blockchain for Policy Transparency and Public Trust

To sell obligation, protection, and public self-assure, present-day healthcare insurance frameworks combine AI and blockchain technologies.

6.8.7.1 Secure Fitness Records Sharing

Blockchain generation ensures unalterable and decentralized health information, facilitating sturdy cooperation among government companies, healthcare centers, and worldwide health businesses.

6.8.7.2 Bias Detection in Policymaking

AI uncovers racial, gender, and economic biases present in insurance technique, thereby ensuring equitable and truly healthcare hints.

6.8.7.3 Public Health Conversation

AI-extra equipment shows social sentiment and traits in incorrect records, allowing government entities to disseminate clean facts—knowledgeable public health messages.

By leveraging predictive analytics, AI, and huge statistics, policymakers are prepared to plot efficient, proactive, and equitable healthcare guidelines that beautify population fitness, optimize resource allocation, and put together for coming near-fitness challenges. These statistics-informed techniques guarantee that healthcare structures stay adaptable, resilient, and proficient in addressing each of the instantaneous and prolonged public health exigencies (Ehn et al., 2021).

6.8.8 Benefits of DSSs in Healthcare

Key benefits of AI and data-driven technologies in healthcare are the amalgamation of AI, predictive analytics, and records—pushed technologies inside the healthcare quarter have profoundly altered affected person care, hospital administration, and decision-making methodologies. These improvements make contributions to better affected person results, expanded operational performance, value financial savings, and evidence-based total decision-making, in the end culminating in a greater powerful and sustainable healthcare paradigm.

The implementation of artificial intelligence (AI) and automation technologies has significantly reduced the administrative costs of healthcare services by streamlining workflows. These benefits extend beyond scheduling and include medical record management, insurance claim processing, and resource allocation. Chatbots and voice recognition systems powered by Natural Language Processing (NLP) assist healthcare professionals in documenting clinical activities, enabling physicians to devote more time for direct patient care. Moreover, AI-enhanced hospital resource management systems optimize staff scheduling, bed occupancy, and equipment usage, ensuring a smooth and well-coordinated hospital environment.

6.8.8.1 Improved Patient Outcomes

AI-driven contraptions facilitate extra diagnostic accuracy, treatment strategizing, and continuous affected character surveillance, culminating in greater particular and timely medical interventions. Sophisticated device studying algorithms help in the early identity of diseases, consisting of the detection of malignancies in imaging research or the prediction of cardiovascular disease danger based on affected character scientific histories. Furthermore, individualized remedy regimens, customized normal with an affected man or woman's genetic profiles and scientific histories, make certain improved fulfillment charges and superior recuperation consequences. Remote affected individual monitoring and AI-enabled wearable era permit real-time tracking of vital fitness parameters, taking into account proactive intervention and decreased health center readmissions.

6.8.8.2 Enhanced Efficiency

The implementation of artificial intelligence and automation technologies has significantly reduced the administrative costs of healthcare services by streamlining workflows. These benefits extend beyond scheduling and include medical record management, insurance claim processing, and resource allocation. Chatbots and voice recognition systems powered by Natural Language Processing (NLP) assist healthcare professionals in documenting clinical activities, enabling physicians to devote more time for direct patient care. Moreover, AI-enhanced hospital resource management systems optimize staff scheduling, bed occupancy, and equipment usage, ensuring a smooth and well-coordinated hospital environment..

6.8.8.3 Cost Reduction

The use of forecast analysis and AI-driven Decision Support Systems plays an important role in incomplete medical examinations, fruitless processes, and being admitted to the hospital, leading to sufficient cost reduction for both health professionals and patients. Through the analysis of broad datasets, the AI is able to identify high-risk patients, which may require initial intervention, and reduces the emergency input and long-term treatment expenses. In addition, AI increases the management of the supply chain, ensuring economically viable procurement and distribution of medical supply, which further reduces operating costs.

6.8.8.4 Data-Driven Decision-Making

Integration of AI and massive data analysis presents evidence-based insights that allow healthcare professionals and decision-makers to interact in further informed and special decision-making perspectives. Such insight plays an important role in identifying public health development, assessing treatment efficiency, and adaptation of resource allocation. In addition, the AI manual units contribute to scientific test research, accelerate drug discovery, and facilitate the active availability of modern treatment to the victims. By collaborating the information on real time and historically affected persons, health services are providers designed to provide further accurate diagnosis, resignation of personal treatment, and powerful health techniques. The incorporation of AI-driven solutions into the healthcare zone, not handiest, complements the exceptional patient care, however, additionally allows the streamlining of health center operations, diminishes charges, and encourages a record-driven paradigm for choice-making. As technological improvements hold, healthcare systems are poised to become increasingly more efficient, proactive, and patient-centric, in the end resulting in progressed fitness effects on a worldwide scale (Dreiseitl and Ohno-Machado, 2002).

6.9 CHALLENGES AND ETHICAL CONSIDERATIONS

Despite the benefits, the implementation of the Decision Support Systems (DSSs) faced many challenges.

6.9.1 Data Quality and Data Integration in Challenges and Health Services in AI

Although AI and data-driven technologies have fundamentally changed the healthcare system, clinical workflows must face many important challenges to ensure their efficiency, reliability, and spontaneous integration. Two primary concerns include challenges with interpretability, which arise when the healthcare system struggles to communicate effectively, and data related to data accuracy and perfection, because poor data quality can lead to wrong medical recommendations and potential risks for patient safety.

6.9.1.1 Interoperability Challenges: Lack of Spontaneous Communication between Systems

One of the most important obstacles in modern healthcare is the difference, which is defined as the ability of different health information systems to exchange and use data effectively. Hospitals, clinics, laboratories, pharmacies, and insurance institutions often appoint electronic health record (EHR) systems as an uneven electronic health record (EHR) system, each characterized by its unique data formats, standards, and protocols. This absence of standardization causes sufficient difficulties with spontaneous sharing of important patient information in the system.

For example, the EHR system of a hospital may store the patient's record in a format that is incompatible with the clinical system of the external laboratory, resulting in a delay in achieving test results, fruitless data registration but potentially achieved. Similarly, the AI-driven decision-making systems can face challenges in recurrent patient data in real time from multiple sources, which reduces their ability to provide accurate and timely insight. Lack of universal data exchange standards in health organizations interferes with efforts and significantly reduces workflakes, and limits the entire capacity of AI-controlled diagnosis and treatment plan. To deal with the challenges related to interoperability, the Healthcare Institute tries to implement standardized contours such as Fast Healthcare Interoperability Resources (FHIR) and Health Level Seven (HL7). These frames facilitate secure and organized data exchange between different healthcare, which increases communication, coordination of patient care, and integration of artificial intelligence (De Andres et al., 2021).

6.9.1.2 Data Accuracy and Completeness: Risks of Poor-Quality Data

The effect of artificial intelligence and future analysis in the healthcare system is deeply preparedness for quality, accuracy, and perfection of data used for training models and prepares recommendations. Inadequate, chronic, or incorrect data can lead to incorrect diagnosis, inappropriate treatment protocols, and incorrect decision-making process.

6.9.1.3 Various Factors Contribute to Suboptimal Data Quality

This includes human errors in data registration, involvement of inaccuracy in the patient's knowledge, post repetition, or absence of clinical documentation. Inconsistent documentation practice, where health professionals record the data analysis, complicated data analysis. The bias that is present in the AI training dataset, where the AI model can be trained on a dataset that inadequately represents a diverse patient population, results in one that leads to health inequalities and crazy predictions. Inaccurate for sensors or equipment, where unclear healthcare providers, Internet of Things (IoT) units, and external surveillance technologies can get incompatible or misconceptions, affecting the AI-powered diagnosis. For example, if an AI model designed to predict cardiovascular diseases is mainly trained on the data of male individuals, it may be inadequate for assessing symptoms in women or young patients, resulting in bias or incomplete recommendations. In a similar vein, if an AI-enhanced medication management system receives flawed allergy information due to incomplete patient records, it could propose hazardous prescriptions, thereby jeopardizing patient safety. To alleviate these risks, healthcare providers and AI developers must prioritize data validation, standardization, and ongoing quality enhancement. The use of data cleaning function, cross reference, and use of AI algorithms are important measures to ensure accurate and reliable health services AI solutions that are able to detect and flag incompatibility. While artificial intelligence and computer technologies have the opportunity to revolutionize health services, challenges such as interoperability barriers and data quality problems require systematic resolution. The installation of universal data exchange standards, the increase of electronic health record (EHR) system compatibility and the warranty for accurate and fair data sets will promote more qualification in AI. By overcoming these challenges, health organizations can fully utilize AI for better patient results, customized operation and evidence-based decisions (Figure 6.4).

6.9.2 Ethical and Legal Concerns

6.9.2.1 Ethical and Legal Challenges in AI-Driven Healthcare Systems

Including artificial intelligence and Decision Support Systems (DSSs) in the healthcare system provides sufficient capacity; however, it faces significant moral and legal challenges at the same time. The patient presents important challenges to protect privacy and data security, algorithm bias and openness, and reduce obligations

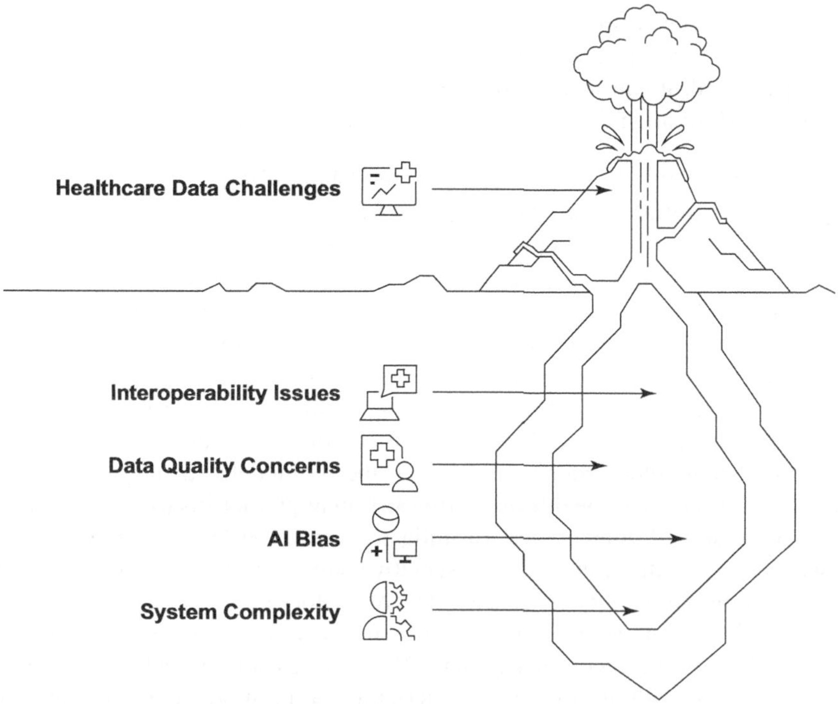

FIGURE 6.4 Challenges in healthcare.

for AI-driven decisions that require careful control to maintain trust, justice, and responsibility in the applications of AI health services.

6.9.2.2 Patient Privacy and Data Security: Ensuring Compliance with HIPAA and GDPR

Given that AI systems manage extensive versions of sensitive health information, privacy protection and strong data security measures are of great importance. Rules such as Health Insurance Portability and Accountability Act (HIPAA) in the United States and General Data Protection Regulation (GDPR) in Europe use strict guidelines for the collection, storage, and spread of patient data from health organizations. AI-MANGO Healthcare System often requires extensive datasets for real-time training and analytical procedures, improving the capacity of data violations, cyber-attacks, and unauthorized access. Whether the patient records are compromised, it can lead to identity theft, insurance fraud, or even important medical misinformation that puts the patient's safety at risk. Given that AI systems manage extensive versions of sensitive health information, privacy protection and strong data security measures are of great importance. Rules such as health insurance portability and liability law (HIPAA) in the United States and General Data Protection Regulation (GDPR) in Europe use strict guidelines for the collection, storage and spread of patient data from health organizations. AI-MANGO Healthcare System often requires extensive datasets for real-time training and analytical procedures, improving the capacity of data violations, cyberattacks, and unauthorized access. Whether the patient records are compromised, it can lead to identity theft, insurance fraud, or even important medical misinformation that puts the patient's safety at risk.

6.9.2.3 Algorithmic Bias and Transparency: Mitigating Discrimination in AI-Driven Decisions

AI algorithms are fundamentally dependent on historical datasets for health services, which can naturally incorporate biases related to race, gender, age, or socioeconomic condition. If these biases are unnatural, AI-produced decision-making can exacerbate existing health inequalities, unequal access to treatment, incorrect diagnoses, or harmful risk assessments. For example, empirical studies have indicated that some AI models employed in medical imaging show better performance on light skin tones compared to dark skin colors, increasing the chances of misdiagnosis in specific demographic groups. Similarly, if the AI model is primarily trained on data derived from urban healthcare settings, it may predict insufficient results for rural or underserved populations. To mitigate biases, the healthcare system must engineer the use of different and representative datasets and subject them to ongoing study for discriminatory tendencies. The regulatory structure should ensure that the AI models present clear decision, and ensure that doctors understand the rationale behind AI-borne recommendations. Mechanisms for the detection of moral AI audits, fair algorithms, and bias are necessary to promote openness and equity within AI-controlled health services (Yang et al., 2018).

6.9.3 Liability Issues

This is to establish responsibility for errors made by Decision Support Systems. One of the most complex legal dilemmas in AI-operated healthcare is related to the determination of responsibility when an AI system provides an erroneous or harmful decision. Decision Support Systems (DSSs) provide assistance to health professionals by offering clinical advice, treatment recommendations, and risk prognoses. However, if such suggestions result in medical errors, incorrect diagnoses, or inappropriate treatments, who holds legal responsibility?

6.9.3.1 Potential Liability Scenarios Encompass

Medical officer: If a doctor follows the recommendation of an incorrect AI and the patient suffers, should the doctor be blamed for relying on the system? Hospital responsibility: If a health institution integrates a deficient AI-controlled DSS, should the organization be held accountable for unfavorable patient outcomes? AI developer responsibility: If an AI system generates incorrect predictions due to suboptimal training data or biased algorithms, should software developers or health professionals be considered responsible?

In order to navigate these complications, the legal framework must clarify whether AI-driven decisions should be regarded as advisory tools or autonomous decisions. Some researchers advocate the "Human-in-the-loop" model, where AI provides recommendations, while the final medical decision is made by human doctors, thus reducing the risk of liability. Additionally, AI interpretation and model verification should be compulsory before deploying AI systems in the clinical environment. Since artificial intelligence (AI) and Decision Support Systems (DSSs) are intertwined with the healthcare system, it is essential to address challenges related to data privacy, bias, and responsibility to maintain trust, equity, and accountability. Increasing data protection protocols, ensuring transparency in the AI mechanisms, and defining clear legal responsibilities will facilitate the mitigation of these risks and promote a safer and moral sound-enhanced health system's ecosystem.

6.9.4 Future Trends in Healthcare DSS

6.9.4.1 Emerging Trends in AI-Driven Decision Support Systems (DSSs) in Healthcare

Artificial Intelligence (AI), Internet of Things (IoT), blockchain technology, and significant technological advancements with integration of personalized medicine contribute significantly to diagnosis, monitoring the patient and data security. These innovations enhance Decision Support Systems (DSSs) by increasing the accuracy of prognosis, enabling real-time health monitoring, facilitating secure data exchange, and providing individualized patient profiles. Artificial intelligence and machine learning are useful to increase deep learning models for medical image analysis and predictive diagnostics. Artificial intelligence (AI) and machine learning (ML) development in medical technology enables rapid and more accurate clinical processes. Deep learning architecture, especially convolutional neural networks (CNN), is increasingly used in analyzing medical imaging, assisting radiologists in detecting tumors, fractures, and non-conformities in X-rays, MRIs, and CT scans with greater accuracy than traditional function (Figure 6.5).

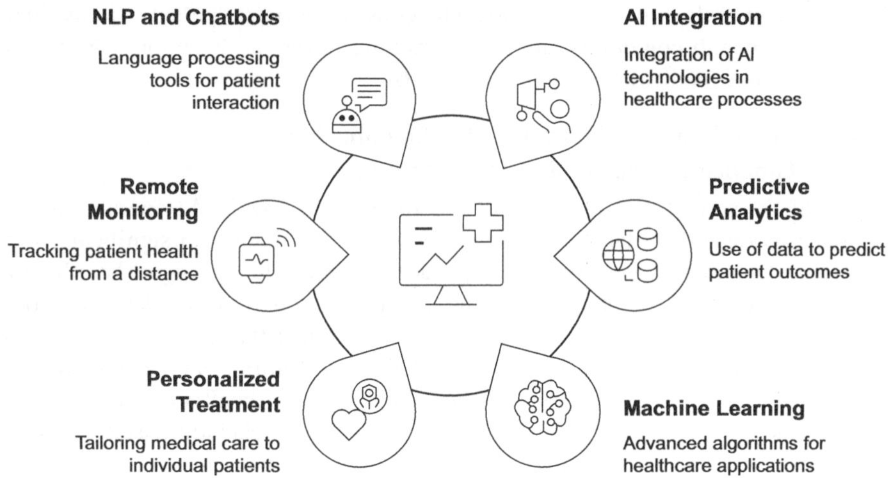

FIGURE 6.5 AI and data-driven technologies in healthcare.

In addition to imaging methods, AI can enhance predictive diagnostics by analyzing electronic health records (EHR), laboratory results, and genetic information to identify patterns associated with pathologies such as cancer, diabetes, and heart disease. By utilizing natural language processing (NLP), AI can gain valuable insights from extensive clinical notes, thereby improving clinical decision-making and identifying facilities for early illness.

AI-enhanced DSS platforms contribute to treatment by suggesting individualized medications based on the basis of individual biomarkers of a patient's specific biomarkers. The continuous development of interpretive AI aims to ensure that the decisions made by these systems remain transparent and intelligent for health services.

6.9.4.2 Integration with IoT and Wearable Devices: Real-Time Monitoring of Patient Health

Through the use of Internet of Things (IoT) portable technology and intelligent medical sensors, the healthcare sector is revolutionized by facilitating real-time monitoring of health. Smartwatch, fitness trackers, electrocardiogram (ECG) screens, and glucose sensors collect real-time data related to heartbeat, blood pressure, blood sugar levels, oxygen saturation, and physical activity. This information is forwarded to AI-operated DSS platforms to monitor chronic conditions, to identify early warning indicators and take preemptive measures before significant health (Sharma et al., 2022). For example, AI-assisted pacemakers and external cardiac monitors can alert physicians to arrhythmia or potential stroke risks in real time. Likewise, intelligent insulin delivery systems modulate insulin administration in accordance with real-time blood sugar measurements, thereby improving diabetes management. By utilizing IoT-enabled remote patient monitoring (RPM) systems, healthcare institutions can decrease hospital readmissions, optimize post-operative care, and offer personalized treatment recommendations grounded in real-time physiological data. This paradigm shift is particularly advantageous for geriatric patients, individuals with chronic health conditions, and those residing in remote locations who necessitate continuous medical oversight (Figure 6.6).

6.9.4.3 Blockchain for Secure Health Data Sharing: Enhancing Security and Transparency

In light of the spread of digital health records and the use of AI-operated analysis, concerns related to data security and privacy have reached a significant turn. Blockchain technology appears to be a panacea for the safe sharing of health data, the management of patient records, and the prevention of fraudulent activities. Blockchain forms a decentralized, tamper-resistant ledger that facilitates encrypted storage and regulates access to patient data. This data guarantees integrity, prevents unauthorized changes, and increases transparency within healthcare transactions. Through the implementation of smart contracts, the blockchain-based decision-based Decision Support System (DSSs) can effectively automate the management of patient consent, ensuring that only authorized institutions have access to medical data.

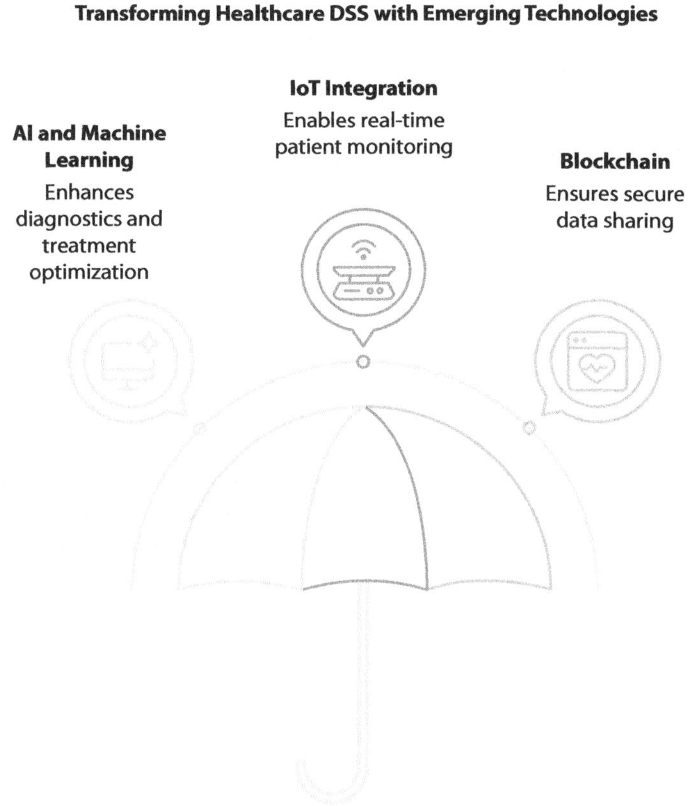

FIGURE 6.6 Transforming healthcare DSSs with emerging technologies.

For example, blockchain can be applied to the drug supply chain to monitor the authenticity of medicines, eliminate counterfeit medications, and ensure the correct storage status for vaccines. In addition, telemedicine platforms utilize blockchain for secure identification verification and medical consultation documentation, reducing data violations and risks associated with cyberattacks. Blockchain assimilation in interoperable health data exchanges ensures that the patient's information can be safely transmitted between hospitals, research institutes, and insurance providers, fostering a cooperative healthcare system to protect the patient's privacy.

Individual medicine and genomics correspond to genetic profiles, bolstered by recent developments in genomic sequencing and AI-driven Decision Support Systems, which facilitate the emergence of personalized medicine, where treatment is tailored to the patient's specific genetic structure, lifestyle, and medical history. The traditional "one-size-fits-all" therapeutic approach is being replaced by the precision medicine methodology, which helps estimate how a person will respond to a specific drug or medical intervention.

AI-enhanced decision-making systems can control genomic data, biomarkers, and epigenetic effects to manage conditions such as cancer, neurodegenerative disorders, and autoimmune diseases. In oncology, AI helps identify tumor profiles to identify tumor aids.

6.9.4.4 Epigenetic Effect of Pharmacogenomics

Decision Support Systems analyze genetic variations affecting drug metabolism and ensure that patients receive the right medication in the right dosage, thereby reducing side effects.

6.9.4.5 Themes Related to Neurocognitive Disorders

AI frameworks evaluate genomic indicators associated with Alzheimer's and Parkinson's diseases, facilitating early intervention and lifestyle adjustments to slow disease reactions. The rapid development of AI, IoT, blockchain, and personalized medicine is basically changing the landscape of Decision Support Systems within healthcare. Deep learning models are refining diagnostic capabilities, IoT devices facilitate real-time patient monitoring, blockchain secures the sharing of health information, and DSS-driven precision medicine is tailoring treatment plans based on genetic insights. As these technologies continue to evolve, they are poised to yield more accurate diagnoses, proactive healthcare interventions, and enhanced patient outcomes, heralding a new epoch of sensible and information-driven healthcare answers.

6.10 CONCLUSION

Support system for the healthcare system is revolutionizing medical practice by aiding clinical decisions, increasing operational efficiency, and furthering public health initiatives. Despite the existence of challenges, advancements in AI, data analysis, and interoperability are charting a course for more efficient and ethical implementation of support systems. The future orbit is located in intelligent, adaptive, and patient-focused technologies that will continue to transform the healthcare system.

REFERENCES

Antoniadi AM, Du Y, Guendouz Y, et al. (2021) Current challenges and future opportunities for XAI in machine learning-based clinical decision support systems: A systematic review. *Appl Sci* 11: 5088. https://doi.org/10.3390/app11115088.

Ben Khalfallah H, Jelassi M, Demongeot J, Bellamine Ben Saoud N (2025) Advancements in predictive analytics: Machine learning approaches to estimating length of stay and mortality in sepsis. *Computation* 13(1). https://doi.org/10.3390/computation13010008

De Andres J, Ten-Esteve A, Harutyunyan A, et al. (2021) Predictive clinical decision support system using machine learning and imaging biomarkers in patients with neurostimulation therapy: A pilot study. *Pain Physician* 24: E1279–E1290.

Divya D, Savita S, Kaur S (2025) Unveiling excellence in Indian healthcare: A patient-centric PRISMA analysis of hospital service quality, patient satisfaction and loyalty. *Int J Pharm Healthc Mark.* https://doi.org/10.1108/IJPHM-05-2024-0043

Dreiseitl S, Ohno-Machado L (2002) Logistic regression and artificial neural network classification models: A methodology review. *J Biomed Inform* 35: 352–359. https://doi.org/10.1016/S1532-0464(03)00034-0.

Ehn M, Derneborg M, Revenäs Å, et al. (2021) User-centered requirements engineering to manage the fuzzy front-end of open innovation in e-health: A study on support systems for seniors' physical activity. *Int J Med Inform* 154: 104547. https://doi.org/10.1016/j.ijmedinf.2021.104547.

Faust O, Acharya UR (2021) Automated classification of five arrhythmias and normal sinus rhythm based on RR interval signals. *Expert Syst Appl* 181: 115031. https://doi.org/10.1016/j.eswa.2021.115031.

Fernandes M, Vieira SM, Leite F, et al. (2020) Clinical decision support systems for triage in the emergency department using intelligent systems: A review. *Artif Intell Med* 102: 101762. https://doi.org/10.1016/j.artmed.2019.101762.

Hamedan F, Orooji A, Sanadgol H, et al. (2020) Clinical decision support system to predict chronic kidney disease: A fuzzy expert system approach. *Int J Med Inform* 138: 104134. https://doi.org/10.1016/j.ijmedinf.2020.104134.

Haque MdR, Islam MdM, Iqbal H, et al. (2018) Performance evaluation of random forests and artificial neural networks for the classification of liver disorder. International Conference on Computer, Communication, Chemical, Material and Electronic Engineering (IC4ME2). IEEE, 1–5. https://doi.org/10.1109/IC4ME2.2018.8465658.

Houssem Ben Khalfallah, Mariem Jelassi, Narjes Bellamine Ben Saoud, Jacques Demongeot (2023a) Chapter 19, 229. https://doi.org/10.1007/978-3-031-40116-9_19.

Houssem Ben Khalfallah, Mariem Jelassi, Narjes Bellamine Ben Saoud, Jacques Demongeot (2023b) Chapter 19–2, 1. https://doi.org/10.1007/978-3-319-12125-3_19-2.

Hussain M, Iacovides I, Lawton T, Sharma V, Porter Z, Cunningham A, et al. (2024). Development and translation of human-AI interaction models into working prototypes for clinical decision-making. Proceedings of the 2024 ACM Designing Interactive Systems Conference, July, pp. 1607–1619. https://doi.org/10.1145/3643834.3660697.

Jammal M, Saab A, Abi Khalil C, Mourad C, Tsopra R, Saikali M, et al. (2025) Impact on clinical guideline adherence of Orient-COVID, a clinical decision support system based on dynamic decision trees for COVID19 management: A randomized simulation trial with medical trainees. *Int J Med Inform* 195: 105772. https://doi.org/10.1016/j.ijmedinf.2024.105772.

Jin Y, Qin C, Huang Y, et al. (2020) Multi-domain modeling of atrial fibrillation detection with twin attentional convolutional long short-term memory neural networks. *Knowl-Based Syst* 193: 105460. https://doi.org/10.1016/j.knosys.2019.105460.

Kannan S (2022) An automated clinical decision support system for predicting cardiovascular disease using ensemble learning approach. *Concurrency Comput Pract Exp* 34: e7007. https://doi.org/10.1002/cpe.7007.

Lyu J, Zhang J (2019) BP neural network prediction model for suicide attempt among Chinese rural residents. *J Affect Disorders* 246: 465–473. https://doi.org/10.1016/j.jad.2018.12.111.

Manta O, Vasileiou N, Giannakopoulou O, Bromis K, Georgas K, Vagenas TP, et al. (2024) TeleRehaB DSS Project: Advancing balance rehabilitation through digital health technologies. 2024 IEEE International Conference on Engineering, Technology, and Innovation (ICE/ITMC), IEEE, June, pp. 1–5. https://doi.org/10.1109/ICE/ITMC61926.2024.10794240

Pappada SM, Owais MH, Cameron BD, et al. (2020) An artificial neural network-based predictive model to support optimization of inpatient glycemic control. *Diabetes Technol Ther* 22: 383–394. https://doi.org/10.1089/dia.2019.0252.

Shafi I, Ansari S, Din S, et al. (2021) Artificial neural networks as clinical decision support systems. *Concurrency Comput Pract Exp* 33: e6342. https://doi.org/10.1002/cpe.6342.

Sharma SK, Vijayakumar K, Kadam VJ, et al. (2022) Breast cancer prediction from microRNA profiling using random subspace ensemble of LDA classifiers via Bayesian optimization. *Multimed Tools Appl* 81: 41785–41805. https://doi.org/10.1007/s11042-021-11653-x.

Yang S, Bian J, Sun Z, et al. (2018) Early detection of disease using electronic health records and Fisher's Wishart discriminant analysis. *Procedia Comput Sci* 140: 393–402. https://doi.org/10.1016/j.procs.2018.10.299.

Ylenia C, Chiara DL, Giovanni I, et al. (2021) A clinical decision support system based on fuzzy rules and classification algorithms for monitoring the physiological parameters of type-2 diabetic patients. *MBE* 18: 2654–2674. https://doi.org/10.3934/mbe.2021135.

Zeng L, Li RYM, Yigitcanlar T, Zeng H (2023) Public opinion mining on construction health and safety: Latent Dirichlet allocation approach. Buildings 13: 2075–5309. https://doi.org/10.3390/buildings13040927.

7 Healthcare Education and XAI
Future Directions

Giray Kolcu and Mukadder Inci Baser Kolcu

7.1 INTRODUCTION AND CONTEXT

Artificial intelligence (AI) is becoming an indispensable part of healthcare and education. Its applications range from clinical decision-making to enhancing educational experiences. However, the "black box" nature of many AI systems presents challenges for understanding and trust, particularly in professional health education, where transparency and accuracy are paramount. Explainable artificial intelligence (XAI) has emerged as a transformative approach to address this issue, offering insights into how AI models make decisions and ensure that these processes are interpretable and reliable.

This chapter explored the potential of XAI in professional health education, focusing on its role in curriculum development, simulation training, diagnostic support systems, interprofessional education, and program evaluation. By integrating XAI into educational frameworks, healthcare educators and students can gain a clearer understanding of AI-driven insights, fostering a more data-driven and transparent learning environment. Using real-world examples, this chapter highlights how XAI can enhance teaching methods, improve decision-making processes, and strengthen collaboration among healthcare professionals.

Explainable artificial intelligence (XAI) provides transparency in the process of learning the logic behind the decisions made by artificial intelligence systems. With this approach, instead of only showing the results of an algorithm, the decision-making process of the algorithm is evaluated, and an attitude toward learning a thinking process is proposed. Therefore, XAI has the potential to play an important role in professional health education when used under an instructor's guidance (Kolcu et al., 2021)

The black box problem is a term used particularly in the context of artificial intelligence and complex systems (Köse, 2022). It refers to a situation in which the inner workings of a system, especially its decision-making processes, are opaque to an external observer. Today's AI models are becoming "black boxes" due to the increase in data processed, especially using deep learning or hybrid machine

DOI: 10.1201/9781003605416-7

learning systems, which creates the need for XAI (Adadi and Berrada, 2018). XAI aims to ensure that the outputs of the AI models are understandable and interpretable. XAI aims to solve the "black box" problem in AI models (Wang et al., 2023). Two main approaches have been proposed to get AI models out of the "black box" situation (Verma et al., 2022). The first is to use inherently explainable models, such as decision trees and linear models. The second is to use existing sophisticated classification techniques (such as deep neural networks) but supplement them with intermediate models that make the model's predictions and/or internal processes understandable (Verma et al., 2022). XAI is an important research area for understanding and explaining the input–output linkages of AI models (Köse, 2022).

7.2 XAI IN PROGRAM DEVELOPMENT

As an example of the use of "explainable artificial intelligence" (XAI) in curriculum development, it can make educational processes more effective, flexible, and innovative within the framework of Kern's six-step curriculum development model (Thomas et al., 2022). Kern's model covers critical stages of training programs, such as needs analysis, goal setting, strategy development, implementation, evaluation, and feedback loop. In this context, XAI has the potential to contribute to a stronger implementation of each phase.

In the needs analysis phase, XAI offers the ability to make sense of big data to analyze students' learning needs in health education. The transparent disclosure of these analyses allows educators to clearly see which areas require improvement (Adadi and Berrada, 2018).

In the goal-setting and strategy development phases, XAI can simulate the outcomes of different scenarios and provide valuable insights into which goals and learning outcomes are likely to be more effective. For example, modeling reveals the skills students need to shape program objectives directly (Wang et al., 2023).

During the implementation phase, XAI-supported tools analyze the performance of educators and students in real time. They provide in-process guidance to both educators and students by explaining the rationale for the training decisions. This enables quick intervention for problems encountered during implementation and a more flexible learning experience (Arun et al., 2021).

In the evaluation and feedback phase, XAI can make sense of the data used to measure the effectiveness of the program and clearly identify its strengths and weaknesses. For example, it can explain why a module does not meet the expected learning outcomes and provide concrete suggestions for program improvement (Jakesch et al., 2023).

The explainability and data analytics provided by XAI support informed, data-driven, and transparent decision-making at every stage of Kern's curriculum development model. In this way, curricula become more student-centered as well as continuously improvable and dynamic.

7.3 POTENTIAL APPLICATIONS

Simulation Training: XAI-powered simulators have great potential in the field of health education. Such simulators use explainable AI algorithms to explain the logic behind decisions made by AI (Adadi and Berrada, 2018). For example, in simulations based on a patient scenario, when students diagnose a disease or create a treatment plan, they encounter a system that explains AI decisions. This system helps students to understand why they choose what they have chosen (Wang et al., 2023). A transparent explanation is provided, showing which data shape the AI's diagnosis and treatment recommendations and which factors come to the fore. These explanations allow students to better understand the decision-making processes and develop their own clinical thinking skills. In addition, students learn the systematic approach of artificial intelligence when evaluating different patient profiles and have the opportunity to compare their own decisions using this model. Such simulations allow students to make mistakes in safer environments and to improve their clinical decision-making skills (Gunning et al., 2019).

7.4 DIAGNOSIS SUPPORT SYSTEMS

AI-based diagnostic support systems guide healthcare professionals in making clinical decisions. XAI plays an important role because students can better assess the accuracy of these recommendations by understanding how AI arrives at diagnostic recommendations (Galdames, 2024). For example, when diagnosing a patient, AI systems analyze data such as various symptoms, test results, and patient history to provide a diagnostic recommendation. XAI provides explanations for the algorithms used in this process and allows students to understand how diagnostic support systems work. Students can follow each step to understand why a recommendation is correct or incorrect. These explanations provide students with clinical thinking skills and a deeper awareness of the limitations and strengths of AI (Galdames, 2024). Thus, students begin to see diagnostic support systems not only as tools but also as part of a decision-making process. Such practices can provide students with in-depth feedback on systematic thinking, critical evaluation, and decision-making processes as well as help them make more confident and informed choices when making clinical decisions (Hussain, 2024).

7.4.1 The Role of Decision Support Systems and XAI in Professional Health Education

Decision support systems are critical tools for improving clinical decision-making in healthcare. These AI-based systems help healthcare professionals quickly and accurately assess the health status of patients. XAI increases the transparency of these systems, enabling healthcare professionals to better understand the recommendations made by AI. For example, when a diagnostic recommendation is made, XAI explains in detail how it was created and how the data were used. These explanations allow healthcare professionals to more accurately assess the logic of AI and the data on which it is based so that they can confidently decide on the accuracy of the proposed diagnoses.

In professional health education, XAI also plays an important role in the development of clinical thinking skills. Decision support systems supported by XAI give students the ability to make informed choices in their decision-making processes (Lee et al., 2017). In this way, students learn how to make more effective decisions in clinical scenarios while simultaneously understanding the logic behind their decisions (Dionne-Odom et al., 2019). In addition, healthcare professionals can better understand the logic of the algorithms and make more reliable clinical decisions (Nilsson and Fagerström, 2018).

XAI-based decision support systems increase user trust in algorithms, enabling them to be used effectively and efficiently (Dalaba et al., 2015). When healthcare professionals transparently see the rationale for the proposed decisions, they have more trust in the AI systems, which increases the effectiveness of the training system (Mathijssen et al., 2020). This approach not only increases the accuracy of individual decisions but also improves the quality and reliability of healthcare (Kihlgren et al., 2016).

Assessment and Evaluation: Assessment and evaluation are important elements of educational programs (Kolcu, 2020). The integration of XAI into assessment and evaluation tools enables the transparent, data-driven, and understandable analysis of student performance (Conjin et al., 2023). In traditional assessment and evaluation systems, student achievements are often measured with superficial results, which are often presented without explanation (Arrieta et al., 2020). However, with the integration of XAI, the assessment processes can be explained in a more in-depth and clear manner. XAI provides students with a full range of data and criteria used to assess student performance, showing which factors play a role in each step (Felzmann et al., 2019).

For example, in a multiple-choice written assessment, an XAI-supported assessment system can explain to students which questions are correct or incorrect, which skills need to be further developed, and which learning outcomes are missing. In this way, students can understand the contribution of their results to their graduation goals rather than just seeing it as a score. They can also learn which questions they have difficulty with and which subjects they need to practice more (Conjin et al., 2023).

XAI also provides instructors with objective and data-driven evaluations. Students' performances were compared and analyzed against large datasets processed by XAI systems, making instructors' decisions more reliable. Educators can identify each student's strengths and weaknesses and communicate this to the student in a tangible way to provide sound feedback. This allows for a more targeted development plan.

Integrating XAI into student performance assessment processes provides instructors with a significant advantage in identifying weaknesses in their instruction (Conjin et al., 2023). The data provided on which skills students lack allows instructors to review their current teaching methods and reshape them if necessary. By analyzing students' learning processes in depth, XAI clarifies the areas in which they are strong and in which they need to improve. Such data enable instructors to provide more targeted and personalized feedback to students. Furthermore, by explaining the factors that influence students' achievement levels, XAI shows which aspects of instructional materials are more effective, thus helping instructors adapt material selection and teaching strategies more efficiently.

The transparency aspect of XAI is an important factor that increases trust in the teaching and assessment processes. Students can evaluate the feedback they receive by understanding the processes behind it, rather than just a score or an overall assessment. This clarity allows students to develop a clearer view of themselves by knowing how the assessments are made and the criteria by which they are scored. This enables students to better track their progress and understand where they need to make efforts.

This transparent communication between students and teachers encourages them to participate more actively in the learning process (Felzmann et al., 2019). Strengthening the interaction between students and instructors in education increases students' motivation and commitment to lessons. Owing to the transparency offered by XAI, students can make sense of the decisions made by their instructors, take more responsibility in this process, and participate more in learning. This approach creates a more dynamic and effective learning environment through a continuous feedback and improvement cycle. As the educational process is continuously shaped and improved through a student-centered approach, students develop a greater sense of ownership in their own learning process and progress more effectively.

The integration of XAI allows for not only assessment of students' performance in a more transparent and understandable way, but also the creation of a learning environment that continuously improves and enhances educational processes. This process encourages instructors to make more informed and data-driven decisions, and students play a more active role in education.

Program Evaluation: Program evaluation is among the important elements of health professional education. It is recommended that training programs be evaluated within the scope of a model. XAI provides an important contribution to the identification of points that can be improved by ensuring the continuous monitoring of training programs. In traditional program evaluation methods, general analyses are typically performed and the results cover a limited period (Kolcu et al., 2020). However, owing to XAI-based systems, each stage of the training process can be continuously monitored, and in-depth analysis can be performed on each component of the program. This allows trainers and program managers to identify and respond quickly to the challenges encountered during the training process. This type of continuous monitoring increases the effectiveness of the program and allows training materials, teaching methods, and strategies to become more efficient over time.

7.4.2 Example: Program Evaluation Using the Kirkpatrick Model

The Kirkpatrick model is a widely used framework for evaluating the effectiveness of training programmes. This model consists of four basic levels: Engagement, Learning, Behavior, and Outcomes. While XAI contributes to each stage of this model, it allows for more in-depth analysis, especially at each level of the training process.

Engagement/Satisfaction: Students' level of engagement and satisfaction with the educational process can be monitored in more detail using XAI. Data can be collected on which modules students interacted with more, which activities they were successful in, and which subjects they had difficulties with. These data can help to measure engagement levels and understand how students are involved in the educational process.

XAI can make the feedback processes more transparent and interactive. Students not only see the feedback they receive as an overall assessment of their performance but also receive explanations about each assessment criterion and the decisions made. This justifies the feedback and provides students with a concrete guide on which areas they need to improve. Supporting feedback processes with XAI helps students see their areas of development more clearly and better direct the educational process according to their own development.

Assessment of Learning: XAI can analyze data to measure how much learning students have achieved, what skills they have developed, and in which areas they need support. This provides information on which subjects instructors need to do more teaching and shows which subjects or modules students are lacking in. XAI can better assess how students apply the knowledge gained in education, and how effective this knowledge is in real-world situations. When educational processes are linked to real-life situations that students may encounter through simulations and practical lessons, XAI reveals how efficiently students can use the knowledge learned. This provides educators with information on which areas need more practice and shows how effectively students apply their theoretical knowledge.

Assessment of Behavior: Changes in students' behavior after training can be monitored using XAI. How students use what they have learned in their professional life, clinical practice, or other areas can be analyzed. In this process, XAI systems provide data that evaluates how students act in practice and the functionality of the knowledge learned.

Assessment of Institutional or National Contributions: XAI can analyze students' educational outcomes and their impact on the overall efficiency of the institution or health system. This is not limited to individual student achievements but also assesses the long-term effects of training on healthcare providers and organizations. For example, factors such as improvement in students' clinical judgment, improvement in the quality of patient care, and contribution to the health system can be examined.

The integration of XAI into program evaluation processes is not limited to students; it can also have a positive impact on institutions and health systems. Continuous monitoring and improvement of training programs enable healthcare providers to receive better training, make better clinical decisions, and deliver services more efficiently. Although training programs are shaped according to the needs of the healthcare system, XAI also contributes to broader data analysis in the healthcare sector. Continuous improvement of training processes can increase the overall efficiency of the health system and enable better-quality patient care.

The integration of XAI into program evaluation processes ensures that education programs have a transparent, effective, and continuously improving structure. In this way, both students and institutions can obtain maximum benefits from the results obtained from education, and significant improvements can be achieved in healthcare services.

Interprofessional Education: XAI can play an important role in interprofessional education, helping professionals to better understand each other's roles, responsibilities, and tasks. Interprofessional education is an area in which different health professionals work together, and communication and collaboration are critical (Vernon et al., 2024). Using XAI in this training not only clarifies the roles and responsibilities of the participants but also increases collaboration within the team (Fedor et al., 2020).

XAI-based systems transparently explain the stages and decisions that each individual contributes to in training scenarios. These descriptions allow participants to better understand the roles that carry which responsibilities and how these responsibilities should work in harmony with other members. For example, in an emergency medicine scenario, the roles of doctors, nurses, dietitians, and physiotherapists can be explained in detail using an XAI-powered platform. These descriptions allow team members to see each other's contributions clearly and understand how they can improve collaboration in carrying out their respective tasks. In interprofessional scenarios, XAI can enhance communication and coordination within teams. The XAI's description of decision-making processes shows how each professional contributes and how these contributions complement each other. Thus, team members respect each other's roles, understand each other better, and collaborate more efficiently to achieve common goals.

XAI-based systems provide feedback at the end of the scenarios and evaluate each individual's training performance in detail. This can show the collaboration skills of each professional and how effectively they fulfill their roles. This approach allows team members to be more involved in the training process and build a stronger interprofessional bond between professionals. In this context, XAI helps team members evaluate each other's contributions more objectively and improve their collaboration skills.

The use of XAI in interprofessional education not only provides an understanding of individual roles but also enhances intra-team coordination and collaboration. Such openness and transparency in training can improve the quality of interdisciplinary healthcare by enabling participants to collaborate more effectively.

7.5 CHALLENGES AND CONCERNS

Ethical Issues: The use of AI in health education raises significant concerns, particularly with respect to privacy, data security, and human centeredness (Najjar, 2024). XAI collects and analyzes sensitive data such as student performance, and ensuring the security of these data is a major responsibility (Köse and Köse, 2024). Furthermore, the sharing and use of personal data must comply with privacy rules and legal regulations often encountered in the healthcare sector. The use of AI-based systems in the educational process requires transparency to ensure that the data of instructors and students are not manipulated in an unauthorized manner. However, it is necessary to carefully consider the implications of XAI's capacity to explain decision processes to users (e.g., whether the decision will create personal or professional security concerns) (Baser et al., 2021). In health education, as teaching processes need to remain human-centered, having AI systems completely take over instructors' decisions could put the human aspects of teaching at risk (Najjar, 2024).

Technical Integration: The integration of XAI systems into existing training tools poses a significant technical challenge (Morandini et al., 2023). While educational institutions often use more traditional manual training processes, integrating XAI-based systems into these infrastructures can be complex and time consuming (Vries et al., 2023). Ensuring compatibility with existing systems requires a new learning process for both educators and students. At the same time, for XAI to produce accurate and reliable results, the algorithms used must be fed with quality data. Technical errors or data gaps during the acquisition, analysis, and processing of data can negatively affect the accuracy and reliability of the XAI systems. Inadequate technological compatibility of the tools used in education or infrastructure deficiencies may prevent the full potential of XAI from being fully utilized (Vries et al., 2023).

Usability: For educators and students, managing the complexity of XAI systems, providing necessary support to users, and creating ease of use pose significant challenges (Jiménez-Luna et al., 2020). The explanations provided by XAI can sometimes be full of technical jargon, making it difficult for users to understand the decision support processes (Tiwari, 2023). User-friendly interfaces and clear guidelines are needed for educators and students to efficiently use such advanced systems. Providing explanations and visual aids in the design of XAI systems to help educators and students understand the inner workings of the system can increase its effectiveness (Tiwari, 2023). It is also important to provide appropriate training materials and user guides to understand the impact of XAI on the users (Belghachi, 2023). Educators need to understand how these systems work and incorporate them into their educational processes to make most of the information provided by XAI.

7.6 FUTURE DIRECTIONS

Interactive Systems: In the future, XAI-based interactive systems are expected to become increasingly important in education. These systems will make learning processes more effective by not only providing real-time feedback to students and instructors but also by providing explainable decision support mechanisms. Real-time feedback enables students to quickly understand and correct their mistakes but also allows educators to monitor students' learning processes in a more dynamic way. XAI-powered interactive systems transparently analyze students' decisions, thoughts, and learning processes so that teaching strategies can be adapted quickly. Furthermore, these systems offer customized training in learning processes, making it possible to deliver content according to students' individual needs.

Collaborative Learning: In interprofessional education, the future role of XAI has great potential to involve team members in decision-making processes.

In healthcare, it is becoming increasingly important for professionals from different disciplines to work together. XAI can enhance collaboration within a team by explaining how each team member contributes to decision-making in collaborative learning environments. Students can learn to collaborate by better understanding the perspectives of individuals in different professional groups. XAI's explanation of decision-making processes allows for more efficient roles and interactions by clearly defining the responsibilities of each professional group. This can improve the quality of interdisciplinary education and enable healthcare professionals to work together more effectively.

Global Access: Another important aspect of XAI is that it facilitates access to global education systems. Providing transparent access to educational materials, analytics, and student data provides opportunities for health professionals and students worldwide. XAI-based systems can create equal opportunities for global health education by overcoming language barriers, cultural differences, and geographical limitations (McDermid et al., 2021). By coming together across geographies and cultural contexts, students and instructors can bridge gaps and become part of a broader learning ecosystem (Baser et al.,2021; Kolcu et al., 2021). Additionally, education provided globally can help evaluate and improve health systems from a broader perspective. By making data and learning materials available globally, XAI can make health education more accessible.

REFERENCES

Adadi Amina, and Mohammed Berrada, 'Peeking Inside the Black-Box: A Survey on Explainable Artificial Intelligence (XAI)', *IEEE Access*, 6 (2018), 52138–60 <https://doi.org/10.1109/access.2018.2870052>

Arrieta Alejandro Barredo, Natalia Díaz-Rodríguez, Javier Del Ser, Adrien Bennetot, Siham Tabik, Alberto Barbado, and others, 'Explainable Artificial Intelligence (XAI): Concepts, Taxonomies, Opportunities and Challenges Towards Responsible AI', *Information Fusion*, 58 (2020), 82–115 <https://doi.org/10.1016/j.inffus.2019.12.012>

Arun Nishanth, Nathan Gaw, Praveer Singh, Ken Chang, Mehak Aggarwal, Bryan Chen, and others, 'Assessing the Trustworthiness of Saliency Maps for Localizing Abnormalities in Medical Imaging', *Radiology Artificial Intelligence*, 3.6 (2021) <https://doi.org/10.1148/ryai.2021200267>

Baser Aysel, Sibel Baktır Altuntaş, Giray Kolcu, and Gökmen Özceylan, 'Artificial Intelligence Anxiety of Family Physicians in Turkey', *Progress in Nutrition*, 23.S2 SE-Special issue_Sports and Health Sciences (2021), e2021275 <https://doi.org/10.23751/pn.v23iS2.12003>

Belghachi Mohammed, 'A Review on Explainable Artificial Intelligence Methods, Applications, and Challenges', *Indonesian Journal of Electrical Engineering and Informatics (IJEEI)*, 11.4 (2023) <https://doi.org/10.52549/ijeei.v11i4.5151>

Conijn Rianne, Patricia Kahr, and Chris J Snijders, 'The Effects of Explanations in Automated Essay Scoring Systems on Student Trust and Motivation', *Journal of Learning Analytics*, 10.1 (2023), 37–53 <https://doi.org/10.18608/jla.2023.7801>

Dalaba Maxwell Ayindenaba, Hengjin Dong, Melkizedeck Leshabari, Rainer Sauerborn, Felix Sukums, Antje Blank, and others, 'Cost of Installing and Operating an Electronic Clinical Decision Support System for Maternal Health Care: Case of Tanzania Rural Primary Health Centres', *BMC Health Services Research*, 15.1 (2015) <https://doi.org/10.1186/s12913-015-0780-9>

Dionne-Odom, J Nicholas, Deborah Ejem, Rachel Wells, Amber E Barnato, Richard A Taylor, Gabrielle Betty Rocque, and others, 'How Family Caregivers of Persons with Advanced Cancer Assist with Upstream Healthcare Decision-Making: A Qualitative Study', *PLoS One*, 14.3 (2019), e0212967 <https://doi.org/10.1371/journal.pone.0212967>

Fedor Emily, MaryCatherine Heighton, and Victoria Freniere, 'Collaboration of Healthcare Professions to Provide Interprofessional Experiences Through the Eyes of Learners', *Health Interprofessional Practice and Education*, 4.1 (2020), 2121 <https://doi.org/10.7710/2641–1148.2121>

Felzmann Heike, Eduard Fosch-Villaronga, Christoph Lutz, and Aurelia Tamò-Larrieux, 'Transparency You Can Trust: Transparency Requirements for Artificial Intelligence Between Legal Norms and Contextual Concerns', *Big Data & Society*, 6.1 (2019) <https://doi.org/10.1177/2053951719860542>

Galdames Iván Suazo, 'From Anatomy to Algorithm: Scope of AI-Assisted Diagnostic Competencies in Health Sciences Education', *International Journal of Medical and Surgical Sciences (IJMSS)*, 11.3 (2024), 1–24

Gunning Dave, Mark Stefik, Jaesik Choi, Tim Miller, Simone Stumpf, and Guang-Zhong Yang, 'XAI—Explainable Artificial Intelligence', *Science Robotics*, 4.37 (2019) <https://doi.org/10.1126/scirobotics.aay7120>

Hussain Aisha K, 'Advances in Artificial Intelligence: Current Trends and Future Directions', *Frontiers in Artificial Intelligence Research*, 1.01 (2024), 1–35

JakeschMaurice,JeffreyTHancock,andM o pH a a м a н,'HumanHeuristicsforAI-Generated Language Are Flawed', *Proceedings of the National Academy of Sciences*, 120.11 (2023) <https://doi.org/10.1073/pnas.2208839120>

Jiménez-Luna José, Francesca Grisoni, and Gisbert Schneider, 'Drug Discovery with Explainable Artificial Intelligence', *Nature Machine Intelligence*, 2.10 (2020), 573–84 <https://doi.org/10.1038/s42256-020-00236-4>

Thomas, P. A., D. E. Kern, M. T. Hughes, S. A. Tackett, and B. Y. Chen (eds.), *Curriculum Development for Medical Education: A Six-Step Approach*. JHU Press, 2022.

Kihlgren, Annica, Fredrik Svensson, Conny Lövbrand, Mervyn Gifford, and Annsofie Adolfsson, 'A Decision Support System (DSS) for Municipal Nurses Encountering Health Deterioration Among Older People', *BMC Nursing*, 15.1 (2016) <https://doi.org/10.1186/s12912-016-0184-0>

Kolcu Giray, 'Çevrimiçi Ölçme Değerlendirme Uygulamalarının Değerlendirilmesi Evaluation of Online Measurement and Evaluation Applications', *Sdü Sağlık Bilimleri Enstitüsü Dergisi*, 11.3 (2020), 330–33 <https://doi.org/10.22312/sdusbed.757416>

Kolcu Giray, Mukadder İnci Başer Kolcu, Sadettin Demir, and Kanat Gülle, 'The Evaluation of Learning Management System in Medical Education in Time of COVID-19: Evaluation of Learning Management System', *Progress in Nutrition*, 22.2-S SE-Original articles (2020), e2020005 <https://doi.org/10.23751/pn.v22i2-S.10443>

Kolcu Giray, Belkıs Can, Aysel Başer, Sibel Baktır Altuntaş, and Gökmen Özceylan, 'Artificial Intelligence in Health Education TT – Sağlik Eğîtîmlerînde Yapay Zeka', *Medical Journal of Süleyman Demirel University*, 28.2 (2021), 355–59 <https://doi.org/10.17343/sdutfd.876439>

Kolcu Giray, Gökmen Özceylan, Aysel Başer, and Sibel Baktır Altuntaş, 'Yapay Zekâ Kaygısı Ölçeğinin Aile Hekimlerinde Geçerlik ve Güvenirliğinin Değerlendirilmesi TT - Evaluation of The Validity and Reliability of the Artificial Intelligence Anxiety Scale in Family Physicians', *Research Journal of Biomedical and Biotechnology*, 2.1 (2021), 20–28 <https://dergipark.org.tr/en/pub/rjbb/issue/63487/870229>

Köse Gamze, 'XAI for Trustworthiness in Medical Tourism', in *Explainable Artificial Intelligence (XAI) in Healthcare*, ed. by Utku Kose, Nilgun Sengoz, Xi Chen, and Jose Antonio Marmolejo Saucedo. Taylor & Francis Group, 2024, pp. 157–68 <https://doi.org/10.1201/9781003426073>

Köse Utku, 'Yorumlanabilir ve Açıklanabilir Yapay Zekâ ve Güncel Konular', in *Yapay Zekâ Ve Büyük Veri Kitap Serisi 4*, ed. by Prof. Dr. Şeref SAĞIROĞLU and Dr. Mustafa Umut DEMİREZEN, 1st ed. Nobel, 2022, pp. 43–80

Lee, Daphne S K, Khatijah Lim Abdullah, Pathmawathi Subramanian, Robert Thomas Bachmann, and Swee Leong Ong, 'An Integrated Review of the Correlation Between Critical Thinking Ability and Clinical Decision-making in Nursing', *Journal of Clinical Nursing*, 26.23–24 (2017), 4065–79 <https://doi.org/10.1111/jocn.13901>

Mathijssen Elke, Bart J F van den Bemt, Sabien Wielsma, F H J van den Hoogen, and Johanna E Vriezekolk, 'Exploring Healthcare Professionals' Knowledge, Attitudes and Experiences of Shared Decision Making in Rheumatology', *RMD Open*, 6.1 (2020), e001121 <https://doi.org/10.1136/rmdopen-2019-001121>

McDermid John, Yan Jia, Zoë Porter, and Ibrahim Habli, 'Artificial Intelligence Explainability: The Technical and Ethical Dimensions', *Philosophical Transactions of the Royal Society a Mathematical Physical and Engineering Sciences*, 379.2207 (2021), 20200363 <https://doi.org/10.1098/rsta.2020.0363>

Morandini Sofia, Federico Fraboni, Enzo Balatti, Aranka Hackmann, Hannah Brendel, Gabriele Puzzo, and others, 'Assessing the Transparency and Explainability of AI Algorithms in Planning and Scheduling Tools: A Review of the Literature', 2023 <https://doi.org/10.54941/ahfe1004068>

Najjar Reabal, 'Digital Frontiers in Healthcare: Integrating MHealth, AI, and Radiology for Future Medical', *A Comprehensive Overview of Telemedicine*, (2024), 307.

Nilsson Lina, and Cecilia Fagerström, 'Decision-Makers and Mediators in a Home Healthcare Digitisation Process: Nurses' Experiences of Implementation and Use of a Decision Support System', *Contemporary Nurse*, 54.4–5 (2018), 511–21 <https://doi.org/10.1080/10376178.2018.1507676>

Tiwari Rudra, 'Explainable AI (XAI) and Its Applications in Building Trust and Understanding in AI Decision Making', *International Journal of Scientific Research in Engineering and Management*, 07.01 (2023) <https://doi.org/10.55041/ijsrem17592>

Verma Sahil, Keegan E Hines, and John P Dickerson, 'Amortized Generation of Sequential Algorithmic Recourses for Black-Box Models', *Proceedings of the Aaai Conference on Artificial Intelligence*, 36.8 (2022), 8512–19 <https://doi.org/10.1609/aaai.v36i8.20828>

Vernon Veronica, Brian W Skinner, Patricia S Devine, Lori Fauquher, and Emily Young, 'Building Interprofessional Competencies Through a Collaborative Prescribing Activity With Osteopathic, Pharmacy, and Physician Assistant Students', *Mededportal*, 2024 <https://doi.org/10.15766/mep_2374-8265.11403>

Vries Bart M de, Gerben J C Zwezerijnen, George L Burchell, Floris H P van Velden, C Willemien Menke-van der Houven van Oordt, and Ronald Boellaard, 'Explainable Artificial Intelligence (XAI) in Radiology and Nuclear Medicine: A Literature Review', *Frontiers in Medicine*, 10 (2023) <https://doi.org/10.3389/fmed.2023.1180773>

Wang Han, Kelvin Chong, Zhiyuan Lin, Xiangrong Yu, and Yi Pan, 'An Explainable Artificial Intelligence-Based Robustness Optimization Approach for Age-Related Macular Degeneration Detection Based on Medical IOT Systems', *Electronics*, 12.12 (2023), 2697 <https://doi.org/10.3390/electronics12122697>

8 Multinational Collaborations and Innovation

Ilhan Uysal and Surbhi Gupta

8.1 INTRODUCTION: BACKGROUND AND DRIVING FORCES

Global healthcare challenges such as pandemics or the ever-increasing need for modernized medicine require comprehensive multinational partnerships and collaboration, with AI facilitating processes. Such challenges require the collaboration of different countries, organizations, and research institutes, and the integration of AI further optimizes such endeavors. Information technology has revolutionized healthcare through the use of algorithms and data analytical tools that enable precise decision-making, promote the speed of drug development, and improve the quality of diagnosing diseases (Yang, 2022; Secinaro et al., 2021; Rathore and Rathore, 2023). For example, AI technologies helped manage the COVID-19 pandemic through data-driven pattern recognition and outbreak prediction (Islam et al., 2021; Chen and See, 2020). Because different types of large datasets can be processed by AI, there is the possibility of early diagnosis and the formulation of more sophisticated treatment plans (Rathore and Rathore, 2023; Davenport and Kalakota, 2019). While AI's predictive success improves decision-making processes in the clinic, the opacity of AI algorithms poses serious issues in trust and responsibility in the use of medicine. This makes explainable AI (XAI) timely, as XAI provides guidance in understanding and justifying the evidence supplied by AI to users and patients.

For understanding explainable artificial intelligence (XAI), there are two major terms: the first one is data and the second is model. The data part is based on the samples and the features and the model part is with a local explanation and a global explanation. Figure 8.1 shows the basic understanding of XAI.

A number of AI systems still operate under the "black box" paradigm whereby their decision-making processes cannot be deciphered by users, including health experts and patients (Allen, 2024; Zhang, Luo et al., 2022; Jung, 2024). This lack of transparency causes ethical problems and poses doubts about the reliability of AI use in the clinic. To this, we respond with explainable artificial intelligence (XAI). Furthermore, XAI is needed not just for clarification but also to ensure that AI use conforms to clinical and ethical requirements. In deep brain stimulation research, for instance, the absence of sufficient explainability is considered one of the obstacles to

DOI: 10.1201/9781003605416-8

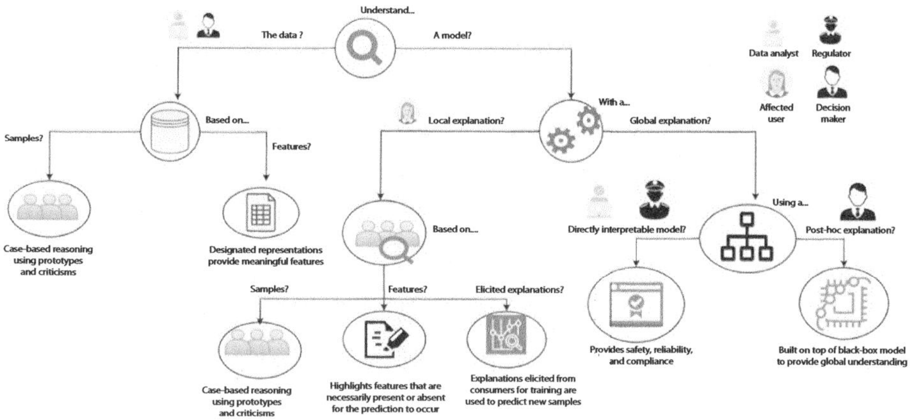

FIGURE 8.1 Understanding of XAI.

applying machine learning models (Allen, 2023). This notion of control leads to the belief that through XAI, healthcare providers will have adequate information about the ways AI systems make decisions, which will allow them to take actions that can enhance patient care (Gupta, 2022; Zhang, Weng et al., 2022). Also, the reliance of healthcare systems on AI to perform essential functions underscores the need for XAI to build the interface between human intelligence and machine intelligence (Gupta and Kumar, 2021).

In AI-enabled healthcare, the foremost concerns include data sharing, policy adherence, and ethical boundaries. The application of artificial intelligence (AI) in healthcare systems (Gupta et al., 2022) promises to transform medical services and research for the better; however, it also creates new hurdles that require international collaboration to overcome. The development of XAI significantly improves these international collaboration inferences because it enhances the interpretability and transparency of AI models. So, through the lens of XAI, healthcare professionals, policymakers, and other experts from different parts of the world are able to understand, authenticate, and rely on the conclusions to which AI systems have arrived (Frassini, 2024; Adus, 2023). Figure 8.2 shows tenets of XAI.

The tenets of XAI are interpretability, explainability, transparency, comprehensibility, justifiability, and accountability. The role of interoperability in alleviating the health information exchange and sharing issue across different systems and organizations is of utmost importance. Administrations save time, effort, and money and enable better healthcare services to be delivered when patients' important information is accessible and shareable by many (Torab-Miandoab et al., 2023; Denhere, 2024; Pournik, 2023). This interoperability is assisted by XAI for AI models to be indeed useful and at the same time explainable, allowing relevant actors to use AI outputs comfortably (Frassini, 2024; Ndlovu et al., 2023). XAI decreases the bias in the AI models as well as the subjectivity of various healthcare jurisdictions, making the use of AI in different countries more dependable (Coleman, 2024; MBA, 2023).

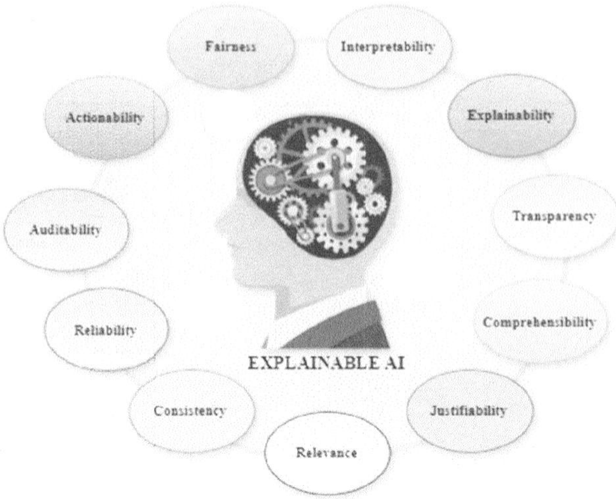

FIGURE 8.2 Tenets of XAI.

In international collaborations in AI, interoperability and the sharing of data are crucial to enhancing the healthcare services of our world. It is XAI that allows the flow of information across the borders of various countries and institutions while respecting the said regions' privacy or laws because AI models are made explainable and compliant with the regulations' stipulations.

XAI also enhances the innovation capability within the healthcare startup ecosystem by offering a framework for building user-centric, ethical AI applications. Those startups employing XAI are able to develop solutions that ensure engagement and transparency, which is vital for fostering trust among users (Adus, 2023; Attaran, 2020). With efforts from every part of the world to create value with healthcare systems by improving patient outcomes and operational efficiency, the need to incorporate XAI into AI-powered healthcare systems becomes more important (Ndlovu et al., 2023; Coleman, 2024). In this regard, this chapter aims to assess the ways XAI is influencing innovation in multinational collaborations, startup frameworks within healthcare, and global healthcare initiatives by making advanced technologies accessible, interpretable, and free from comprehensive ethical boundaries.

This chapter focuses on the impact of explainable artificial intelligence on data sharing, the enhancement of AI-powered medical research (Gupta and Gupta, 2022), and international collaboration in drug development and public health. In addition, it will discuss how XAI is leading innovation in healthcare startups' use of AI technology in different countries in a just and open manner. There is almost no aspect of modern regulation, case studies, and trends analysis that does not describe how XAI is changing healthcare collaborations internationally, and what are the prospects for these changes to be done ethically regarding the application of medicine and artificial intelligence. XAI integrated into international healthcare collaborations is a major development toward the implementation of artificial intelligence-driven solutions in different countries. By mitigating algorithmic bias, border, and security regulatory gaps, XAI permits the integration of healthcare systems around the globe. This improves the confidence given to AI systems applications and the trust of developing the scalable global healthcare systems in the future. In addition, XAI gives powerful ability to the stakeholders of healthcare systems including policymakers, clinicians, and programmers of artificial intelligence to work together to improve the AI use for the benefit of the patients. Multinational collaborations can apply AI to understanding disease, treatment, and public health monitoring through explainable and interpretable AI-driven insights. In the end, XAI emerges as a vital catalyst for worldwide healthcare innovation by ensuring the transparency, accountability, and compliance of AI technologies with ethical and regulatory standards. Those multilateral enterprises that adopt XAI will be best placed to foster sustainable, patient-centered, and technologically advanced healthcare services as the application of AI in healthcare continues to grow.

8.2 IMPORTANCE OF MULTINATIONAL COLLABORATIONS IN HEALTHCARE

The deepening sophistication of global healthcare issues leads to the requirement for multinational cooperation to foster innovation, enhance outcomes, and provide fair access to advanced medical technologies and procedures. Catastrophic health events such as pandemics or the emergence of uncommon diseases alongside the increased interest in AI-assisted diagnostics emphasize the need for effective globalization. No single entity, whether it be a government or an organization, possesses sufficient resources to address these challenges single-handedly, making the pooling of resources, data, and establishing standardized AI-centered healthcare systems vital (Chan and Petrikat, 2023). These efforts are not only restricted to pandemics but also play pivotal roles for uncommon diseases, global health emergencies, and AI-based personalized medicine. XAI enables multinational partnerships to provide transparency and trust in the application of AI while improving interoperability between various stakeholders and healthcare systems (Varnosfaderani, 2024). The most challenging issue regarding international cooperation on healthcare AI lies in the different enforcement policies and laws of different nations. The European GDPR, US HIPAA, and other countries' specific legislations on data protection are significant obstacles for many organizations (Javanmard, 2024; Anyanwu, 2024). These legal frameworks are intended to maintain patient confidentiality as well as to control the use of artificial intelligence ethically; however, they often result in problems with data availability and interoperability (Kamalendar et al., 2024). XAI accounts for this by offering compliant interpretable artificial intelligence models. Using XAI transparency, organizations can legally operate from several jurisdictions and be compliant with responsible AI legislation (Varnosfaderani, 2024).

In regard to international cooperation in healthcare, the most challenging issue has always been the sharing of information across national borders. Sharing health data at an institutional level is crucial for furthering medical research and AI-based diagnostics and predicting disease outcomes (Krishnan, 2023). On the other hand, ethical considerations, data security concerns, and even organizational reluctance to share private patient data often impede data sharing (Anyanwu, 2024). Collaboration beyond country borders is made easier with XAI because data-driven decisions are made explainable, auditable, and comply with privacy regulations. XAI shifts the paradigm by allowing organizations to collaboratively train AI models without exposing sensitive data due to the implementation of privacy-preserving AI techniques like federated learning and differential privacy (Husnain, 2023). Despite the increased privacy protection from decentralized AI model training through federated learning, there are still issues such as financial expenditure, standardization of AI models, and the computational burden of the AI models.

In addition to mitigating ethical compliance and the misuse of artificial intelligence, "XAI" works toward improving the productivity of AI solutions in multinational healthcare collaborations. XAI aids in ensuring trust and the consolidation of AI-powered healthcare systems by allowing relevant stakeholders from different countries to interpret the results provided by the artificial intelligence systems. Because explainable AI can clearly state the reasons for decisions made by the AI, it is easier to remove biases in the models and ensure that the outputs are fair and representative of all population groups (Vuong et al., 2019). This is particularly relevant for global health efforts, where the introduction of unproportionate AI technologies that lack proper validation across many demographic groups only serves to deepen the existing gaps in access and outcomes of healthcare services (Dai and Tayur, 2022). Enabling stakeholders, including, healthcare providers, patients, and policymakers, to trust the rationale of the decisions made allows these parties to work effectively together to solve key global health issues (Gupta and Koul, 2025).

In summary, the nexus of multinational cooperation, harmonization of regulations, and the XAI principles is important for tackling the global healthcare dilemma. In most healthcare settings, the global adoption of AI will make its explainability absolutely essential for fostering trust, regulatory compliance, and patient satisfaction. Further studies should devise new flexible XAI models that would increase the AI system's interpretability across different borders. Also, creating unified metric standards for XAI evaluation in healthcare would simplify the systems' integration for various countries in AI technology. Making systems more transparent will help foster trust and enable better cooperation. Thus, XAI can efficiently transform the future of global healthcare collaboration and stimulate development in the industry. Figure 8.3 shows federated AI model training process.

8.3 XAI AS A CATALYST FOR INNOVATION IN HEALTHCARE

The integration of AI into contemporary medicine makes it necessary to maintain accountability and systematization in AI technologies for medical purposes. This is where XAI comes in; it helps multinational research collaborations build trust, enables different healthcare systems to work together, and helps mitigate the biases that may arise in AI models when used over different populations. This part examines how XAI fosters healthcare innovations by improving the interpretability of

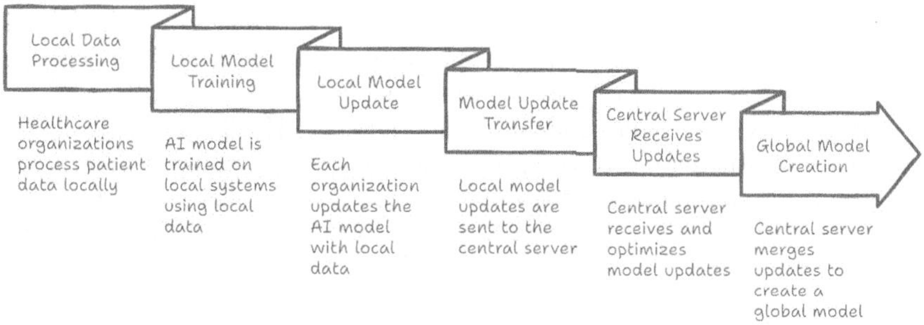

FIGURE 8.3 Federated AI model training process.

healthcare AI systems, thereby encouraging objective decision-making and ensuring equity across different nations in the use of AI.

8.3.1 How XAI Enhances Transparency in Multinational Research Projects

Collaborative research conducted across national borders is an important strategy for developing innovation in healthcare, particularly in precision medicine, AI-assisted diagnostics, and drug discovery. One notable issue is the lack of trust when it comes to using AI models for decision-making in government healthcare systems. A considerable number of AI systems function as "black boxes" where they make decisions without providing reasons that can be understood by healthcare practitioners, policymakers, or patients. The absence of transparency makes it complicated to validate the AI-generated recommendations, thus hampering the deployment of intelligent systems in multinational healthcare projects (Adamidi et al., 2021; Duell et al., 2022). With the use of XAI, autonomous systems can be made transparent, which helps in coordinating the efforts of research and regulatory institutions and healthcare providers in various countries so that the use of AI complies with accepted medical and ethical standards (Suraci et al., 2022; Olorunsogo, 2024). XAI seeks to solve these problems through AI models that can explain their predictions using human language (Uysal and Kose, 2024). There are also some techniques like SHAP (Shapley Additive Explanations), LIME (Local Interpretable Model-agnostic Explanations), and attention in neural networks that scan and explain the features that led to the model's decision while enabling accountability and, hence, trust in AI's assistance (Parashar, 2024; Elshawi et al., 2020).

Moreover, peer review and regulatory approval processes for AI-based medical applications are enhanced with XAI-driven transparency. The FDA (the United States), EMA (Europe), and PMDA (Japan) are known to require pre-clinical explainability in AI models with the aim of governing their reliability before clinical use (Akpan et al., 2022; Dwivedi, 2023). The adoption of XAI techniques within international XAI research initiatives allows for easier regulatory compliance, which lowers approval times and increases the speed at which AI-powered healthcare solutions can be used globally (Lokare, 2024; Rawal, 2024). This is especially critical as there is greater reliance on AI in the provision of quality care services and efficient operational management in the healthcare sector (Khan, 2023).

Integrating XAI into Multinational Collaborations in Healthcare makes it easier to build trust, transparency, and compliance with regulatory requirements. XAI not only improves the credibility of AI solutions but also fosters collaboration by addressing difficulties arising from the black-box aspect of AI. This situation encourages stakeholders to actively participate in contributing to solving healthcare problems. Figure 8.4 shows aspects of enhancing AI transparency in healthcare.

8.3.2 Interoperability of AI Systems in Global Health Networks

Achieving interoperability in global healthcare is of utmost importance for facilitating information flow and the use of AI in various healthcare entities, geographical locations, and legal contexts. AI systems developed in one country may not be directly transferable to another country due to variations in medical regulations, availability of healthcare services, and the healthcare population's profile. Such non-uniformity makes it difficult to implement AI solutions and work collaboratively on healthcare projects involving multiple nations (Lekkala, 2023; Brown et al., 2022).

XAI has a role in achieving interoperability by providing standardized and explainable AI models that are sufficient for validation and adaptation to different ecosystems. Healthcare practitioners and data scientists can use the AI's interpretable decisions to understand how healthcare systems function with an AI model and modify the AI model to make it more suitable for other systems (Guo et al., 2020).

Several initiatives are leveraging XAI to enhance interoperability in multinational healthcare networks:

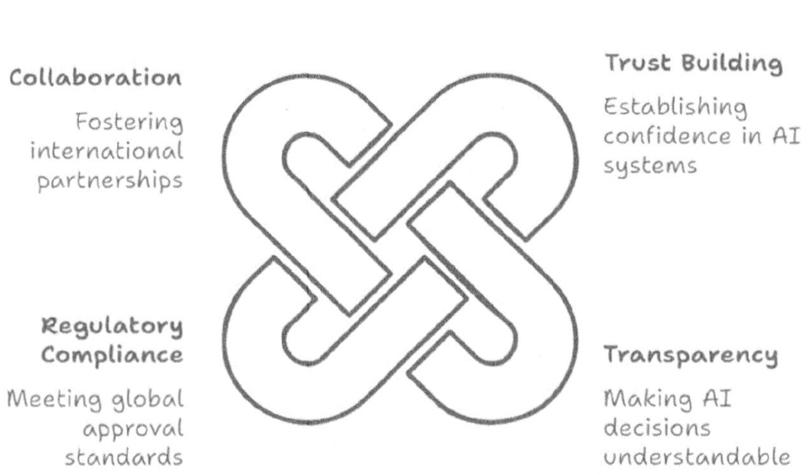

FIGURE 8.4 Enhancing AI transparency in healthcare.

- **FHIR (Fast Healthcare Interoperability Resources) and HL7 Standards**: Enable AI features to be integrated into electronic health records (EHRs) and provide processes through which explainable AI can be embedded in various platforms (Williams et al., 2023; Arshad, 2024). The FHIR standard enables the exchange of health information in both human and machine-readable form, which is important for AI functionality (Tabari, 2024).
- **Global AI Consortia**: Like the Global Digital Health Partnership (GDHP) and the WHO AI for Health Initiative are working on developing governance frameworks for AI with a focus on interoperability and explainability of medical technologies (Hillmer, 2024; Sasse and Fluck, 2023). The goal is to achieve a "mixed-mode" strategy where local policies are followed, but global policies are also advanced.
- **Multicenter Clinical Trials**: Utilizing XAI models ensures that AI-driven diagnostics and treatment recommendations are validated across various patient populations and healthcare settings (Asan and Choudhury, 2021; Naseem et al., 2020). This validation is essential for ensuring that AI tools are effective and safe for diverse groups of patients, thereby enhancing their applicability in different healthcare environments.

The incorporation of XAI into global AI systems allows healthcare networks to improve international collaboration, implement better telemedicine services, and guarantee that AI medical insights are transparent and consistent across regions (Bahmani et al., 2021; Giansanti, 2022). This integration not only promotes trust among stakeholders but also facilitates the efficient use of AI technologies in addressing global health challenges (Stroud et al., 2025; Nong and Ji, 2025).

In summary, the integration of artificial intelligence into healthcare systems calls for a new regulatory approach. XAI has the most important role to play in the promotion of interoperability for the successful adoption of AI into global healthcare systems. Through explainability and standardization, XAI has the potential to tear down barriers set by disparate healthcare systems and regulatory frameworks, to the benefit of global patient care and outcomes. Figure 8.5 focuses on enhancing global health AI interoperability.

8.3.3 Addressing Bias and Fairness in Multinational AI Models

AI bias is an imperative concern in AI-enabled healthcare technologies because it can lead to unpleasant treatment suggestions, unfavorable misdiagnoses, or inequality in the results of patients. Several factors contribute to bias in AI systems:

- **Unrepresentative Training Data**: A considerable number of AI applications are trained using data that is biased toward particular groups and hence is ineffective for the less represented population. For example, AI systems based on data from higher-level hospitals often fail in community

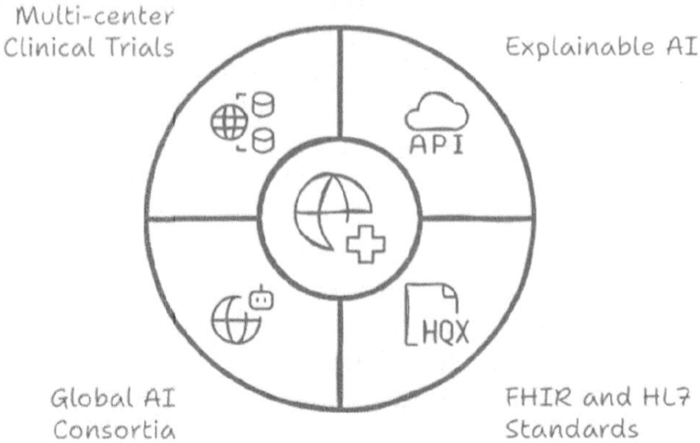

FIGURE 8.5 Enhancing global health AI interoperability

clinics and result in biased care for patients from different cultures (Zhang and Zhang, 2023).

- **Cultural and Socioeconomic Variability***:* Differing patients' health conditions and their stimuli and the extent to which they can receive medical care can affect AI-based recommendations and their effectiveness. This AI system reliance poses the risk of widening the gap in the provision of services since it accounts for the reality of very few people from diverse populations (Giordano et al., 2021; Liu and Wu, 2022).
- **Algorithmic Bias**: Certain models of artificial intelligence systematically discriminate against some groups in healthcare because of the way they use demographic characteristics in the feature selection process. One possible instance is where AI systems emphasize some population's demographic factors while the health needs of such populations are nonexistent. This scenario results in an unjust allocation of suggestive treatment options (Ferrara, 2023; Kerasidou, 2021).

XAI fosters the neutrality of biases by making AI processes easy to follow and open to scrutiny as well as enabling audit trails to be established. With this, researchers can identify, evaluate, and rectify biases prior to deploying models in real-life healthcare settings. Some of the main areas that XAI bias mitigation strategies work on includes:

- **Feature Importance Analysis***:* SHAP (Shapley Additive Explanations) and Integrated Gradients are XAI techniques that enable the user to evaluate how each variable impacts the predictions of the AI model, which then assists in the evaluation of what biases in the model's reasoning may exist (Familoni, 2024; Vincy et al., 2024). After analyzing the outcomes, developers can make changes to eliminate biases that AI decisions may project in the model.

- **Bias Detection Frameworks**: Toolkits that enable AI fairness such as IBM AI Fairness 360 and Google's What-If Tool allow researchers check if an AI is making biased predictions and incorporate XAI principles to confirm that the system uses XAI to predict where the bias is concentrated (Jagtiani, 2024; Chellappan, 2024). Such tools help organizations verify and eliminate biases prior to deployment.
- **Ethical AI Audits***:* Explainable AI models are required to be audited continuously by some other form of authority, which enables these systems to ensure compliance with non-discrimination and fairness rules concerning discrimination in the health sector (Kerasidou, 2021; Cary, 2024). Audits help ensure accountability and that AI systems develop to a level where they adhere to ethical norms.

For equitable healthcare in different parts of the world, it is important to maintain balance with multinational AI models. The incorporation of XAI into AI-based medical systems can help enhance the inclusivity of the models and guarantee unbiased medical information irrespective of geographic, ethnic, or socioeconomic boundaries for the populations in need (Elendu, 2023; Zhang et al., 2020). Reinforcing these AI models with trust improves the patients' faith in these advanced technologies and enables better health results across varying populations. Figure 8.6 stresses on ensuring fairness in AI healthcare models.

8.4 MULTINATIONAL HEALTHCARE COLLABORATIONS USING XAI

The growing use of AI in healthcare has fostered international collaborations that improve medical research, drug discovery, and public health monitoring. However, a major challenge in global AI deployment is the lack of transparency and interpretability of these models. XAI plays a crucial role by making AI-driven healthcare solutions more trustworthy, interpretable, and ethically sound. XAI enables researchers, policymakers, and healthcare professionals to understand and validate AI models, facilitating their adoption across diverse regulatory environments. This section

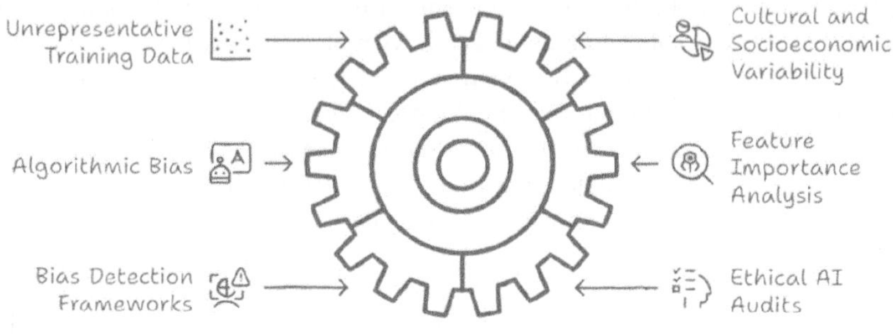

FIGURE 8.6 Ensuring fairness in AI healthcare models.

examines how XAI supports global healthcare initiatives, enhances collaboration in drug discovery and personalized medicine, and improves public health monitoring.

8.4.1 Global AI-Driven Healthcare Initiatives

Notable global AI-driven healthcare initiatives utilizing XAI:

- **WHO AI for Health Initiative**: As part of the WHO AI for Health Initiative, the WHO has developed AI governance frameworks that center on XAI. This approach fosters trust by ensuring that AI-powered diagnostics and treatment recommendations are ethical and transparent. The initiative provides support for AI explainability in developing countries so that AI solutions are appropriate for under-resourced healthcare systems. The WHO's focus on XAI is critical for fostering trust and ensuring that AI technologies are effectively integrated into diverse healthcare systems (Rehburg, 2024; Mello et al., 2022).
- **The Global Digital Health Partnership (GDHP)**: Within this AI XAI framework, this international collaboration seeks the development of interoperable AI healthcare systems that would also enhance transparency and trust by patients in AI-generated medical information. The GDHP aims at establishing a digital health framework that incorporates ethical use of AI while enabling cross-border data exchange (Ejjami, 2024). By focusing on interoperability, the GDHP ensures that the deployment of AI technologies in healthcare can be done in many different environments.
- **The European Health Data Space (EHDS)**: This program works on developing an integrated ecosystem of health data driven by AI in the European Union while offering explainability of AI and regulation under the scope of GDPR and the AI Act. The aim of EHDS is to support the member states in the secure sharing of health data and AI enablement for research undertakings and patient care (Huang et al., 2022; Lai et al., 2020). By providing interoperability standards and AI explainability, the EHDS alleviates some of the major obstacles AI technologies face.

The integration of XAI into comprehensive AI healthcare programs enhances transparency, trust, and ethical behavior within multinational collaborations in the healthcare sector. One of the areas where XAI makes a most notable contribution is in programs aimed at rapid disease detection, where AI models process extensive amounts of health data to forecast epidemics, recognize at-risk populations, and suggest necessary interventions. These programs use XAI to make accessible the processes by which the AI-generated predictions are made, so that public health stakeholders and physicians can act on them without skepticism (Koo et al., 2024; Stroud, 2024).

Another fundamental aspect of XAI's contribution is its support for the interjurisdictional validation of AI models. In multinational healthcare studies, algorithms for medical diagnosis and treatment recommendation have AI at their core and are subsequently used in different countries with varying degrees of healthcare system sophistication, patient population, and clinical practices. Medical practitioners from different countries would find it almost impossible to determine whether an AI model is making sound decisions, which can be deemed reliable, neutral, and relevant to a wide range of populations. XAI makes sure that models provide explainable outputs so that the users of the AI system can assess the reasoning of the AI, enhance the generalizability of the model, and reduce the likelihood of biases that are considered harmful to certain patient populations (Banerjee et al., 2022; Giordano et al., 2021).

Moreover, compliance with regulations is one of the main problems of multinational AI healthcare ventures because every country has its own ethical and legal policies regarding the use of AI in medicine. The FDA (the United States), EMA (Europe), and WHO have general requirements on transparency and responsibility of the given medical solutions operating through AI. XAI provides interpretable models of AI that enable the fulfillment of ethical requirements and assist regulatory bodies in evaluating the equity, trustworthiness, and safety of healthcare applications driven by artificial intelligence (Montani and Striani, 2019; Makubhai, 2023). This explainability not only accelerates the approval process on the regulations but also enhances the trust and acceptance of the processes among healthcare personnel and the patients.

The integration of XAI in large-scope AI healthcare projects enables multinational companies to guarantee the absence of bias and unethical practices in the implementation of AI-powered medical solutions. This promotes broad acceptance and compliance with numerous health systems, enabling innovations in artificial intelligence to be adopted worldwide without compromising the safety of patients, equity, and trust (Makubhai, 2023; Sharma, 2023a).

8.4.2 Collaborative Research in Drug Discovery and Personalized Medicine

To further expedite the creation of new therapies, multinational drug companies and research organizations are looking to AI technology in drug discovery. AI models analyze several chemical compounds, molecular interactions, and genomic analyses using qualitative analysis to flag drug candidates more effectively than traditional methods. The AI techniques used have by far the greatest impact, and the most significant hurdle for them is the black-box characterization of many AI-driven models that make drug discovery automatic and raise questions about reproducibility and the validity of AI outcomes (Singh, 2023; Kimta, 2024).

How XAI is transforming drug discovery and personalized medicine;

- **Interpretable AI Models for Drug Target Identification**: XAI methods like SHAP and LIME allow users to understand what molecular features are responsible for enabling predicted drug efficacies. By elucidating AI-driven drug target selection through explanation, XAI mitigates ethical concerns related to automated decision-making and increases acceptance by regulatory bodies (Mouchlis et al., 2021; Cherney, 2023). In order to win the trust of governance bodies and stakeholders, it is paramount to ensure that processes of drug discovery are transparent and accountable, and this is what calls for the interpretation of AI models (Flathmann, 2024).

- **Personalized Treatment Optimization**: The software which uses AI technologies is capable of devising personalized treatment plans for patients according to their genetic makeup and family medical history. For example, XAI can provide physicians with explanations for why an AI-suggested treatment seems appropriate for a specific patient, which guarantees that AI-made decisions are not blindly given (Singh, 2023; Kimta, 2024). This is important during the adoption of AI in medicine, as it aids healthcare personnel to arrive at choices that reflect the situation of the patient individually.
- **Multinational Drug Research Collaborations**: Pfizer and Novartis, AstraZeneca, and many other pharmaceutical companies teamed up with international universities and biotech startup companies for new drug development utilizing AI. Junior (2024) and Hongsong et al. (2022) note that XAI improves participatory transparency by making it possible to explain AI predictions on drug effectiveness' results, thus facilitating the approval process by regulatory agencies for new medications. The integration of XAI into drug discovery increases the ease with which new international collaboratives trust AI results, enhances clinical decision-making, and accelerates drug approval processes while maintaining equity and good order (Cherney, 2023; Zhang Yue et al., 2022).

To close, the adoption of XAI into AI-powered drug discovery adds value by improving model AI transparency and interpretability, aiding personalized medicine, and promoting collaboration within international pharmaceutical research. With the constant evolution of the industry, adoption of XAI will be imperative in solving the issues AI poses in drug discovery while ensuring new treatments are effective and not biased.

8.4.3 AI-Powered Public Health Monitoring

AI-driven health monitoring is useful in outbreak detection, epidemiologic forecasting, and healthcare resource optimization in multi-national settings. Nevertheless, AI models must be explainable if public health stakeholders are to accept and rely on AI recommendations.

The adoption of explainable artificial intelligence (XAI) in large-scale AI applications in healthcare is crucial in building transparency, trust, and ethical responsibility in multinational healthcare systems. One of the areas where XAI has greatly impacted is early disease detection and surveillance. AI systems capture and process global health event data, social media activities, and other relevant phenomena to detect abnormal trends suggestive of impending disease outbreaks. BlueDot and HealthMap are examples of platforms that incorporate XAI in providing explainable assessments of outbreak risks to help public health agencies address the reasons for AI predictions (Mienye et al., 2024). XAI enables epidemiologists, policymakers, and other healthcare practitioners to identify disease hotspots with more confidence and facilitates them to respond swiftly and effectively to the potential spread of diseases.

Apart from early recognition, XAI plays a critical role in anticipating epidemiological trends where models powered by artificial intelligence predict disease spread, vaccine efficacy, and public health policy impacts. These models depend on a variety of advanced statistical techniques and algorithms from machine learning, which are notoriously hard to explain. Attention mechanisms in deep learning models are a form of XAI that allows healthcare professionals and epidemiologists to appreciate the reasons behind AI predictions, allowing them to verify the trustworthiness of the AI forecast (Phadatare & Naik, 2023). By articulating why certain variables were considered more important, for example population density, mobility, and vaccination coverage, XAI enables policymakers to rely on the data provided for public health decisions.

XAI is influential in addressing the challenges of a pandemic and optimizing resource allocation. Governments, as well as healthcare organizations, used AI-based models to estimate the needed ICU resources, ventilators, and the containment measures' efficacy ratio during COVID-19. Decision-makers had issues on trusting AI recommendations because of the model's lack of explainability. The incorporation of XAI allowed decision-makers to appreciate the AI projections made on hospitalization rates, infection curves, and mobility limits. This provided more accurate resource allocation and lessened the burden on healthcare systems and improved the response to the pandemic overall (Miyachi, 2024; Linardatos et al., 2020).

Global cooperation is equally critical in health monitoring to complement national efforts in disease surveillance and outbreak management. Coordination among institutions such as the Global Outbreak Alert and Response Network (GOARN) and the Centers for Disease Control and Prevention (CDC) is focused on the deployment of XAI-enabled public health surveillance systems in different regions. XAI nurtures confidence in global health agencies by ensuring that AI models provide interpretable findings into disease modeling as well as enabling coordination of disease response in real time. Such trust is needed especially for managing epidemics across borders, where AI assistance must be transparent enough to allow the requisite sharing of information, response planning integration, and public health decision-making (Hrnjica and Softic, 2020).

Health security is enhanced globally by enabling reliable and well-justified AI-driven systems for epidemiological forecasting, pandemic response, and building trust in XAI-integrated public health warning systems. It is also essential for XAI to strengthen public health monitor systems as AI continues to take a center stage in "reshaping" the field. Multinational collaborations in healthcare will put in action more dependable and pragmatic AI-controlled disease monitoring systems. Coordination, harmonization, and ethical application of AI in global healthcare initiatives will call for greater collaboration through the use of XAI (So, 2020).

8.5 THE ROLE OF XAI IN HEALTHCARE STARTUPS AND INNOVATION ECOSYSTEMS

XAI transforms the healthcare startup ecosystem by creating new avenues for innovation. Moreover, it deals with trust, transparency, and regulatory issues effectively. For all healthcare XAI-integrated startups, the added value is not just improving decision-making for medical specialists but also enhancing the level of patient trust and proxy approval. This part analyzes the ways in which XAI accomplishes innovation in healthcare startups, how investors are influencing the AI revolution in healthcare, and the problems and approaches to scaling AI-enabled solutions internationally.

8.5.1 Fostering Innovation in the Healthcare Startup Ecosystem

Most emerging economies have poor quality healthcare services. Adopting dual strategies of investing in essential health infrastructure and technology (such as AI) can augment healthcare access. AI technology is able to make automated interactions with doctors, medical records computerization, and doctor's recommendations to patients. Because of these factors, there is much scope for new business initiatives for the development of innovative solutions in diagnosis and monitoring, personalized medicine, drug discovery, and even, patient monitoring. However, the utilization of some self-learning models of AI meets the challenge of transparency, interpretability, relatability, and explainability. Durán and Jongsma (2021) suggested that these models function as "black boxes." Healthcare professionals are not willing to employ AI systems which, to all appearances, they cannot comprehend.

With regard to the problem in question, XAI is helpful because it provides explainable and interpretable AI models. By providing transparency in AI decision-making, startups can gain trust from the medical professionals and other parties such as regulators. For instance:

- **AI-Assisted Diagnostics Startups**: AI-assisted diagnostics startups use XAI to demonstrate medical features contributing to diagnoses, allowing doctors to validate recommendations – a step critical for trust-building, as emphasized by Winter & Carusi (2022) and Frank et al. (2021)
- **Pharmaceutical Startups**: Allen (2023) explains how these companies leverage XAI to enhance the accuracy of identifying molecular structures that, with greater than usual probability, will be successively accepted. It also dramatically improves the efficiency of justifying the selection of candidates to stakeholders and regulatory bodies. The reason for this is that clear explanations of why specific compounds are subjected into consideration are provided.
- **Telemedicine and Remote Patient Monitoring Companies**: Islam et al. (2021) highlighted the use of interpretable recommendation provision by AI-powered virtual consultations by these companies. The level of trust

that can be afforded to AI recommendations is accompanied by the level of explanation provided by the AI. These companies are therefore able to boost acceptance from patients and healthcare providers.

With the incorporation of XAI, healthcare startups can now have a competitive edge, raise adoption rates, and create AI models compliant with medical standards (Sharma, 2023b). This strategic use of explainability improves the credibility of the AI solutions, as well as the patient outcomes and efficiency of healthcare services. Figure 8.7 shows integration of explainable AI in healthcare startups.

8.5.2 Investment Trends in AI-Driven Healthcare

The increased interest in artificial intelligence solutions for healthcare has attracted considerable funding from multinational venture capital (VC) firms, accelerators, and corporate investors. Yet, in an industry that is becoming more controlled, investors are favoring early-stage companies that embed explainability and regulatory compliance in their AI solutions. Because it guarantees healthcare providers' transparency and trust, which simplifies regulatory processes, XAI has become one of the primary factors of differentiation, adding value to investors' portfolios and increasing the attractiveness of XAI-driven startups Shah (2024).

The funding of regulatory-compliant AI systems is one of the most prominent AI healthcare investment trends. Investors are eager to support startups targeting AI-based solutions that comply with significant regulations like the FDA's Good Machine Learning Practice (GMLP) rules, GDPR, and HIPAA. Supported by XAI, these startups can showcase ethical and transparent AI usage, aligning with regulations and increasing the likelihood of funding (Nilsén et al., 2022). Furthermore, healthcare AI accelerators and incubators, like Google's Digital Health Lab, the MIT Hacking Medicine Initiative, and Rock Health, place XAI at the forefront and aid in developing its practical applications in medicine. These programs provide financing, expert guidance, and access to the healthcare system to guarantee that AI developments are clinically useful and socially responsible (Priestley and Simperl, 2022).

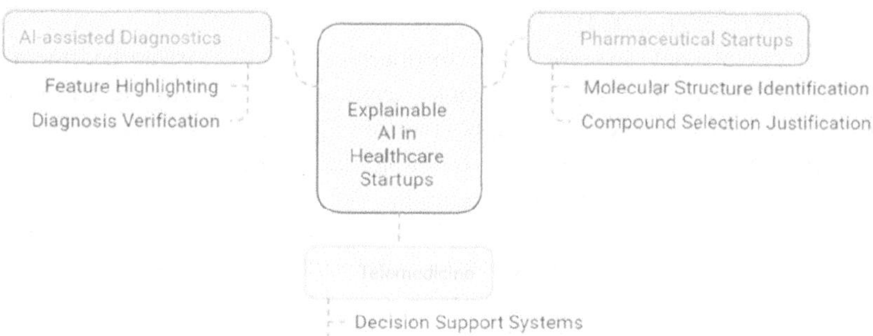

FIGURE 8.7 Integration of explainable AI in healthcare startups.

The development of strategic partnerships with healthcare providers represents another emerging investment opportunity in XAI healthcare startups. These investors are supporting new developments with direct links to hospitals, medical research centers, and healthcare organizations, so that AI model development is compatible with clinical processes and healthcare system standards. XAI is especially important in this case because it enables healthcare professionals to validate and interpret findings generated by AI before the application of AI tools in patient care. This level of explainability helps reduce risk and increases confidence in AI-derived medical decisions (Pradhan et al., 2021).

Furthermore, there is a shift toward greater concern regarding explainable artificial intelligence in drug discovery and genomics, particularly coming from investors with a focus on precision medicine. Investors have shown great interest in AI-powered startups that use XAI for drug discovery, biomarker discovery, and treatment optimization. This space is more sensitive than the other because regulatory authorities need to ensure adequate levels of safety and efficacy for the AI-assisted drug discovery processes. XAI models allow pharmaceutical companies to explain the selection of the drug candidates, how AI predicts treatment responses, and how clinical outcomes are optimized (Temsah, 2023).

Startups in the healthcare sector that XAI invests in receive funding commensurate with compliant regulatory solutions that mitigate risks of implementing unexplainable innovative AI technology. With rising skepticism toward trusting AI, healthcare startups that show commitment to explainable AI ethics and transparency will position themselves as leading AI-centric healthcare providers (Rodríguez et al., 2023).

8.5.3 Scaling AI Solutions Across Borders

The growth potential for AI-centric healthcare startups as they expand internationally is, however, dampened by the existence of legal, operational, and socio-cultural barriers to the acceptability of foreign healthcare services. XAI allows for easier worldwide adoption of AI-powered healthcare services by ensuring transparency, relevance, and compliance with varying regulations. The ability of XAI to provide trustable interpretation of AI-powered decision-making helps to gain regulatory approval, improve system interoperability, and foster confidence in disparate stakeholders (Adithyan et al., 2024).

The next key obstacle is achieving interoperability with existing healthcare systems. The integration of AI models must occur with ease into electronic health records (EHRs), clinical decision support systems (CDSS), and even telemedicine services, which may utilize different technologies. Various standards like FHIR or HL7 are essential for the proper functioning of AI solutions in different healthcare infrastructures. This is made possible through XAI, which helps integrate AI into healthcare systems and providers by granting them the necessary transparency toward AI's decision-making (Inacio, 2024).

Cultural and ethical issues constitute barriers as much as the more practical issues of regulation or technology do. Attitudes toward automated decision-making, trust in technology, and even concerns about privacy differ from culture to culture, which impacts how healthcare givers and receivers relate to AI-oriented tools. In providing an explanation for different users, XAI enables interfaces that cater to diverse groups – patients, doctors, and regulators – to help ensure the output of AI-powered recommendations is actionable, appropriate, and considerate of the local healthcare system (Kilintzis et al., 2021)

Startups need to take several important steps to effectively scale AI-driven healthcare solutions in different countries. Validation of AI models is the primary one, which has to be performed on local datasets of patients in every new market in which a startup is planning to operate. XAI contributes to this by determining how populations differ in their experience with and the performance of AI models, enabling startups to adjust their models to remove biases before deploying them at scale. Also, working with multinational healthcare providers like global hospitals, insurance companies, and pharmaceutical companies allows the startups to practice and improve their AI solutions in differing regulatory conditions, making the solutions more flexible. In addition, explainability can itself be a market differentiator; startups marketing themselves as providers of Trustworthy AI who focus on XAI might be able to obtain faster regulatory and market acceptance (Choudhury and Asan, 2020).

Through the use of XAI to address the intricacies of regulations, interoperability, and transparency, healthcare startups are able to effectively venture into international markets and implement their AI solutions at scale. Furthermore, with the use of XAI, compliance is guaranteed, trust is established across borders, and the adoption of AI into global healthcare systems is accelerated, resulting in improved patient outcomes and more efficient healthcare delivery across the globe (Guiñez-Molinos et al., 2023).

8.6 FUTURE TRENDS AND CHALLENGES IN GLOBAL AI COLLABORATIONS

Even though healthcare-focused AI startups have great promise, their international expansion faces challenges such as market regulations, interoperability, and cultural acceptance of AI in healthcare. XAI provides a major leap in the global scaling of AI-powered healthcare solutions. With its adaptive, flexible, and attentive AI models, XAI guarantees compliance with various healthcare regulatory legislations. Jawaid (2023) argues that XAI's ability to provide explanation and understanding in healthcare solutions facilitates regulatory acceptance, interoperability of systems, and builds trust in stakeholders from different geographic areas.

One of the primary challenges in scaling AI healthcare solutions internationally is regulatory differences. The same X-ray or ultrasound might be performed by different doctors around the world, yet the regulations on a physician's treatment or diagnostic works differ widely through the boundaries of countries. Requiring different healthcare AI systems to operate at the various national levels significantly restricts their scalability. A system that can get FDA approval AI model will need significant reworking to receive EMA or NMPA approval (Ejjami, 2024). XAI streamlines the process of complying with differing regulations by automating the provision of sufficient explanation of AI model actions that would receive compliance assessment by regulatory bodies (Namli, 2024).

A further key issue is integration with existing health systems. AI models must integrate with electronic health records, clinical decision support systems, and telemedicine software which might use different technologies. AI solutions must be able to work in different healthcare environments for a variety of reasons and Fast Healthcare Interoperability Resources and HL7 standards are essential for this. XAI supports this integration by providing information on how the systems make decisions, thus, resolving the problem of different healthcare providers adopting AI-powered systems while assuring there is uniformity in patient management (Farah, 2024).

Apart from legal and technological issues, social and moral factors are equally important within the framework of AI adoption. The degree of acceptance of automated decision-making, trust in AI, or data privacy is not universal and differs from one culture to the other which influences interactions between healthcare personnel, patients, and AI systems. XAI addresses the issue by allowing for different and tailored explanations for different user categories (patients, doctors, and policy-makers) so that recommendations from the system are contextually relevant and applicable in the local healthcare system (Naik et al., 2022).

In order to scale healthcare solutions enabled by AI, companies must implement a set of critical measures. Localized AI model validation is vital as startups have to validate their models in every new market that they are trying to enter using local patient datasets to guarantee accuracy, fairness, and relevancy. Explainable AI is significant in this step as it explains how the performance of an AI model is affected by its population, hence allowing a startup to optimize their algorithms prior to widespread adoption and remove biases. Also, partnering with global healthcare providers, such as global hospitals or insurance and pharmaceutical companies, allows startups to pilot and improve AI solutions across varying regulatory frameworks, leading to broader applicability. Also, XAI serves as a competitive advantage; marketing an XAI solution positions a startup as a credible AI sponsor and helps garner faster regulatory approvals and market adoption (Huang, 2024).

The use of XAI as a tool to handle regulatory challenges, facilitate efficiency in different systems, and heighten transparency allows healthcare businesses to successfully access international markets and scale their AI-driven solutions globally. With the use of advanced and explainable artificial intelligence, businesses can ensure compliance, foster international trust, and accelerate the adoption of AI in healthcare systems worldwide, ultimately improving patient outcomes and making healthcare service delivery more efficient globally (Lee and Yoon, 2021).

REFERENCES

Adamidi, E., Mitsis, K., and Nikita, K. (2021). Artificial intelligence in clinical care amidst covid-19 pandemic: A systematic review. *Computational and Structural Biotechnology Journal*, 19, 2833–2850. https://doi.org/10.1016/j.csbj.2021.05.010

Adithyan, N., Chowdhury, R. R., Padmavathy, L., Peter, R. M., and Anantharaman, V. V. (2024). Perception of the adoption of artificial intelligence in healthcare practices among healthcare professionals in a tertiary care hospital: A cross-sectional study. *Cureus*, 16(9), e69910. https://doi.org/10.7759/cureus.69910

Adus, S. (2023). Exploring patient perspectives on how they can and should be engaged in the development of artificial intelligence (AI) applications in health care. *BMC Health Services Research*, 23(1). https://doi.org/10.1186/s12913-023-10098–2

Akpan, A., Nkubli, F., Mbazor, J., Luntsi, G., and Udeme, O. (2022). XAI methods for precision medicine in medical decision support systems. In *Explainable artificial intelligence in medical decision support systems* (pp. 471–487). https://doi.org/10.1049/pbhe050e_ch17

Allen, B. (2023). Discovering themes in deep brain stimulation research using explainable artificial intelligence. *Biomedicines*, 11(3), 771. https://doi.org/10.3390/biomedicines11030771

Allen, B. (2024). The promise of explainable AI in digital health for precision medicine: A systematic review. *Journal of Personalized Medicine*, 14(3), 277. https://doi.org/10.3390/jpm14030277

Anyanwu, E. (2024). Artificial intelligence in healthcare: A review of ethical dilemmas and practical applications. *International Medical Science Research Journal*, 4(2), 126–140. https://doi.org/10.51594/imsrj.v4i2.755

Arshad, K. (2024). *Leveraging clinical data treasures: Integration of an AI platform into clinical it.* https://doi.org/10.3233/shti240619

Asan, O., and Choudhury, A. (2021). Research trends in artificial intelligence applications in human factors health care: Mapping review. *JMIR Human Factors*, 8(2), e28236. https://doi.org/10.2196/28236

Attaran, M. (2020). Blockchain technology in healthcare: Challenges and opportunities. *International Journal of Healthcare Management*, 15(1), 70–83. https://doi.org/10.1080/20479700.2020.1843887

Bahmani, A., Alavi, A., Buergel, T., Upadhyayula, S., Wang, Q., Ananthakrishnan, S., … Snyder, M. (2021). A scalable, secure, and interoperable platform for deep data-driven health management. *Nature Communications*, 12(1). https://doi.org/10.1038/s41467-021-26040-1

Banerjee, S., Alsop, P., Jones, L., and Cardinal, R. (2022). Patient and public involvement to build trust in artificial intelligence: A framework, tools, and case studies. *Patterns*, 3(6), 100506. https://doi.org/10.1016/j.patter.2022.100506

Brown, S., Berman, G., Logan, J., Sadler, D., Moudgil, R., Patel, B., … Teske, A. (2022). Leveraging innovation, education, and technology for prevention and health equity: Proceedings from the cardiology oncology innovation ThinkTank 2021. *Frontiers in Cardiovascular Medicine*, 9. https://doi.org/10.3389/fcvm.2022.982021

Cary, M. (2024). Empowering nurses to champion health equity and be fair: Bias elimination for fair and responsible AI in healthcare. *Journal of Nursing Scholarship*, 57(1), 130–139. https://doi.org/10.1111/jnu.13007

Chan, C., and Petrikat, D. (2023). Strategic applications of artificial intelligence in healthcare and medicine. *Journal of Medical and Health Studies*, 4(3), 58–68. https://doi.org/10.32996/jmhs.2023.4.3.8

Chellappan, R. (2024). *From algorithms to accountability: The societal and ethical need for explainable AI.* https://doi.org/10.21203/rs.3.rs-5277731/v1

Chen, J., and See, K. (2020). Artificial intelligence for covid-19: Rapid review. *Journal of Medical Internet Research*, 22(10), e21476. https://doi.org/10.2196/21476

Cherney, R. (2023). Qualify AI drug discovery tools through FDA istand program to model responsible drug discovery AI and mitigate dual use concerns. *Journal of Science Policy and Governance*, 22(03). https://doi.org/10.38126/jspg220302

Choudhury, A., and Asan, O. (2020). Role of artificial intelligence in patient safety outcomes: Systematic literature review. *JMIR Medical Informatics*, 8(7), e18599. https://doi.org/10.2196/18599

Coleman, B. (2024). The world federation of chiropractic global patient safety task force: A call to action. *Chiropractic and Manual Therapies*, 32(1). https://doi.org/10.1186/s12998-024-00536-1

Dai, T., and Tayur, S. (2022). Designing AI-augmented healthcare delivery systems for physician buy-in and patient acceptance. *Production and Operations Management*, 31(12), 4443–4451. https://doi.org/10.1111/poms.13850

Davenport, T., and Kalakota, R. (2019). The potential for artificial intelligence in healthcare. *Future Healthcare Journal*, 6(2), 94–98. https://doi.org/10.7861/futurehosp.6-2–94

Denhere, P. (2024). Evaluating and addressing interoperability constraints in health information systems for enhanced healthcare delivery in Zimbabwe. *Journal of Computer and Communications*, 12(07), 133–154. https://doi.org/10.4236/jcc.2024.127010

Duell, J., Fan, X., and Seisenberger, M. (2022). Towards polynomial adaptive local explanations for healthcare classifiers. In *Lecture notes in computer science* (pp. 411–420). Springer International Publishing. https://doi.org/10.1007/978-3-031-16564-1_39

Durán, J. M., and Jongsma, K. R. (2021). Who is afraid of black box algorithms? On the epistemological and ethical basis of trust in medical AI. *Journal of Medical Ethics*, 47(5), 329–335. https://doi.org/10.1136/medethics-2020-106820

Dwivedi, G. (2023). Rmsxai: Arginine methylation sites prediction from protein sequences using machine learning algorithms and explainable artificial intelligence. *Discover Applied Sciences*, 6(7), 329. https://doi.org/10.21203/rs.3.rs-3363024/v1

Ejjami, R. (2024). AI-driven healthcare in France. *International Journal for Multidisciplinary Research (IJFMR240322936)*, 6(3), 1–27.

Elendu, C. (2023). Ethical implications of AI and robotics in healthcare: A review. *Medicine*, 102(50), e36671. https://doi.org/10.1097/md.0000000000036671

Elshawi, R., Sherif, Y., Al-Mallah, M., and Sakr, S. (2020). Interpretability in healthcare: A comparative study of local machine learning interpretability techniques. *Computational Intelligence*, 37(4), 1633–1650. https://doi.org/10.1111/coin.12410

Familoni, B. (2024). Ethical frameworks for AI in healthcare entrepreneurship: A theoretical examination of challenges and approaches. *International Journal of Frontiers in Biology and Pharmacy Research*, 5(1), 057–065. https://doi.org/10.53294/ijfbpr.2024.5.1.0032

Farah, L. (2024). Suitability of the current health technology assessment of innovative artificial intelligence-based medical devices: Scoping literature review. *Journal of Medical Internet Research*, 26, e51514. https://doi.org/10.2196/51514

Ferrara, E. (2023). Fairness and bias in artificial intelligence: A brief survey of sources, impacts, and mitigation strategies (preprint). *Science*, 6(1), 3. https://doi.org/10.2196/preprints.48399

Flathmann, C. (2024). Empirical impacts of independent and collaborative training on task performance and improvement in Human-AI teams. *Proceedings of the Human Factors and Ergonomics Society Annual Meeting*, 68(1), 1447–1453. https://doi.org/10.1177/10711813241274425

Frank, D., Elbæk, C., Børsting, C., Mitkidis, P., Otterbring, T., and Borau, S. (2021). Drivers and social implications of artificial intelligence adoption in healthcare during the COVID-19 pandemic. *PLoS One*, 16(11), e0259928. https://doi.org/10.1371/journal.pone.0259928

Frassini, J. (2024). Civ-mil integration in the transformation of the EU healthcare network: A dual-gain strategy. *Journal of Integrated Care*, 32(3), 252–269. https://doi.org/10.1108/jica-08-2023-0065

Giansanti, D. (2022). The regulation of artificial intelligence in digital radiology in the scientific literature: A narrative review of reviews. *Healthcare*, 10(10), 1824. https://doi.org/10.3390/healthcare10101824

Giordano, C., Brennan, M., Mohamed, B., Rashidi, P., Modave, F., and Tighe, P. (2021). Accessing artificial intelligence for clinical decision-making. *Frontiers in Digital Health*, 3. https://doi.org/10.3389/fdgth.2021.645232

Guiñez-Molinos, S., García, F., Sierra, J., Cabada, J., and Díaz, J. (2023). Computer-supported collaborative design of standardized clinical cases: Algorithm development and validation. *JMIR Medical Informatics*, 11, e45315–e45315. https://doi.org/10.2196/45315

Guo, Y., Hao, Z., Zhao, S., Gong, J., and Yang, F. (2020). Artificial intelligence in health care: Bibliometric analysis. *Journal of Medical Internet Research*, 22(7), e18228. https://doi.org/10.2196/18228

Gupta, S. (2022). Automated diagnosis of breast cancer: An ensemble approach. In P. Verma, C. Charan, X. Fernando, and S. Ganesan (Eds.), *Advances in data computing, communication and security*. Lecture Notes on Data Engineering and Communications Technologies (Vol. 106). Springer. https://doi.org/10.1007/978-981-16-8403-6_18

Gupta, S., and Gupta, M. K. (2022). Computational prediction of cervical cancer diagnosis using ensemble-based classification algorithm. *The Computer Journal*, 65(6), 1527–1539.

Gupta, S., Gupta, M. K., and Kumar, R. (2022). A novel multi-neural ensemble approach for cancer diagnosis. *Applied Artificial Intelligence*, 36(1), 2018182.

Gupta, S., and Koul, A. (2025). AI-based image processing techniques for the automatic segmentation of human organs. In *Advances in computers* (Vol. 136, pp. 207–248). Elsevier.

Gupta, S., and Kumar, M. (2021). Prostate cancer prognosis using multi-layer perceptron and class balancing techniques. In *Proceedings of the 2021 Thirteenth International Conference on Contemporary Computing* (pp. 1–6). Association for Computing Machinery.

Hillmer, T. (2024). *Advancing healthcare research through live-data integration: Implementing IEEE 11073 and FHIR in clinical environment*. https://doi.org/10.3233/shti240661

Hongsong, F., Gao, K., Chen, D., Shen, L., Robison, A., Ellsworth, E., … Wei, G. (2022). Machine learning analysis of cocaine addiction informed by dat, sert, and net-based interactome networks. *Journal of Chemical Theory and Computation*, 18(4), 2703–2719. https://doi.org/10.1021/acs.jctc.2c00002

Hrnjica, B., and Softic, S. (2020). Explainable ai in manufacturing: A predictive maintenance case study. In *Advances in production management systems: Towards smart and digital manufacturing* (pp. 66–73). https://doi.org/10.1007/978-3-030-57997-5_8

Huang, J., Wang, J., Ramsey, E., Leavey, G., Chico, T., and Condell, J. (2022). Applying artificial intelligence to wearable sensor data to diagnose and predict cardiovascular disease: A review. *Sensors*, 22(20), 8002. https://doi.org/10.3390/s22208002

Huang, X. (2024). Reviewing researches on artificial intelligence – driven education and teaching from 2014 to 2023: A citespace-based visual analysis. *Frontiers in Educational Research*, 7(1). https://doi.org/10.25236/FER.2024.070102

Husnain, A. (2023). Ai's healing touch: Examining machine learning's transformative effects on healthcare. *Journal of World Science*, 2(10), 1681–1695. https://doi.org/10.58344/jws.v2i10.448

Inacio, P. (2024). Integrating laboratory testing results at point-of-care in hospital@home care settings: A FHIR-based approach. https://doi.org/10.3233/shti240055

Islam, M., Poly, T., Alsinglawi, B., Li, L., Chien, S., Liu, J., … Jian, W. (2021). Application of artificial intelligence in covid-19 pandemic: Bibliometric analysis. *Healthcare*, 9(4), 441. https://doi.org/10.3390/healthcare9040441

Jagtiani, P. (2024). *A concise framework for fairness: Navigating disparate impact in healthcare ai (preprint)*. https://doi.org/10.2196/preprints.63465

Javanmard, S. (2024). Revolutionizing medical practice: The impact of artificial intelligence (AI) on healthcare. *Open Access Journal of Applied Science and Technology*, 2(1), 01–16.

Jawaid, S. (2023). *Artificial intelligence in healthcare delivery and control side effects.* https://doi.org/10.20944/preprints202312.1138.v1

Jung, J. (2024). Evaluating the effectiveness of explainable artificial intelligence approaches (student abstract). *Proceedings of the Aaai Conference on Artificial Intelligence*, 38(21), 23528–23529. https://doi.org/10.1609/aaai.v38i21.30458

Junior, D. (2024). Artificial intelligence in antibiotic discovery against superbugs. *International Journal for Research in Applied Science and Engineering Technology*, 12(2), 401–403. https://doi.org/10.22214/ijraset.2024.58345

Kamalendar, R. K., Sai, C. T., and Srikanth, P. S. (2024). Ai and ERP for predictive supply chain management and quality assurance in healthcare. *IJFMR*, 6(5). https://doi.org/10.36948/ijfmr.2024.v06i05.29762

Kerasidou, A. (2021). Ethics of artificial intelligence in global health: Explainability, algorithmic bias and trust. *Journal of Oral Biology and Craniofacial Research*, 11(4), 612–614. https://doi.org/10.1016/j.jobcr.2021.09.004

Khan, A. (2023). *A systematic literature review of Explainable Artificial Intelligence (XAI) in Software Engineering (SE).* https://doi.org/10.21203/rs.3.rs-3209115/v1

Kilintzis, V., Alexandropoulos, V., Beredimas, N., and Maglaveras, N. (2021). *A methodology for an auto-generated and auto-maintained hl7 FHIR owl ontology for health data management.* https://doi.org/10.3233/shti210824

Kimta, A. (2024). *Artificial intelligence in the pharmaceutical sector of india: Future prospects and challenges.* https://doi.org/10.21203/rs.3.rs-3878145/v1

Koo, T. H., Zakaria, A. D., Ng, J. K., and Leong, X. B. (2024). Systematic review of the application of artificial intelligence in healthcare and nursing care. *Malaysian Journal of Medical Sciences*, 31(5), 135–142. https://doi.org/10.21315/mjms2024.31.5.9

Krishnan, G. (2023). Artificial intelligence in clinical medicine: Catalyzing a sustainable global healthcare paradigm. *Frontiers in Artificial Intelligence*, 6. https://doi.org/10.3389/frai.2023.1227091

Lai, M., Brian, M., and Mamzer, M. (2020). Perceptions of artificial intelligence in healthcare: Findings from a qualitative survey study among actors in france. *Journal of Translational Medicine*, 18(1). https://doi.org/10.1186/s12967-019-02204-y

Lee, D., and Yoon, S. (2021). Application of artificial intelligence-based technologies in the healthcare industry: Opportunities and challenges. *International Journal of Environmental Research and Public Health*, 18(1), 271. https://doi.org/10.3390/ijerph18010271

Lekkala, L. (2023). Integration of mobile computing and cloud computing in healthcare. *Voice of the Publisher*, 09(03), 119–128. https://doi.org/10.4236/vp.2023.93012

Linardatos, P., Papastefanopoulos, V., and Kotsiantis, S. (2020). Explainable AI: A review of machine learning interpretability methods. *Entropy*, 23(1), 18. https://doi.org/10.3390/e23010018

Liu, T., and Wu, J. (2022). The ethical and societal considerations for the rise of artificial intelligence and big data in ophthalmology. *Frontiers in Medicine*, 9. https://doi.org/10.3389/fmed.2022.845522

Lokare, R. (2024). Transparent precision: Explainable AI empowered breast cancer recommendations for personalized treatment. *IAES International Journal of Artificial Intelligence (IJ-AI)*, 13(3), 2694. https://doi.org/10.11591/ijai.v13.i3.pp2694-2702

Makubhai, S. (2023). Prevention in healthcare: An explainable AI approach. *International Journal on Recent and Innovation Trends in Computing and Communication*, 11(5), 92–100. https://doi.org/10.17762/ijritcc.v11i5.6582

MBA, B. (2023). Surmounting barriers to healthcare data and information: International case studies. *Telehealth and Medicine Today*, 8(4). https://doi.org/10.30953/thmt.v8.428

Mello, B., Rigo, S., Costa, C., Righi, R., Donida, B., Bez, M., … Schunke, L. (2022). Semantic interoperability in health records standards: A systematic literature review. *Health and Technology*, 12(2), 255–272. https://doi.org/10.1007/s12553-022-00639-w

Mienye, I. D., Obaido, G., Jere, N., Mienye, E., Aruleba, K., Emmanuel, I. D., … Ogbuokiri, B. (2024). A survey of explainable artificial intelligence in healthcare: Concepts, applications, and challenges. *Informatics in Medicine Unlocked*. https://doi.org/10.20944/preprints202408.1702.v1

Miyachi, Y. (2024). *Evidence-based XAI of clinical decision support systems for differential diagnosis: Design, implementation, and evaluation*. https://doi.org/10.1101/2024.07.18.24310609

Montani, S., and Striani, M. (2019). Artificial intelligence in clinical decision support: A focused literature survey. *Yearbook of Medical Informatics*, 28(01), 120–127. https://doi.org/10.1055/s-0039-1677911

Mouchlis, V., Afantitis, A., Serra, A., Fratello, M., Papadiamantis, A., Aidinis, V., … Melagraki, G. (2021). Advances in de novo drug design: From conventional to machine learning methods. *International Journal of Molecular Sciences*, 22(4), 1676. https://doi.org/10.3390/ijms22041676

Naik, N., Hameed, B., Shetty, D., Swain, D., Shah, M., Paul, R., … Somani, B. (2022). Legal and ethical consideration in artificial intelligence in healthcare: Who takes responsibility? *Frontiers in Surgery*, 9. https://doi.org/10.3389/fsurg.2022.862322

Namli, T. (2024). A scalable and transparent data pipeline for AI-enabled health data ecosystems. *Frontiers in Medicine*, 11. https://doi.org/10.3389/fmed.2024.1393123

Naseem, M., Akhund, R., Arshad, H., and Ibrahim, M. (2020). Exploring the potential of artificial intelligence and machine learning to combat covid-19 and existing opportunities for lmic: A scoping review. *Journal of Primary Care and Community Health*, 11. https://doi.org/10.1177/2150132720963634

Ndlovu, K., Mars, M., and Scott, R. (2023). Validation of an interoperability framework for linking mHealth apps to electronic record systems in Botswana: Expert survey study. *JMIR Formative Research*, 7, e41225. https://doi.org/10.2196/41225

Nilsén, P., Svedberg, P., Nygren, J., Frideros, M., Johansson, J., and Schueller, S. (2022). Accelerating the impact of artificial intelligence in mental healthcare through implementation science. *Implementation Research and Practice*, 3. https://doi.org/10.1177/26334895221112033

Nong, P., and Ji, M. (2025). Expectations of healthcare ai and the role of trust: Understanding patient views on how AI will impact cost, access, and patient-provider relationships. *Journal of the American Medical Informatics Association*, 32(5), 795–799. https://doi.org/10.1093/jamia/ocaf031

Olorunsogo, T. (2024). Ethical considerations in ai-enhanced medical decision support systems: A review. *World Journal of Advanced Engineering Technology and Sciences*, 11(1), 329–336. https://doi.org/10.30574/wjaets.2024.11.1.0061

Parashar, G. (2024). *Improving explainability in machine learning: A cluster-driven approach to feature importance*. https://doi.org/10.21203/rs.3.rs-5454576/v1

Phadatare, T. S., and Naik, P. (2023). AI based disease prediction. *International Journal of Advanced Research in Science, Communication and Technology*, 621–628. https://doi.org/10.48175/ijarsct-12094

Pournik, O. (2023). *Interoperable e-health system using structural and semantic interoperability approaches in carepath*. https://doi.org/10.3233/shti230571

Pradhan, K., John, P., and Sandhu, N. (2021). Use of artificial intelligence in healthcare delivery in india. *Journal of Hospital Management and Health Policy*, 5, 28. https://doi.org/10.21037/jhmhp-20-126

Priestley, M., and Simperl, E. (2022). Open innovation programmes related to data and AI: How do the entrepreneurial orientations of startups align with the objectives of public funders?. *Data and Policy*, 4. https://doi.org/10.1017/dap.2022.8

Rathore, F., and Rathore, M. (2023). The emerging role of artificial intelligence in healthcare. *Journal of the Pakistan Medical Association*, 73(7), 1368–1369. https://doi.org/10.47391/jpma.23–48

Rawal, P. (2024). Cancer detection and treatment using explainable AI. *International Journal of Scientific Research and Modern Technol*, 3(9), 1–8. https://doi.org/10.38124/ijsrmt.v3i9.47

Rehburg, F. (2024). *How interoperability can enable artificial intelligence in clinical applications*. https://doi.org/10.3233/shti240485

Rodríguez, J., Ramírez-Montoya, M., Fernández, M., and Lara, F. (2023). Use of chatgpt at university as a tool for complex thinking: Students' perceived usefulness. *Journal of New Approaches in Educational Research*, 12(2), 323–339. https://doi.org/10.7821/naer.2023.7.1458

Sasse, J., and Fluck, J. (2023). *An annotation workbench for semantic annotation of data collection instruments*. https://doi.org/10.3233/shti230074

Secinaro, S., Calandra, D., Secinaro, A., Muthurangu, V., and Biancone, P. (2021). The role of artificial intelligence in healthcare: A structured literature review. *BMC Medical Informatics and Decision Making*, 21(1). https://doi.org/10.1186/s12911-021-01488-9

Shah, N. (2024). *Optimizing healthcare delivery: Investigating key areas for ai integration and impact in clinical settings*. https://doi.org/10.20944/preprints202402.1694.v1

Sharma, A. (2023a). Ensuring patient safety and trust: The critical importance of regulatory compliance in healthcare. *Journal of Pharmaceutical Research International*, 35(18), 1–15. https://doi.org/10.9734/jpri/2023/v35i187390

Sharma, A. (2023b). The influence of artificial intelligence technologies in healthcare systems and rise in their applications. *Ip International Journal of Forensic Medicine and Toxicological Sciences*, 8(3), 88–93. https://doi.org/10.18231/j.ijfmts.2023.020

Singh, S. (2023). *Artificial intelligence and machine learning in pharmacological research: Bridging the gap between data and drug discovery*. Cureus. https://doi.org/10.7759/cureus.44359

So, C. (2020). *What emotions make one or five stars? understanding ratings of online product reviews by sentiment analysis and xai*. Artificial Intelligence in HCI: First International Conference, AI-HCI 2020, Held as Part of the 22nd HCI International Conference, HCII 2020, Copenhagen, Denmark, pp. 412–421. https://doi.org/10.1007/978-3-030-50334-5_28

Stroud, A. (2024). *Patient information needs for transparent and trustworthy artificial intelligence in healthcare*. https://doi.org/10.1101/2024.07.02.24309850

Stroud, A., Minteer, S., Zhu, X., Ridgeway, J., Miller, J., and Barry, B. (2025). Patient information needs for transparent and trustworthy cardiovascular artificial intelligence: A qualitative study. *PLoS Digital Health*, 4(4), e0000826. https://doi.org/10.1371/journal.pdig.0000826

Suraci, C., Angelis, V., Lofaro, G., Giudice, M., Marrara, G., Rinaldi, F., … Araniti, G. (2022). The next generation of ehealth: A multidisciplinary survey. *IEEE Access*, 10, 134623–134646. https://doi.org/10.1109/access.2022.3231446

Tabari, P. (2024). State-of-the-art fast healthcare interoperability resources (FHIR)–based data model and structure implementations: Systematic scoping review. *JMIR Medical Informatics*, 12, e58445. https://doi.org/10.2196/58445

Temsah, M. (2023). Chatgpt and the future of digital health: A study on healthcare workers' perceptions and expectations. *Healthcare*, 11(13), 1812. https://doi.org/10.3390/healthcare11131812

Torab-Miandoab, A., Samad-Soltani, T., Jodati, A., and Rezaei-Hachesu, P. (2023). Interoperability of heterogeneous health information systems: A systematic literature review. *BMC Medical Informatics and Decision Making*, 23(1). https://doi.org/10.1186/s12911-023-02115-5

Uysal, İ., and Kose, U. (2024). Explainability and the role of digital twins in personalized medicine and healthcare optimization. In U. Kose, N. Sengoz, X. Chen, and J. A. Marmolejo Saucedo (Eds.), *Explainable Artificial Intelligence (XAI) in Healthcare* (pp. 141–156). CRC Press.

Varnosfaderani, S. (2024). The role of AI in hospitals and clinics: Transforming healthcare in the 21st century. *Bioengineering*, 11(4), 337. https://doi.org/10.3390/bioengineering11040337

Vincy, S. J., Agarwal, S., Mathialagan, C., Shantanu, K., Subramanian, S. S., Rao, D. S., and Dey, P. (2024). *Exploring allied health professionals' perceptions and knowledge of artificial intelligence in healthcare.* https://doi.org/10.52783/jchr.v14.i2.3660

Vuong, Q., Hồ, M., Vuong, T., La, V., Nghiem, K., Tran, B., … Ho, R. (2019). Artificial intelligence vs. natural stupidity: Evaluating ai readiness for the vietnamese medical information system. *Journal of Clinical Medicine*, 8(2), 168. https://doi.org/10.3390/jcm8020168

Williams, E., Kienast, M., Medawar, E., Reinelt, J., Merola, A., Klopfenstein, S., … Niehaus, S. (2023). A standardized clinical data harmonization pipeline for scalable AI application deployment (FHIR-DHP): Validation and usability study. *JMIR Medical Informatics*, 11, e43847. https://doi.org/10.2196/43847

Winter, P., and Carusi, A. (2022). 'If you're going to trust the machine, then that trust has got to be based on something': validation and the co-constitution of trust in developing artificial intelligence (AI) for the early diagnosis of pulmonary hypertension (PH). *Science & Technology Studies*, 35(4), 58–77. https://doi.org/10.23987/sts.102198

Yang, C. (2022). Explainable artificial intelligence for predictive modeling in healthcare. *Journal of Healthcare Informatics Research*, 6(2), 228–239. https://doi.org/10.1007/s41666-022-00114-1

Zhang, H., Lu, A., Abdalla, M., McDermott, M., and Ghassemi, M. (2020). *Hurtful words: Quantifying biases in clinical contextual word embeddings.* CHIL '20: Proceedings of the ACM Conference on Health, Inference, and Learning. Association for Computing Machinery, pp. 110–120. https://doi.org/10.1145/3368555.3384448

Zhang, J., and Zhang, Z. (2023). Ethics and governance of trustworthy medical artificial intelligence. *BMC Medical Informatics and Decision Making*, 23(1). https://doi.org/10.1186/s12911-023-02103-9

Zhang, Yiming, Weng, Y., and Lund, J. (2022). Applications of explainable artificial intelligence in diagnosis and surgery. *Diagnostics*, 12(2), 237. https://doi.org/10.3390/diagnostics12020237

Zhang, Yue, Luo, M., Wu, P., Wu, S., Lee, T., and Bai, C. (2022). Application of computational biology and artificial intelligence in drug design. *International Journal of Molecular Sciences*, 23(21), 13568. https://doi.org/10.3390/ijms232113568

9 Investigation on Deployment of XAI in Healthcare through Augmented Analytics and Augmented Artificial Intelligence

Moushumi Barman and Abhijit Bora

9.1 INTRODUCTION

Artificial intelligence (AI) is transforming healthcare by improving diagnostics, treatment, and healthcare delivery. Using advanced algorithms and machine learning models, AI enhances the accuracy and efficiency of medical processes, helping healthcare professionals make informed decisions. It supports early disease detection, such as identifying conditions like cancer and cardiovascular diseases through medical imaging, and enables personalized treatment plans based on patient data. AI tools, including Convolutional Neural Networks (CNNs), excel in interpreting imaging data, while Natural Language Processing (NLP) improves the management of unstructured medical records. In treatment, AI promotes personalized medicine by analyzing patient-specific genomic, phenotypic, and clinical data to recommend tailored therapies, reducing trial-and-error approaches. AI also accelerates drug discovery and clinical trials by identifying potential candidates more efficiently. In healthcare delivery, AI enhances operational efficiency and patient engagement. Virtual assistants and chatbots provide immediate responses to health queries and assist with chronic disease management. Predictive analytics helps hospitals allocate resources effectively, reduce waiting times, and anticipate patient needs, further improving the quality of care (Topol, 2019). AI integration into medical practice presents significant challenges related to transparency, trust, and ethical considerations. Transparency and trust is a primary concern is the opacity of AI algorithms, which often function as "black boxes." This lack of transparency makes it difficult for healthcare professionals and patients to understand how AI systems arrive

 DOI: 10.1201/9781003605416-9

at their decisions, potentially eroding trust in these technologies. Ensuring that AI models are interpretable and their decision-making processes are clear is essential for fostering trust among users (Zhang & Zhang, 2023). Ethical considerations in AI healthcare applications include issues of bias and fairness. AI systems can inherit biases present in their training data, leading to unequal treatment across different demographic groups. For instance, an AI model trained predominantly on data from one ethnicity may perform poorly when diagnosing diseases in other ethnicities, resulting in misdiagnoses or subpar care. Addressing these biases is crucial to ensure equitable healthcare delivery (Mahendra, 2024). Additionally, the delegation of critical healthcare decisions to AI systems raises concerns about accountability. Determining responsibility when AI systems make errors is complex, as it involves developers, healthcare providers, and the AI systems themselves. Establishing clear accountability frameworks is vital to maintain trust and ensure ethical practices in AI applications. To ensure trustworthiness in medical AI, a multidisciplinary approach is necessary. This includes improving data quality, enhancing algorithmic transparency, and implementing robust ethical governance frameworks. Engaging stakeholders from technology, law, and healthcare sectors can help develop standards that promote trustworthiness in medical AI (Zhang & Zhang, 2023).

Explainable artificial intelligence (XAI) focuses on making AI systems transparent and understandable to humans. Unlike traditional "black box" models, XAI clarifies how AI algorithms reach specific conclusions, enhancing trust and accountability. This transparency is particularly important in fields like healthcare, where AI-driven decisions can significantly affect patient outcomes. XAI aims to improve the interpretability of AI systems by explaining their reasoning processes. This helps users validate and understand how specific outcomes are generated. For clinicians, this understanding is crucial for assessing the reliability and relevance of AI recommendations in diagnostics and treatment planning. XAI also plays a role in identifying and addressing biases within AI models, supporting fairness and ethical practices in healthcare applications. In healthcare, explainability is essential for building trust in AI systems used in critical decision-making. Without clear explanations, medical professionals may misinterpret or overly depend on AI, potentially leading to negative consequences. Regulatory standards also require transparency to ensure compliance with ethical and medical guidelines. Incorporating XAI into healthcare systems fosters trust, supports ethical practices, and improves the quality of patient care. Studies have highlighted the importance of XAI in healthcare. Research from 2023 underlined the need for XAI methods in deploying AI models effectively, emphasizing that transparency and interpretability are crucial for clinicians to use AI-based recommendations confidently (Saranya & Subhashini, 2023; Sadeghi et al., 2023).

Figure 9.1 represents the framework of XAI, which integrates interpretability into machine learning workflows. Input data is fed into the ML model to generate predictions while simultaneously being processed by an XAI method to create explanations for the model's decisions. These predictions and explanations are made accessible through a user interface, enabling stakeholders such as data scientists, domain experts, and business managers to interpret and utilize the model's outputs

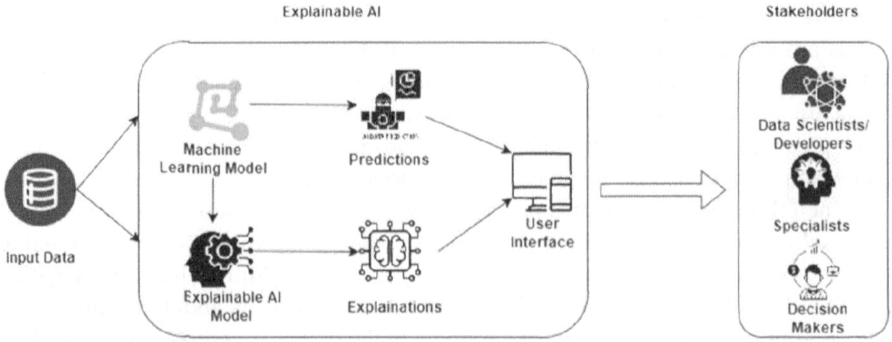

FIGURE 9.1 Framework of explainable AI.

effectively. The goal is to enhance transparency, build trust, and ensure informed decision-making by providing insights into how and why the model produces specific predictions.

9.2 RELATED WORK

The integration of XAI within augmented reality (AR) is an emerging field that aims to enhance the transparency and interpretability of AI systems in immersive environments. Xu et al. (2023) proposed the XAIR framework, addressing the “when,” “what,” and “how” of providing AI explanations in AR settings. The framework is based on a multidisciplinary literature review, a large-scale survey of over 500 end-users, and workshops with experts. Its utility was validated through studies with designers and end users, offering guidelines for effective XAI design in AR (Xu et al., 2023). Wheeler and Carroll (2023) explore how extended reality (XR) can be utilized to make AI systems more transparent and trustworthy. They discuss the potential of XR in providing intuitive explanations of AI processes, thereby enhancing user’s trust and understanding. Maathuis et al. (2025) conduct a systematic survey on the integration of XAI in XR environments. They categorize existing approaches and identify challenges and opportunities in the field, providing a comprehensive overview for researchers and practitioners (Maathuis et al., 2025). The examination of recent advancements in interpretability methods for complex AI models, such as deep learning and reinforcement learning, addresses the challenges faced in ensuring transparency, fairness, and trustworthiness. The study also discusses various use cases across industries like healthcare, finance, and autonomous systems. Looking ahead, it emphasizes the need for further research to enhance XAI’s scalability, reliability, and integration into real-world decision-making processes (Saranya et al., 2023). Arrieta et al. (2019) provide an extensive overview of XAI, including definitions, taxonomies, and challenges. Their work serves as a critical reference point for understanding how XAI can be implemented responsibly across different applications, potentially extending to AR (Arrieta et al., 2019). Angelov et al. (2021) offer an analytical review of XAI, discussing its importance, methodologies, and future research directions. Their insights are valuable for integrating XAI into complex systems, such as those involving AR (Angelov et al., 2021). Hussain et al. (2021) discuss XAI from an engineering viewpoint, highlighting its applications in safety-critical systems. Their perspective is pertinent when considering the integration of XAI in AR applications that require high reliability and user trust (Hussain et al., 2021). The author delves into the significance of XAI, its application domains, and the challenges faced in its implementation. Understanding these aspects is crucial for effectively applying XAI in AR environments (Ullah et al., 2024). Although focused on healthcare, this review (2024) discusses various XAI methods and their applicability, providing insights that can be translated to AR applications in medical fields (Sadeghi et al., 2024). Sun et al. (2024) review XAI in medical applications, emphasizing the need for transparency and trust in AI systems. Their findings are relevant for AR applications in healthcare, where explainability is paramount (Sun et al., 2024). Table 9.1 shows an overview of recent literature on XAI integration in AR and XR.

9.3 EXPLAINABLE ARTIFICIAL INTELLIGENCE

XAI identifies AI systems capable of being understood by humans because their decision-making processes are elucidated. XAI systems stand in stark contrast to the traditional "black-box" models that work independently without disclosing any of their core logic. Unlike these models, XAI strives to show how specific insights are derived from AI models. Such transparency is important when trust has to be built, ensuring ethical usage, and the application of AI into other fields like healthcare, finance, and law is being facilitated (Hamida et al., 2024).

9.3.1 CHARACTERISTICS OF XAI

XAI models are designed to be transparent, enabling users to understand how inputs are processed to produce outputs. This transparency helps identify potential biases or errors within the model. The interpretability of XAI ensures that its outputs can be understood by humans, allowing users to follow the model's logic and rationale, which is crucial for building trust and effective interaction with AI systems (Minh et al., 2022). Additionally, XAI provides justifiable decisions by offering clear reasons for its outputs, enabling users to evaluate the fairness and validity of the results, especially in domains with significant ethical or legal considerations. Reliability is enhanced through explanations that support better debugging and validation, ensuring consistent performance. XAI also provides user-centric explanations, tailoring them to the user's expertise, offering detailed insights for experts and simplified explanations for non-experts. Moreover, XAI helps ensure compliance with industry regulations that require automated decisions to be explainable by providing necessary insights into its decision-making processes. Compliance with Regulations: In certain industries, regulations require that automated decisions be explainable. XAI

TABLE 9.1
An Overview of Recent Literature on XAI integration in AR and XR

Authors	Techniques Used	Dataset Used	Challenges
Xu et al. (2023)	XAIR framework: Addressing the "when," "what," and "how" of AI explanations in AR settings.	Survey of 500+ end-users, multidisciplinary literature review, workshops with experts.	Scalability of design principles, adaptability across diverse AR applications, and ensuring user-friendly explanations.
Wheeler and Carroll (2023)	Use of extended reality (XR) for intuitive explanations of AI processes.	Not explicitly mentioned.	Ensuring trust and transparency while balancing technical depth and simplicity in XR explanations.
Maathuis et al. (2025)	Systematic survey categorizing XAI approaches in XR environments.	Survey and analysis of existing literature.	Integration of XAI into real-world XR systems, scalability, and addressing industry-specific challenges.
Arrieta et al. (2019)	Definitions, taxonomies, and challenges of XAI.	Comprehensive review of prior studies.	Developing universally accepted standards for XAI implementation across domains, including AR.
Angelov et al. (2021)	Analytical review of XAI methodologies and future research directions.	–	Integration into complex systems like AR, scalability of methods, and ensuring real-time explainability.
Hussain et al. (2021)	XAI in safety-critical systems, focusing on engineering aspects.	–	Reliability, trust in safety-critical applications, and maintaining high levels of explainability in AR.

ensures compliance by providing necessary insights into decision-making processes. Figure 9.2 describes the characteristics of XAI. Explainable artificial intelligence (XAI) in healthcare refers to AI systems designed to provide clear, understandable insights into their decision-making processes. Unlike traditional "black box" models, XAI aims to make AI outputs transparent, enabling healthcare professionals to comprehend, trust, and effectively utilize AI-driven recommendations in clinical settings (Hamida et al., 2024).

Following is the significance of XAI in healthcare (Kumar et al., 2025):

(1) **Trust and Adoption**: Clinicians are more likely to adopt AI tools that offer transparent reasoning, as these foster trust in the system's outputs. A lack of explainability can hinder the integration of AI into medical practice.

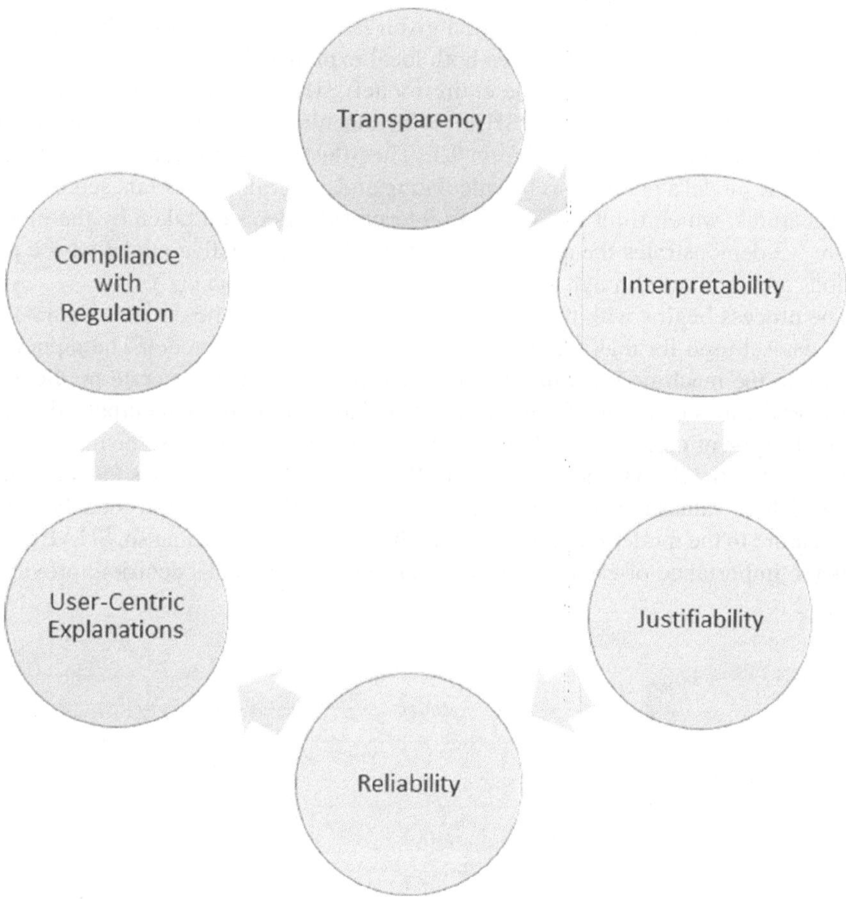

FIGURE 9.2 Characteristics of XAI.

(2) **Ethical and Legal Compliance**: Explainability is crucial for informed consent, certification processes, and liability considerations, ensuring that AI applications adhere to ethical standards and legal requirements.
(3) **Improved Patient Outcomes**: By understanding AI-driven insights, healthcare providers can make more informed decisions, potentially leading to better patient care and outcomes.

Various XAI techniques are employed in healthcare, including model-agnostic methods like Shapley Additive Explanations, which elucidate the contributions of individual features to a model's predictions. It has been particularly effective in areas such as breast cancer detection and risk prediction.

9.3.2 Shapley Additive Explanations (SHAP)

SHAP is an XAI technique based on game theory. For this approach, machine learning models are comprehended through a given feature's importance value, which is labeled as the Shapley value. It gives both local explanations (for individual predictions) and global insights (over the entire model), which increases trust and transparency in complicated models. SHAP with machine learning integration model workflow is demonstrated in Figure 9.3. The illustration represents how SHAP explains the model's predictions by calculating and assigning important scores to the input features, which limit the ability to interpret the decision taken by the model. Figure 9.3 demonstrates the application of SHAP in a predictive model whose predictions are obtained through a surrogate explanation function $g(z')$.

The process begins with the data source, represented by the database icon. This is the dataset used for making predictions or for training the model. The input data is fed into the machine learning model, which processes it to generate predictions. These predictions can range from classification labels to regression outputs, depending on the type of model and task. Parallel to the prediction process, the input data is also passed to the SHAP framework. SHAP computes Shapley values for each input feature. These values are derived from game theory and represent the contribution of each feature to the model's output for a specific prediction. By doing so, SHAP quantifies the importance of each feature in influencing the model's decision, providing

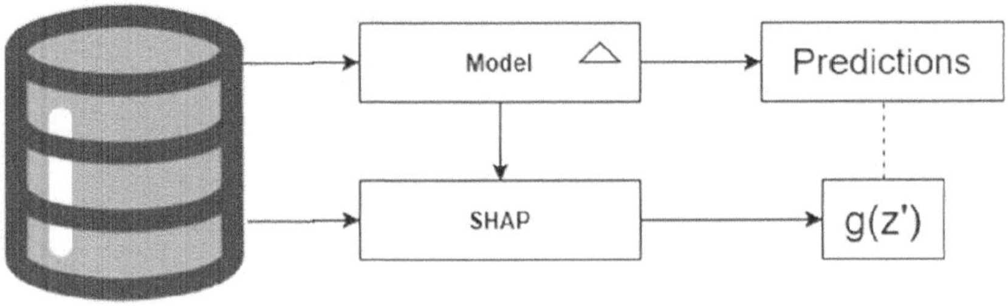

FIGURE 9.3 SHAP pipeline: data, model predictions, and feature explainability.

both local explanations (specific to individual predictions) and global insights (across all predictions). SHAP uses an explanation model denoted as $g(z')$, which is a simplified representation of the original machine learning model. This explanation function approximates the model's behavior while preserving the local fidelity of the predictions. It ensures that the generated explanations are both accurate and interpretable, enabling users to understand why a specific prediction was made.

9.3.3 Local Interpretable Model-Agnostic Explanations

Local Interpretable Model-Agnostic Explanations (LIME) is a technique used in explainable artificial intelligence (XAI) to explain specific predictions of a sophisticated, opaque machine learning model. LIME, through the use of a linear regression model as a local approximation of the black box model, helps understand what contributes to a given prediction.

Figure 9.4 illustrates the workflow of LIME (Local Interpretable Model-Agnostic Explanations), a method to interpret machine learning model predictions. It begins with Sample Selection, where perturbed samples are generated by modifying the features of the instance being explained. These samples are then passed through a Data Shuffling process to create a diverse dataset. Next, the Model Prediction step evaluates these samples using the original machine learning model to understand its behavior. A Sample Weighting mechanism assigns higher weights to samples closer to the original instance in feature space, typically using a kernel function. A simpler, interpretable model is then trained on these weighted samples in the Weighted Explainable step, aiming to approximate the complex model's behavior locally. Finally, the Explain Instance step uses this interpretable model to provide feature-level explanations for the prediction, helping users understand the contributions of various features to the output. This approach ensures locally faithful and model-agnostic explanations.

9.4 AUGMENTED ANALYTICS

Augmented analytics leverages advanced technologies such as AI and machine learning (ML) to enhance decision-making processes by automating data analysis

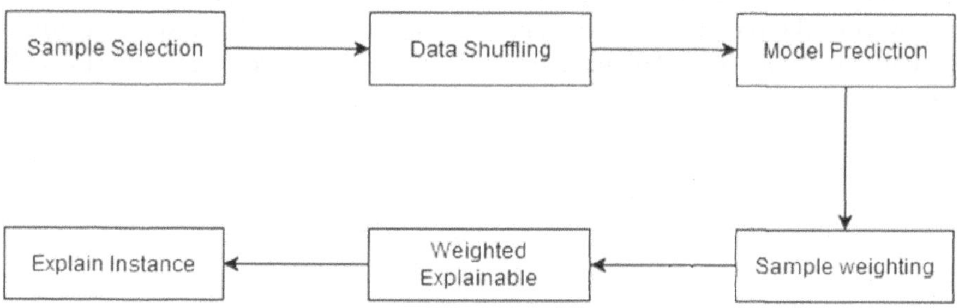

FIGURE 9.4 Flow of generating model explanations through LIME.

and insight generation. By integrating AI into business intelligence (BI) platforms, organizations can automate data preparation, insight discovery, and explanation, enabling users to explore and analyze data more effectively. This approach not only accelerates the analytics process but also democratizes data insights, allowing users without deep technical expertise to make informed decisions. The application of artificial intelligence and machine learning in augmented analysis is fundamentally transforming healthcare decision-making, patient outcomes, and organizational efficiency. Through the combination of data preparation, analysis, and visualization automation, augmented analytics allows healthcare practitioners to analyze data and produce actionable insights quickly and accurately. One prominent example of augmented analytics in healthcare is using predictive analytics to prevent diseases. AI algorithms can analyze patient data such as medical history and lifestyle profiles to identify high-risk individuals, enabling providers to implement timely interventions and personalized care plans. This not only promotes patient health but also helps lower the costs of healthcare associated with advanced disease management. Clinical decision support systems (CDSSs) are also improved with the application of augmented analytics. These systems apply dozens of patient records and clinical guidelines data so that, at the point of patient care, the most appropriate clinical recommendations are provided automatically. This enhances the accuracy of diagnosis and the effectiveness of the resulting treatment, hence improving patient outcomes. Augmented analytics is also making a considerable difference in operational optimization within healthcare facilities. The study of patient flow, resource use, and staff allocation enables healthcare managers to develop and implement plans to rectify identified shortcomings.

As an example, predictive models are capable of predicting patient admissions, which leads to improved resource distribution and lower wait times. Patient engagement and personalized medicine are further supported by augmented analytics. Healthcare providers can provide customized health recommendations and track patient compliance with treatment plans using data from wearable devices and electronic health records. Patients adopting treatment plans become easier through enhanced engagement as a result of this tailored approach. Although helpful, the use of augmented analytics in healthcare is restricted by issues such as privacy and security of data. Organizations need to be ethically responsible by ensuring HIPAA regulations are followed in safeguarding patients' sensitive data. Protecting data from breaches requires sophisticated security controls and strong data governance frameworks. The problems of interoperability are also a challenge since healthcare data exists in many silos. Augmented analytics cannot provide meaningful insights unless relevant data is pulled from multiple known sources. These include normalization of data and usage of interoperable systems. New advances like the integration of AI-based analytic tools, greater emphasis on patient care, and broadened telehealth reach give hope to the future of augmented analytics in healthcare. With these improvements, the efficiency, personalization, and accessibility of healthcare delivery will change over time.

9.5 AUGMENTED ARTIFICIAL INTELLIGENCE

Augmented artificial intelligence (AI) refers to the integration of AI systems with human decision-making to enhance human abilities rather than replace them. Unlike traditional AI, which operates autonomously, augmented AI systems work alongside humans to assist with complex tasks, providing insights, suggestions, and data-driven recommendations. The goal is to empower humans with better decision-making tools and improve productivity, creativity, and efficiency. Figure 9.5 describes how augmented artificial intelligence enhances human decision-making by combining AI's computational capabilities with human expertise, fostering collaboration and improved outcomes through iterative data preparation, exploration, and knowledge discovery. Augmented AI can be seen in various sectors, such as healthcare, where it assists doctors in diagnosing diseases by analyzing medical images and suggesting possible treatments. In business, it helps professionals by automating repetitive tasks, analyzing large datasets, and offering predictive analytics to guide strategic decisions. The collaboration between AI and humans enables more informed and faster decisions while reducing errors that could occur with either pure human or AI-driven decision-making alone.

One of the advantages of augmented AI is its ability to learn and adapt to user preferences and needs over time. It continuously refines its suggestions based on new data and feedback, making it a dynamic tool for evolving tasks. However, it is essential to maintain a balance between human control and AI capabilities to ensure ethical use and accountability, as over-reliance on AI may result in loss of human judgment or decision-making autonomy. Augmented AI is expected to become an essential component in many industries, making systems smarter and enabling humans to focus on higher-level cognitive tasks. By augmenting rather than

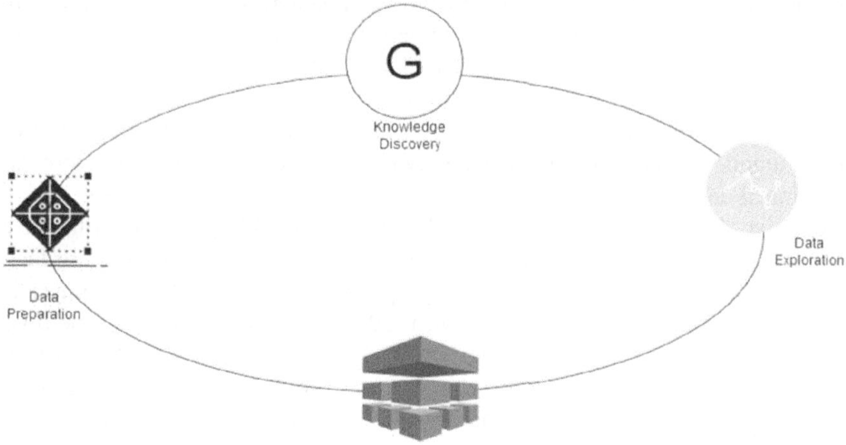

FIGURE 9.5 An overview of augmented artificial intelligence.

replacing human intelligence, it holds the potential to drive innovation and improve the quality of life across various domains.

9.6 APPLICATIONS OF XAI IN HEALTHCARE

XAI refers to AI methods that offer transparency and interpretability, allowing humans to understand the reasoning behind model decisions. In healthcare, XAI has gained significant attention as it addresses the challenge of trusting and understanding complex ML models, especially in life-critical applications such as diagnosis, treatment planning, and medical decision-making (Sindiramutty et al., 2024). XAI techniques are essential in healthcare to provide interpretable results that can be explained to healthcare professionals, patients, and regulatory bodies. Moreover, trust in AI models is vital to ensure safety, compliance with ethical standards, and patient satisfaction (Mariappan, 2025).

As previously mentioned, XAI techniques are helpful in the diagnosis of medical conditions as well. Saliency maps, layer-wise relevance propagation, and attention mechanisms are all examples of XAI techniques where a specific area or region of an image that contributed to the model's decision can be indicated. These techniques are aimed at making the models trained using deep learning algorithms easier for medical professionals to validate the diagnoses made by the machines. Clinicians have limited trust in AI-enabled models relative to their counterparts on account of these models hyper-focusing on images, such as depicting X-rays and MRIs. A deep learning model that is capable of detecting tumors would provide higher trustworthiness if this model was able to display which parts of the images were focused on to make model decisions (Jung et al., 2025).

Personalized Treatment Recommendations: It is another crucial application of XAI in healthcare. AI models are often used to predict the most effective treatment plans based on patient data such as medical history, genetics, and demographic information. With XAI techniques, clinicians can understand why a certain treatment was recommended by the AI model. For instance, the model might show that the decision was based on a patient's genetic predisposition or previous medical history, allowing healthcare professionals to ensure that the treatment aligns with the patient's unique needs. This also helps in avoiding biases that may arise from using AI in clinical decision-making.

Predictive Analytics in Healthcare: The risk of predicting a heart ailment can be improved with cholesterol levels, blood pressure, and age as contributing factors adjusted via XAI. The coalition of the varying components would enable physicians to intercede for better patient progression. Predictive models will always be invaluable for forecasting patient outcomes, potential disease progression, and even risk complications. Interpretability of these predictions is essential for clinicians to leverage such predictions in order to enhance or construct medical strategies aimed at improving outcomes.

Clinical Decision Support Systems (CDSSs): These tools play an important role in XAI, assisting clinicians in making clinical decisions. With the integration of AI, CDSSs can support diagnosis, treatment planning, and patient monitoring. XAI ensures that the reasoning behind a recommendation is clear, which is crucial for clinical accountability and patient safety. For instance, if an AI model suggests a particular treatment protocol, the reasoning behind it must be transparent to ensure that clinicians understand the justification, allowing them to make informed decisions.

AI in Drug Discovery: It is also being leveraged in drug discovery, and XAI can be vital in this field by explaining why certain molecular structures are more likely to bind to a target protein or how a drug might work within a biological system. Understanding the reasoning behind these predictions can help biologists and chemists identify potential new drugs more quickly and efficiently. XAI helps ensure that the process is not only effective but also safe, as any mistakes in drug discovery can have significant consequences.

Ethical and Regulatory Concerns: As AI technologies become more integrated into healthcare, ethical and regulatory concerns regarding accountability, transparency, and fairness are becoming more prominent. XAI can help address these issues by providing clear explanations for decisions made by AI systems. This is crucial for ensuring that AI in healthcare is used ethically, particularly with respect to privacy, bias, and informed consent. XAI can help ensure that decisions are based on fair criteria, minimizing the risk of discrimination or bias against certain demographic groups. The application of XAI in healthcare offers a path toward more transparent, trustworthy, and effective AI systems. It enhances the interpretability of complex AI models, making them more accessible and useful to healthcare professionals. By providing clear, understandable explanations, XAI can foster trust in AI, leading to its broader adoption in clinical settings. As AI continues to play an increasing role in healthcare, the integration of XAI will be critical to ensuring that these technologies are both effective and ethically sound.

9.7 CONCLUSIONS

The integration of XAI in healthcare through augmented analytics and augmented artificial intelligence is reshaping the landscape of medical practice and research. By enhancing the transparency and interpretability of complex AI systems, XAI empowers clinicians, researchers, and other stakeholders to make more informed, accurate, and ethical decisions. Augmented analytics leverages XAI to uncover actionable insights from vast healthcare data, while augmented artificial intelligence ensures that AI-driven predictions and recommendations are comprehensible and trustworthy. This synergy between XAI, augmented analytics, and augmented AI is enabling significant advancements in diagnostics, treatment personalization, predictive analytics, clinical decision support, and drug discovery. Importantly, XAI addresses critical ethical and regulatory challenges, fostering accountability, reducing biases, and promoting fairness in AI-driven healthcare solutions. As AI continues to evolve, the role of XAI in making these technologies more transparent, accessible, and reliable will be pivotal. By bridging the gap between sophisticated AI systems and human understanding, XAI ensures that augmented intelligence in healthcare is not only innovative but also patient-centered and ethically sound.

REFERENCES

Angelov, P. P., Soares, E. A., Jiang, R., Arnold, N. I., & Atkinson, P. M. (2021). Explainable artificial intelligence: An analytical review. *WIREs Data Mining and Knowledge Discovery*, *11*(5), e1424. https://doi.org/10.1002/widm.1424

Arrieta, A. B., Díaz-Rodríguez, N., Ser, J. D., Bennetot, A., Tabik, S., Barbado, A., García, S., Gil-López, S., Molina, D., Benjamins, R., Chatila, R., & Herrera, F. (2019). *Explainable Artificial Intelligence (XAI): Concepts, Taxonomies, Opportunities and Challenges toward Responsible AI* (arXiv:1910.10045). arXiv. https://doi.org/10.48550/arXiv.1910.10045

Hamida, S. U., Chowdhury, M. J. M., Chakraborty, N. R., Biswas, K., & Sami, S. K. (2024). Exploring the landscape of Explainable Artificial Intelligence (XAI): A systematic review of techniques and applications. *Big Data and Cognitive Computing*, *8*(11), Article 11. https://doi.org/10.3390/bdcc8110149

Hussain, F., Hussain, R., & Hossain, E. (2021). *Explainable Artificial Intelligence (XAI): An Engineering Perspective* (arXiv:2101.03613). arXiv. https://doi.org/10.48550/arXiv.2101.03613

Jung, I.-C., Schuler, K., Zerlik, M., Grummt, S., Sedlmayr, Ṁ., & Sedlmayr, B. (2025). Overview of basic design recommendations for user-centered explanation interfaces for AI-based clinical decision support systems: A scoping review. *Digital Health*, *11*. https://doi.org/10.1177/20552076241308298

Kumar, A., Hora, H., Rohilla, A., Kumar, P., & Gautam, R. (2025). Explainable artificial intelligence (XAI) for healthcare: Enhancing transparency and trust. In P. J. S. Gonçalves, P. K. Singh, S. Tanwar, & G. Epiphaniou (Eds.), *Proceedings of Fifth International Conference on Computing, Communications, and Cyber-Security* (pp. 295–308). Springer Nature. https://doi.org/10.1007/978-981-97-7371-8_23

Maathuis, C., Cidota, M. A., Datcu, D., & Marin, L. (2025). Integrating explainable artificial intelligence in extended reality environments: A systematic survey. *Mathematics*, *13*(2), Article 2. https://doi.org/10.3390/math13020290

Mahendra, S. (2024, December 12). *Ethical Concerns in AI Healthcare Applications*. Artificial Intelligence. https://www.aiplusinfo.com/blog/ethical-concerns-in-ai-healthcare-applications/

Mariappan, R. (2025). Extensive review of literature on explainable AI (XAI) in healthcare applications. *Recent Advances in Computer Science and Communications*, *18*(1), E200324228159. https://doi.org/10.2174/0126662558296699240314055348

Minh, D., Wang, H. X., Li, Y. F., & Nguyen, T. N. (2022). Explainable artificial intelligence: A comprehensive review. *Artificial Intelligence Review*, *55*(5), 3503–3568. https://doi.org/10.1007/s10462-021-10088-y

Saranya, A., & Subhashini, R. (2023). A systematic review of explainable artificial intelligence models and applications: Recent developments and future trends. *Decision Analytics Journal*, *7*, 100230. https://doi.org/10.1016/j.dajour.2023.100230

Sadeghi, Z., Alizadehsani, R., Cifci, M. A., Kausar, S., Rehman, R., Mahanta, P., Bora, P. K., Almasri, A., Alkhawaldeh, R. S., Hussain, S., Alatas, B., Shoeibi, A., Moosaei, H., Hladik, M., Nahavandi, S., & Pardalos, P. M. (2023). *A Brief Review of Explainable Artificial Intelligence in Healthcare* (arXiv:2304.01543). arXiv. https://doi.org/10.48550/arXiv.2304.01543

Sadeghi, Z., Alizadehsani, R., Cifci, M. A., Kausar, S., Rehman, R., Mahanta, P., Bora, P. K., Almasri, A., Alkhawaldeh, R. S., Hussain, S., Alatas, B., Shoeibi, A., Moosaei, H., Hladík, M., Nahavandi, S., & Pardalos, P. M. (2024). A review of explainable artificial intelligence in healthcare. *Computers and Electrical Engineering*, *118*, 109370. https://doi.org/10.1016/j.compeleceng.2024.109370

Sindiramutty, S. R., Tee, W. J., Balakrishnan, S., Kaur, S., Thangaveloo, R., Jazri, H., Khan, N. A., Gharib, A., & Manchuri, A. R. (2024). Explainable AI in healthcare application. In *Advances in Explainable AI Applications for Smart Cities* (pp. 123–176). IGI Global Scientific Publishing. https://doi.org/10.4018/978-1-6684-6361-1.ch005

Sun, Q., Akman, A., & Schuller, B. W. (2024). Explainable artificial intelligence for medical applications: A review. *ACM Transactions on Computing for Healthcare*. https://doi.org/10.1145/3709367

Topol, E. J. (2019). High-performance medicine: The convergence of human and artificial intelligence. *Nature Medicine*, *25*(1), 44–56. https://doi.org/10.1038/s41591-018-0300-7

Ullah, N., Khan, J. A., De Falco, I., & Sannino, G. (2024). Explainable artificial intelligence: Importance, use domains, stages, output shapes, and challenges. *ACM Computing Surveys*, *57*(4), 94:1–94:36. https://doi.org/10.1145/3705724

Wheeler, R., & Carroll, F. (2023). An explainable AI solution: Exploring extended reality as a way to make artificial intelligence more transparent and trustworthy. In *Proceedings of the International Conference on Cybersecurity, Situational Awareness and Social Media: Cyber Science 2022; 20–21 June; Wales* (pp. 255–276). Singapore: Springer Nature Singapore.

Xu, X., Yu, A., Jonker, T. R., Todi, K., Lu, F., Qian, X., Evangelista Belo, J. M., Wang, T., Li, M., Mun, A., Wu, T.-Y., Shen, J., Zhang, T., Kokhlikyan, N., Wang, F., Sorenson, P., Kim, S., & Benko, H. (2023). XAIR: A framework of explainable AI in augmented reality. In *Proceedings of the 2023 CHI Conference on Human Factors in Computing Systems* (pp. 1–30). https://doi.org/10.1145/3544548.3581500

Zhang, J., & Zhang, Z. (2023). Ethics and governance of trustworthy medical artificial intelligence. *BMC Medical Informatics and Decision Making*, *23*(1), 7. https://doi.org/10.1186/s12911-023-02103-9

10 Generative Artificial Intelligence and Generative Adversarial Networks (GAN)

Ayhan Arisoy

10.1 INTRODUCTION

10.1.1 WHAT IS GENERATIVE ARTIFICIAL INTELLIGENCE?

Generative AI consists of algorithms capable of creating new and meaningful content by learning from datasets. These models produce realistic and original outputs based on learned data distributions, rather than only analysing existing data. Generative AI works based on deep learning architectures and is often realised through techniques such as Generative Adversarial Networks (GANs), Transformer-based Models, and Diffusion Models (Goodfellow et al., 2014; Vaswani et al., 2017). For example, a model can create a work of art or a language model can produce a natural dialogue text.

Generative AI has undergone significant development with advances in machine learning and deep learning. One of the most important breakthroughs in this field was the GAN architecture proposed by Ian Goodfellow and his team in 2014 (Goodfellow et al., 2014). GANs have revolutionised realistic content production by enabling two models called generator and discriminator to work in a competitive structure. In the following years, Transformer-based Models in language and image generation, especially GPT (Generative Pretrained Transformer) and BERT (Bidirectional Encoder Representations from Transformers), have increased the potential of generative artificial (Radford et al., 2019).

Recently, more complex architectures, such as Diffusion Models, have overcome some of the limitations of GANs and offered the possibility of generating content with higher accuracy and diversity (Ho et al., 2020). These developments have enabled the rapid advancement of generative artificial intelligence in both theoretical and applied fields.

Productive artificial intelligence offers innovative solutions in many sectors today.

DOI: 10.1201/9781003605416-10

Image Generation: Generative artificial intelligence is used to produce realistic visuals in fields such as art, design, and advertising. For example, systems such as DeepArt and DALL-E can create artistic images or designs (Ramesh et al., 2021).

Natural Language Processing (NLP): Models such as ChatGPT and GPT-4 are used in a wide range of applications such as dialogue systems, text generation, and translation (Ahmadova, 2024). These models provide effectiveness in various fields ranging from customer service to academic writings.

Music Composition: Generative artificial intelligence is used in the music industry to create new melodies. OpenAI's MuseNet and Google's Magenta projects demonstrate the power of this technology in music composition (Huang et al., 2018).

Medical Analyses: Generative artificial intelligence offers innovative solutions in areas such as medical imaging, disease diagnosis, and drug discovery. In particular, GANs play an important role in the development of low-resolution medical images and biomedical simulations (Shen et al., 2017).

Productive artificial intelligence has rapidly taken its place in many fields as a complementary technology to human creativity. Its development has supported technological innovations and practical applications, leading to productivity and efficiency gains across industries. However, challenges such as ethical issues and the potential for misinformation show that this technology needs to be developed responsibly.

10.1.2 A Short Overview of GANs

Generative Adversarial Networks (GANs) are recognised as a groundbreaking innovation in the field of generative artificial intelligence. GANs are powerful models that can generate realistic and creative content by learning data distributions. In various domains such as image rendering, video generation, and natural language processing, GANs enable the generation of original content (Goodfellow et al., 2014). In particular, the use of GANs has had a wide impact in applications such as synthetic data generation and enhancement of low-resolution images (Das, 2019). In addition, GANs are also widely used in virtual reality, gaming, and entertainment industries (Harper, 2020).

GANs were first proposed by Ian Goodfellow and his team in 2014 and quickly gained popularity in the field of machine learning. The original GAN architecture is based on two basic components, a generator and a discriminator. These two networks work competitively against each other. While the generator tries to generate content similar to the data distribution, the discriminator tries to distinguish whether this content is real or artificial (Goodfellow et al., 2014). Figure 10.1 illustrates the basic architecture of a Generative Adversarial Network (GAN), consisting of a generator and a discriminator. The generator aims to produce realistic samples from random noise, while the discriminator is trained to distinguish between the generated samples and real data. This process is carried out within the framework of minimax game theory and the performance of both networks improves over time thanks to this competition (Sharma et al., 2024).

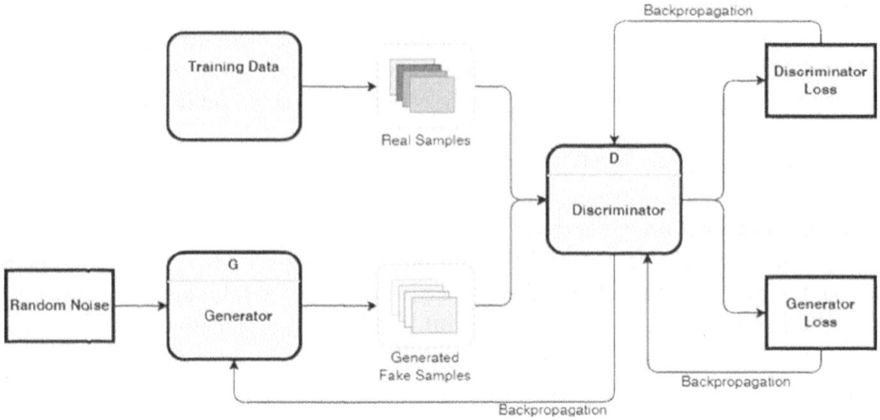

FIGURE 10.1 Simple GAN architecture.

Although the original GAN model works especially with low-resolution data, the derivatives developed in the following years, such as DCGAN (Deep Convolutional GAN) and WGAN (Wasserstein GAN), have enabled the generation of much more complex and high-resolution content (Dale, 2022).

10.2 THEORETICAL FOUNDATIONS

10.2.1 Mathematical Background of Generative Models

The mathematical basis of generative models is based on the ability to learn probability distributions and to sample from these distributions. These models work to understand the hidden distribution behind the dataset and generate new data samples by mimicking this distribution (Carbone, 2024). Probability distributions represent the space in which data are generated, and generative models learn this space, especially with the help of methods such as maximum likelihood estimation and Bayesian theory (Wang, 2020).

Bayes' theory is an important tool for calculating posterior probabilities and plays a central role in models such as Variational Autoencoders (VAEs). VAEs use Bayesian approximations and approximate inference methods to estimate the posterior probability. This allows generative models to model probabilistic distributions based on observed data (Böhm & Seljak, 2020).

Deep learning-based generative models often use neural networks to learn the distributions in the dataset. In particular, Autoencoders (AEs) and Variational Autoencoders (VAEs) are two basic models commonly used in generative AI.

Autoencoders (AEs) convert high-dimensional data into a compressed form of coding (latent space) and reconstruct it with the help of this compressed representation. However, traditional autoencoders are not productive because they can only reconstruct the input and cannot generate new samples (Nikolenko, 2021).

Variational Autoencoders (VAEs) are an improved version of autoencoders. VAEs offer a more flexible and generative structure by using metrics such as Kullback–Leibler divergence to model a probability distribution over the latent space. This method makes it possible to randomly sample from the latent space to generate new samples (Ehrhardt & Wilms, 2022). VAEs also enable the convergence of the learned distribution to the dataset through log-likelihood-based optimisation methods (Bergamin, 2024). Figure 10.2 presents the architecture of a Variational Autoencoder (VAE), which consists of an encoder, a latent space with a probabilistic distribution, and a decoder. The encoder maps input data to a latent representation by learning mean and variance, while the decoder reconstructs data samples by generating outputs from the latent space distribution.

Mathematical Basis: VAEs are optimised with the following objective function:

$$\mathcal{L} = \mathbb{E}_{q(z|x)}\left[\log p(x|z)\right] - D_{KL}\left(q(z|x)\|p(z)\right).$$

Here, $q(z|\,x)$ is the posterior distribution and DKL is the Kullback–Leibler distance. This structure allows the model to better understand the distribution of the latent field.

10.2.2 Comparison of VAEs and GANs

Both models are widely used in the field of generative artificial intelligence but have different advantages. These different advantages are shown in Table 10.1.

10.2.3 Basic Operation Principle of GANs

Generative Adversarial Networks (GANs) are one of the most remarkable innovations among generative artificial intelligence models. GANs consist of two neural networks, Generator and Discriminator, which work in adversarial competition against each other. The *generator* takes random input vectors (e.g., from a Gaussian distribution) and generates fake (generated) data samples. The *discriminator* tries to distinguish whether these data are real or fake (Goodfellow et al., 2014).

This competitive process is optimised by the discriminator providing feedback to the generator. The generator tries to fool the discriminator to make sure that the data it generates resembles real data, while the discriminator tries to detect this fake

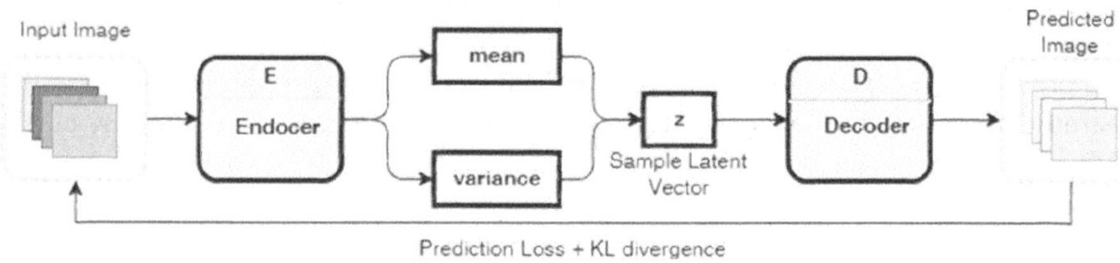

FIGURE 10.2 Variational Autoencoders (VAEs) architecture.

TABLE 10.1
Comparison of VAEs and GANs

Features	Variational Autoencoders (VAEs)	Generative Adversarial Networks (GANs)
Probabilistic approach	Based on Bayesian foundations, uncertainty modelling.	Based on game theory, offers a deterministic structure.
Productive quality	It produces more diversified but lower resolution content.	It produces content in high resolution, but diversity may be limited.
Education challenge	It has a more stable training process.	Training problems such as mode collapse can be seen.

data. This mutual learning loop enables GANs to learn realistic distributions of data (Gui et al., 2023).

The optimisation of GANs is done using two separate loss functions for the generator and discriminator. These functions are defined in the framework of minimax game theory and are formulated as follows:

$$\min_{G}\max_{D} V(D,G) = \mathbb{E}_{x\sim Pdata(x)}\left[\log \mathrm{D}(x)\right] + \mathbb{E}_{\mathrm{z}\sim \mathrm{pz(z)}}\left[\log(1 - \mathrm{D(G(z))})\right]$$

Here:

$D(x)$): Discriminator's estimate of real data (probability of being real).

$G(z)$: Generator's generation of fake data.

$p$data(x): Distribution of real data.

pz: Random input distribution providing input to the generator.

The generator tries to minimise log(1-$D(G(z))$), while the discriminator tries to maximise log$D(x)$ and log(1-$D(G(z))$). This creates a tug of war between the two models and iteratively improves the training process (Arjovsky et al., 2017).

The working principle of GANs is closely related to the minimax strategy used in game theory. Generator and discriminator can be considered two opposing players in a game. While the discriminator tries to learn to correctly distinguish between real and fake data, the generator aims to generate data that is realistic enough to deceive the discriminator.

This is within the framework of game theory:

Nash Equilibrium refers to the point at which the performances of the generator and discriminator reach equilibrium against each other. At this point, the discriminator predicts the generated data as real and fake with 50% probability because the generator has made the fake data very similar to the real data (Goodfellow et al., 2014).

It is not always easy to achieve this equilibrium during the training process, especially problems such as *mode collapse* can create difficulties during the training of GANs (Nowozin et al., 2016).

10.3 BEYOND THE ORIGINAL GAN ARCHITECTURE: ADVANCED GAN ARCHITECTURES

10.3.1 DCGAN (Deep Convolutional GAN)

Deep Convolutional GAN (DCGAN) is considered an important step in the evolution of GANs. It improves on Ian Goodfellow's original GAN architecture, using convolutional neural networks instead of fully connected layers. In this way, it has become possible to produce high-resolution and realistic images (Ramesh et al., 2021). DCGAN has also increased training stability by using techniques such as Batch Normalisation and has been widely used on visual datasets. This model has had groundbreaking results, especially in areas such as art and game development (Hicsonmez et al., 2020). Figure 10.3 illustrates the architecture of Deep Convolutional Generative Adversarial Networks (DCGANs), which consist of a generator and a discriminator built using deep convolutional layers. The generator employs transposed convolutions to synthesise realistic images from random noise, while the discriminator uses standard convolutional layers to differentiate between real and generated images.

10.3.2 WGAN and WGAN-GP

Wasserstein GAN (WGAN) is a solution to the instability problems of GANs in the training process. It provides a more stable learning process during training by using the Wasserstein loss function instead of the loss function of the original GAN. WGAN aims to make training slower but more stable (Arjovsky et al., 2017). However, the weight trimming method has some limitations due to the requirement of a Lipschitz continuous function.

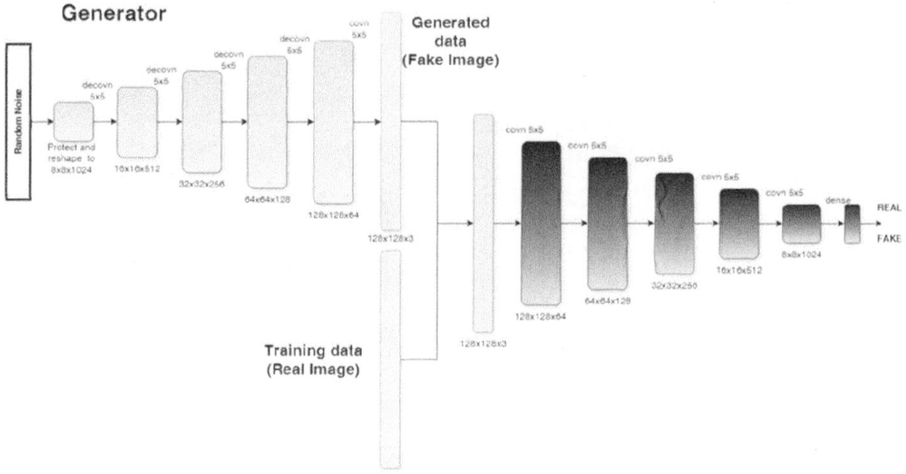

FIGURE 10.3 Deep Convolutional GAN architecture,

WGAN-GP (Wasserstein GAN with Gradient Penalty) was developed to solve this problem. WGAN-GP provides more efficient and accurate results by using gradient penalty to fulfil the Lipschitz condition (Gulrajani et al., 2017). It has been observed that WGAN-GP provides high performance especially in sensitive areas such as biomedical imaging and chemistry (Gulrajani et al., 2017).

10.3.3 StyleGAN and StyleGAN2

StyleGAN is another revolution in GAN architectures. Developed by NVIDIA, StyleGAN is specifically designed for the generation of complex data such as high-resolution and realistic human faces. This model can be controlled using a method called style mapping and provides the ability to create images in different styles (Karras et al., 2019). Figure 10.4 illustrates the architecture of StyleGAN, which introduces style-based synthesis and adaptive instance normalisation (AdaIN) for high-quality image generation. The generator consists of a mapping network that transforms latent vectors into style representations and a synthesis network that progressively generates images through adaptive style modulation. The discriminator evaluates the realism of generated images, ensuring high-fidelity outputs with fine-grained details.

StyleGAN2 is an improved version of the original StyleGAN. This model introduces architectural changes to reduce artefacts during training and achieve more consistent results. In particular, the performance of the model has been improved with innovations such as path length regularisation (Karras et al., 2020). StyleGAN2 has a wide range of applications in areas such as virtual reality and game development (Achicanoy et al., 2021).

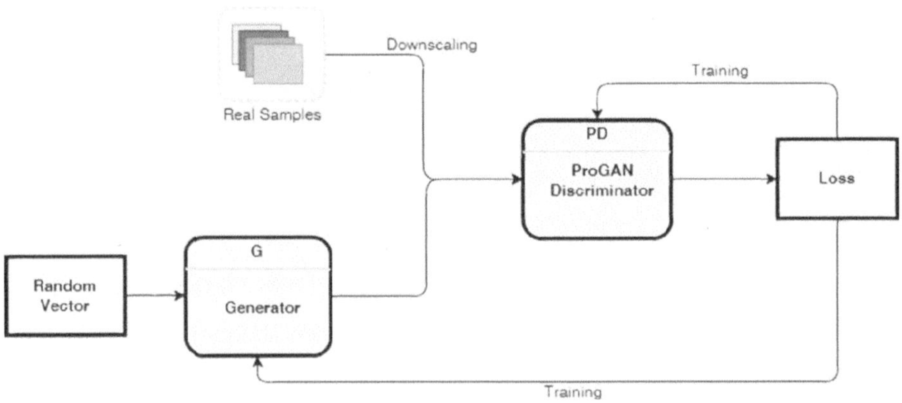

FIGURE 10.4 StyleGAN architectures.

10.3.4 Conditional GANs (cGANs): Conditional Generation

Conditional GANs (cGANs) are a variation of Generative Adversarial Networks, which allow the generated data to depend on certain conditions (e.g., class labels or text annotations). cGANs increase the controllability of the model's outputs by providing an additional condition input for the generator and discriminator (Mirza & Osindero, 2014).

Mathematically, the loss function is defined as follows:

$$\min_G \max_D V(D,G) = \mathbb{E}_{x\sim Pdata(x)}\left[\log D(x \mid y)\right] + \mathbb{E}_{z\sim pz(z)}\left[\log(1 - D(G(z \mid y)))\right]$$

Here y denotes conditional information. cGANs have been widely used in applications such as image completion and text-to-image matching (Isola et al., 2017). For example, the Pix2Pix architecture has demonstrated the power of cGANs in image-to-image conversion (Goodfellow et al., 2020). Figure 10.5 illustrates the architecture of Conditional Generative Adversarial Networks (cGANs), which extend traditional GANs by incorporating conditional information, such as class labels or additional input data. The generator takes both random noise and conditional information as input to generate context-specific samples, while the discriminator learns to distinguish between real and generated samples while considering the same conditional information.

10.3.5 CycleGAN: Two-Way Conversion

CycleGAN can perform transformations between unlabelled data by providing a bidirectional transformation mechanism. For example, it can transform one image

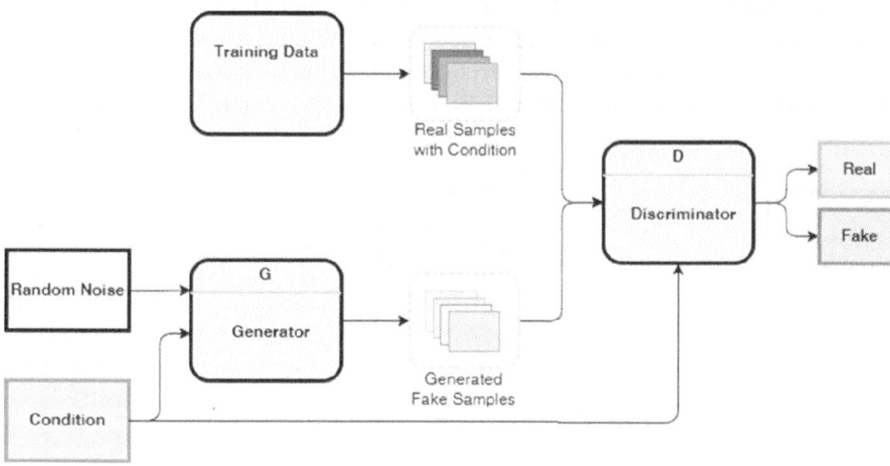

FIGURE 10.5 cGAN architectures.

to another (replacing a horse photo with a zebra). This model works with a pair of GANs and uses a loss function called cycle consistency loss:

$$\mathcal{L}_{\text{cyc}}(G,F) = \mathbb{E}_{\text{x}\sim\text{Pdata}(x)}[\| F(G(x)) - \text{x} \|_1]$$

This allows the model to reconstruct the original data after a transformation (Zhu et al., 2017). CycleGAN is used in many fields such as medical image analysis and art style transfer (Sharma et al., 2024). Figure 10.6 illustrates the architecture of CycleGAN, which enables unpaired image-to-image translation by learning a bidirectional mapping between two domains. It consists of two generators that transform images from one domain to another and two discriminators that evaluate the realism of the generated images. The model employs cycle consistency loss to ensure that an image translated to the target domain can be mapped back to its original form, preserving structural consistency.

10.3.6 BigGAN: GAN Training on Large-Scale Datasets

BigGAN is designed to increase the scalability of GAN architectures. It is particularly notable for its capacity to generate high-resolution images. This model has been trained on large datasets and has shown superior performance in Inception Score (IS) and Fréchet Inception Distance (FID) metrics (Brock et al., 2018). BigGAN uses techniques such as careful hyperparameter selection and orthogonal regularisation for the generator architecture. Although BigGAN's achievements are often based on large-scale computing resources, it has been effectively applied in areas such as biomedical imaging and remote sensing (Golfe et al., 2023).

Advanced GAN architectures have overcome the limitations of the original GAN architecture, providing both higher quality and more diverse generative capabilities. These models are widely used not only in academic research but also in industrial applications. In particular, models such as StyleGAN and StyleGAN2 are pioneers in studies where visual quality is maximised. cGAN, CycleGAN, and BigGAN have extended the GAN architecture and introduced major innovations in both scientific research and commercial applications. BigGAN, in particular, has revolutionised

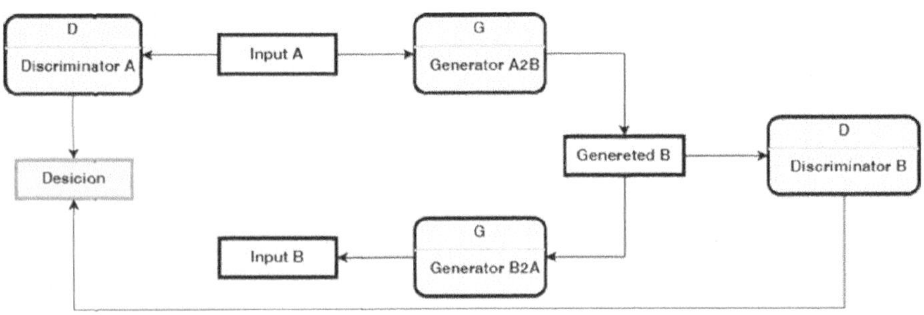

FIGURE 10.6 CycleGAN architecture.

high-resolution images. CycleGAN provides flexibility in unsupervised transformation. In the future, the applicability of these models to larger datasets and complex problems will increase. A comparison of the features, advantages, and limitations of advanced GAN architectures is shown in Table 10.2.

10.4 APPLICATIONS OF GENERATIVE ARTIFICIAL INTELLIGENCE

Generative AI, as a breakthrough technology in data-driven content generation, has a wide range of applications in both academic and industrial fields. These models are used to produce new and realistic content by learning data distributions. In the arts and creative industries, generative AI is used in areas such as digital art, animation, and music composition, offering new creative processes (Takale et al., 2024). For example, models such as DALL-E generate high-quality visuals from text descriptions, while AIVA and MuseNet learn various music genres to create original music compositions (Alabi, 2024). These technologies accelerate production processes while increasing the creative potential of individuals and businesses.

TABLE 10.2
Features, Advantages, and Limitations of Advanced GAN Architectures

Model	Highlights	Advantages	Limitations
DCGAN	Integration with CNN architecture, batch normalisation	Significant improvements in image quality	Limited to complex datasets
WGAN	Wasserstein distance, critic use	Training stability, mode collapse solution	The training period can be longer
WGAN-GP	Adding penalties to gradient norms	More stable training, extended data distribution	High calculation cost
StyleGAN	Style-based structure, progressive growing	Outstanding achievement in image detail	The training period is quite long
StyleGAN2	Improved normalisation, reduction of artefacts	Highest quality image synthesis	Requires very large data and computation
cGAN	Conditional production produces outputs associated with the input	Image-to-image conversion, text-to-image generation	Restrictions subject to conditions
CycleGAN	Unsupervised bidirectional conversion, use of cycle consistency	Style transfer, medical imaging	Limited in complex transformations
BigGAN	High-resolution production of large-scale datasets	Advertising, art, object recognition	High calculation cost

In the field of health and biotechnology, generative artificial intelligence is used in critical functions such as medical image analysis and drug discovery. GAN-based models improve the quality of medical images such as MRI and X-ray, increasing diagnostic accuracy, while artificial intelligence systems that design molecules accelerate the process of new drug discovery (A. Chen et al., 2024). In the field of education, generative language models such as ChatGPT make learning more interactive by providing support to students and facilitating processes such as automatic content creation for teachers (Boscardin et al., 2024). Generative AI is shaping the future technological transformation as a pioneering tool not only in improving existing data and processes but also in developing innovative methods.

10.4.1 Applications of Generative Artificial Intelligence in Art and Creative Industries

Generative artificial intelligence is revolutionising the field of digital art and animation. The models perform functions such as creating original visuals that inspire artists and facilitating complex design processes. While DALL-E converts users' text descriptions into visuals, tools such as Runway ML enable automation in animation and video editing processes (Alabi, 2024). For example, time-consuming tasks such as character design or background creation in animation projects are accelerated by generative AI models (Ranjan et al., 2024).

These models not only create works of art but also offer innovative workflows for artists and designers. In the field of digital art, GANs are used to create a variety of content such as abstract artworks, complex patterns, and realistic landscapes. Style transfer technologies offer artists freedom of creative expression by transforming one art style into another (Takale et al., 2024). These applications are widely used in fashion design, digital advertising, and the entertainment industry (Choi, 2015).

Artificial intelligence has the capacity to produce original melodies and harmonies, opening a new era in music composition. Models such as MuseNet and AIVA create user-specific compositions by learning and combining different music genres. These systems are used in a wide range of applications from film soundtracks to advertising jingles (Takale et al., 2024). Moreover, generative AI models support cultural and historical music studies by imitating the styles of past composers.

The impact of generative AI in the music industry is not only limited to speeding up the composition process. At the same time, models such as OpenAI Jukebox are transforming the processes of sound synthesis and editing. For example, new songs can be produced by adapting an AI-generated composition to an artist's voice (Dasgupta et al., 2023). In addition to facilitating creative processes, this technology offers professional-level production tools to amateur musicians.

10.4.2 Applications of Generative Artificial Intelligence in Health and Biotechnology

Generative AI is transforming healthcare by introducing significant innovations in medical imaging and diagnostics. These models are used in processes such as quality enhancement, noise removal, and missing data completion of magnetic resonance imaging (MRI), computed tomography (CT), and X-ray images (A. Chen et al., 2024). In particular, Generative Adversarial Networks (GANs) stand out as an effective tool for making medical images clearer and more detailed. For example, GAN-based systems accelerate the decision support processes of radiologists in the early diagnosis of serious diseases such as cancer (Li et al., 2023).

These models also support research with synthetic data generation in medical fields where missing data problem is common. The use of synthetic data improves the model training process and ensures the protection of patient data without raising ethical concerns (Gulrajani et al., 2017). For example, CycleGAN models transform between different imaging modalities (MRI and PET) and integrate information from one modality into the other (Gutiérrez, 2024).

Artificial intelligence revolutionises drug discovery processes and accelerates the discovery of new drug molecules. Reinforcement learning and GAN-based models are used to generate potential molecules in drug design and predict their interactions with biological targets (Gayam, 2023). This process shortens the drug development time and significantly reduces costs. For example, platforms such as Insilico Medicine have created innovative molecules for new cancer treatments and minimised laboratory tests in this process (Gangwal et al., 2024).

Furthermore, Diffusion Models and Variational Autoencoders (VAEs) enable more accurate and comprehensive modelling of drug candidates. These models can not only increase biological relevance but also design optimised molecules to minimise side effect profiles (Viswa et al., 2024). For example, DeepChem is used as an effective tool for the prediction of chemical properties and targeted drug design.

Generative AI has groundbreaking potential in healthcare and biotechnology. Accelerating medical imaging processes and optimising drug discovery processes are just some of the important contributions this technology offers. In the future, these applications will become more widespread, enabling more personalised and efficient solutions in the healthcare sector.

10.4.3 Applications of Generative AI in Education and Language Technologies

Generative language models are widely used in education to support learning and personalise individual learning experiences. Models such as ChatGPT are notable for their ability to simplify complex topics, summarise text, and provide personalised feedback. These technologies are used not only to answer students' questions but also to develop skills such as creative writing, language learning and problem solving (Creely, 2023; Law, 2024). For example, in a language learning platform,

ChatGPT can create dialogue scenarios for students in real time and give immediate feedback to their mistakes (Thorne, 2024).

The educational implications of these models also help teachers to optimise their classroom activities. Generative AI can offer suggestions to teachers by analysing the individual needs of students, thus enabling the development of more effective teaching strategies (Abunaseer, 2023). However, it is emphasised that the risk that generative language models may produce misleading information should be controlled by careful supervision and continuous review of the accuracy of educational materials (Alasadi & Baiz, 2023).

Generative artificial intelligence offers great potential in the automatic generation of educational materials. In particular, it provides fast and accurate preparation of resources such as exam questions, summaries, course content, and visual materials. OpenAI Codex and similar models can provide solutions while creating problem sets in programming education (Pack & Maloney, 2023). Moreover, the generation of complex questions and solution steps in disciplines such as mathematics and science relieves the burden of teachers and provides students with customised learning materials (Bengesi et al., 2024).

These applications personalise learning processes by supporting individual learning pace. For example, automatic generation of visual-based materials can be particularly useful for students who prefer visual learning. However, it is important to evaluate the pedagogical suitability of the materials produced by AI to support education with human supervision (Noroozi et al., 2024).

10.5 GENERATIVE AIS: TECHNICAL CHALLENGES AND ETHICAL DEBATES

Although generative AI models offer high-performance content generation, they face significant technical challenges. In particular, data quality, computationally intensive training processes, and lack of transparency are some of the main challenges (Ashraf, 2024). For example, training deep learning-based generative models requires large datasets and costly computational resources. In addition, the lack of transparency in the decision-making processes of the models leads to significant problems in explainability and auditability (Luk et al., 2024).

In addition, the performance of generative AI models is highly dependent on the quality of the datasets used. The use of low-quality or biased data can bias model outputs and lead to misinformation generation. In particular, hallucination in language models reduces the reliability of this technology (Kirova et al., 2023). This situation requires the development of additional systems to verify the outputs of the models and increase their reliability.

Generative artificial intelligence raises serious ethical debates. Problems such as bias in models and the production of fake content raise concerns in terms of societal impacts (Kumar et al., 2023). For example, the potential for these technologies to be used for fake news, deepfakes, and misinformation dissemination threatens both individual rights and public trust (Parra Bautista et al., 2024). Moreover, the extensive use of these models raises legal uncertainties regarding data privacy and intellectual property rights.

In addition, the impact of AI on automation processes may lead to a reshaping of the workforce. While some sectors are concerned about job losses, new jobs are expected to emerge (Madaan et al., 2024). Moreover, considering ethical principles in the design of productive AI can make systems more reliable and human-centered. For this, AI governance and regulations are recommended (Pack & Maloney, 2023).

10.5.1 Challenges in Training of GANs

Generative Adversarial Networks (GANs) have emerged as a powerful tool in generative artificial intelligence applications in recent years. However, technical difficulties encountered during the training of GANs are one of the major obstacles affecting the performance of these models. Among these challenges, mode collapse, unbalanced training, and high computational costs are particularly notable.

Mode collapse is a problem that GANs often face. In this case, the generator model learns only part of the data distribution and fails to generate different types of data. For example, a GAN may focus on generating only cat images instead of a variety of animal species (Wiatrak et al., 2019). This problem occurs because the discriminator's feedback to the generator is inadequate or biased, reducing the diversity of the generated data (Kodali et al., 2017). Alternative architectures such as Wasserstein GAN (WGAN) and Mode Regularised GAN (MR-GAN) have been developed to avoid mode collapse (Arjovsky et al., 2017).

The competitive nature between the generator and discriminator in GANs can cause these two components to learn at different speeds. This imbalanced training can result in the discriminator learning too fast and not providing enough information to the generator, or the generator starting to "cheat" the discriminator (Jabbar et al., 2021). Such an imbalance can lead to training becoming unstable. For example, algorithms such as Loss-Sensitive GAN (LS-GAN) aim to reduce the impact of such instabilities by optimising loss functions (Welfert et al., 2024).

The training process of GANs is a challenging process that requires large datasets and high computational power. In particular, deep network structures and complex loss functions significantly extend the training time. This creates a serious burden in terms of both cost and energy consumption (Durall et al., 2020). Methods such as "Transfer Learning" or "Collaborative-GAN" are used to speed up training processes. These approaches aim to reduce computational costs by providing training with less data (Megahed & Mohammed, 2024).

The difficulties encountered in training GANs have required researchers to develop innovative solution-oriented algorithms. Training these models to be more balanced, efficient, and diverse is critical for future AI applications.

While generative AI offers innovative solutions to many sectors with its capacity to generate content using deep learning techniques, it also brings along various ethical issues. In particular, deepfake and misinformation generation, copyright violations, and negative impacts on society have caused these technologies to be widely discussed.

Deepfake technology is one of the most remarkable and controversial applications of generative artificial intelligence. Its capacity to create realistic images and videos leads to dangers such as media manipulation and misinformation dissemination (Alanazi et al., 2024). Deepfake content, especially on political figures and public figures, has the effect of misleading the public and undermining public trust (Parra Bautista et al., 2024). The spread of such content poses challenges for social media platforms and legal regulations. The spread of misinformation can have negative impacts on individuals as well as on democratic processes and social cohesion (Reichwein, 2024).

The use of existing content by generative models for education raises serious issues of copyright and intellectual property rights. In particular, when a model learns from artworks or music and generates similar content, it creates legal uncertainties about who owns this content (Al-kfairy et al., 2024). The reproduction of copyrighted material by generative AI may violate the rights of the original creators, which may lead to legal disputes (Singh, 2023).

Generative AI has wide-ranging impacts, such as spreading misinformation, contributing to economic imbalances and increasing social polarisation (Zlateva et al., 2024). Moreover, economic consequences, such as job losses, can create injustices in society at a broader scale. For example, processes automated by productive AI threaten the job security of individuals working in creative industries (Moreno, 2024). Drawing the ethical boundaries of these technologies across society is seen as a critical area in AI governance.

The ethical issues of generative AI technologies require not only technical solutions but also legal regulations and social awareness programmes. Regulating deepfakes, establishing clear legal frameworks on copyrights, and addressing the negative impacts on society are critical for a more reliable and ethical use of these technologies.

10.6 FUTURE PERSPECTIVES OF GANS AND GENERATIVE AI

Generative Adversarial Networks (GANs) and generative artificial intelligence are considered to be at the forefront of technological innovation. Making GANs more stable and efficient in the future will be possible by optimising the training processes. In particular, advanced architectures such as Wasserstein GAN (WGAN) and Progressive GAN aim to produce more realistic content by reducing problems such as mode collapse (Balasubramaniam et al., 2024). In addition, multimodal models are planned to be developed by increasing the capacity of GANs to integrate different data types. Such models will be more effective in complex tasks such as generating text or audio along with visuals (Dasgupta et al., 2023).

Generative AI will lead to large-scale transformations, especially in areas such as healthcare, education, creative industries, and finance. For example, synthetic medical data generation with the help of GANs can be used in modelling rare diseases and drug discovery processes. In addition, applications such as the creation of realistic characters and environments in virtual reality and gaming industries aim to enhance the user experience (Hughes et al., 2021). In addition, the wider use of generative models will also entail significant responsibilities in terms of data privacy and ethical issues. Therefore, the development of AI governance and continuous monitoring of societal impacts are necessary (Saxena & Cao, 2021).

The future of GANs and productive AI will be shaped by both technical and societal innovations. More efficient architectures and the expansion of application areas will enable more effective and widespread use of these technologies. However, the establishment of ethical and regulatory frameworks will ensure that these technologies are used for the benefit of society.

10.6.1 The Future of GANs and Generative AI

Quantum computing has the potential to play an important role in the future of generative AI. In particular, the parallel computing capabilities of quantum computers can improve the performance of GANs and other generative models. Hybrid models such as Quantum GAN (QGAN) can enable more efficient content generation on more complex datasets by combining quantum computing techniques with GAN architectures (Ahmed, 2023). However, quantum-based Variational Quantum Circuits (VQC) promise to go beyond traditional methods by offering the ability to learn wider ranges of data distributions (Novo Diaz, 2023).

Quantum computing can also reduce training times and improve energy efficiency, especially on high-dimensional datasets. For example, quantum-based Diffusion Models can make significant contributions to more complex content creation processes (C. Chen et al., 2024). These developments pave the way for generative AI applications in advanced fields such as medical imaging and chemical simulations.

Generative AI models that go beyond GANs offer new approaches to generative content production. In particular, Diffusion Models have the potential to provide more stable training processes and more realistic results compared to GANs. Diffusion Models reduce errors and produce more detailed content by modelling data distributions step by step (Shu et al., 2024). These methods are becoming widespread, especially in applications that require precision, such as medical image processing and chemical compound design.

Mode collapse and training imbalances, which are weaknesses of GANs, are largely overcome by Diffusion Models. Moreover, alternative methods such as Transformer-based generative models and Latent Diffusion Models (LDM) produce more effective results on multimodal datasets (Celik & Eltawil, 2024). The development of these technologies can be used in a wide range of applications such as metaverse applications, artificial reality content generation, and autonomous systems.

The future of GANs and other generative models is being reshaped by the integration of quantum computing and alternative methods. The development of models that can process more complex datasets will enable these technologies to be used more broadly in areas such as healthcare, chemistry, art, and education. However, issues such as energy efficiency, ethics, and data privacy also need to be considered to increase the applicability of these technologies.

10.6.2 GANs and New Research Directions of Generative AI

Training GANs is a process that requires large datasets and high computational power. Therefore, optimisation techniques have been extensively studied to improve energy efficiency and reduce carbon footprint. For example, architectures such as Energy-Based GANs (EBGANs) aim to minimise unnecessary computation by using energy-based loss functions (Zhao et al., 2017). Similarly, the integration of new technologies such as quantum computing into GANs can enable faster and more energy-efficient training processes (Kasgari et al., 2021).

Another approach to increase efficiency is to facilitate the training of GAN models on low-cost hardware. Lightweight GAN architectures provide energy efficiency by offering reduced memory usage and faster training times (Saxena et al., 2023). The development of such architectures supports making AI accessible to a wider audience.

Although large amounts of data are required for training GANs, significant progress has been made toward developing effective models for data scarce situations. Few-Shot GANs and Zero-Shot GANs are innovative methods that offer the capacity to produce high-quality content in limited data scenarios (Abdollahzadeh et al., 2023). In particular, these models, which are trained with small amounts of data, make significant contributions in areas where data scarcity is common, such as biomedical imaging and simulation of rare diseases (Gangwal & Lavecchia, 2024).

In addition, data augmentation techniques improve the performance of GAN models. For example, methods such as Wasserstein GAN with Gradient Penalty (WGAN-GP) provide both accuracy and diversity by optimising training with less data (Gao et al., 2020). This makes training processes faster and more cost-effective.

Research on the energy efficiency and low-data training of GANs makes it possible for these technologies to reach wider application areas. The development of more efficient architectures will both reduce the environmental impact of generative AI and make it more accessible in various sectors.

10.7 DISCUSSION AND CONCLUSION

10.7.1 Current State of Generative Artificial Intelligence

Generative AI has seen groundbreaking applications in various sectors, especially with the development of technologies such as Large Language Models (LLMs) and Generative Adversarial Networks (GANs). These models are used in a wide range of fields such as language processing, image generation, and even biomedical research (Ye et al., 2024). For example, models such as ChatGPT can be used in fields as diverse as customer service to education, while GANs are emerging as an important tool for creating new content in areas such as visual art and medical imaging (Sengar et al., 2024).

Current research is expanding the range of applications of generative AI and developing new methods to improve model performance. In particular, techniques such as data augmentation and multimodal learning enable these models to be used in much more complex tasks (Cao et al., 2023).

Despite its great potential, generative artificial intelligence faces some limitations. In particular, the high cost and energy consumption of training processes is a significant barrier to the sustainability of these technologies (Zhao et al., 2017). Moreover, the lack of accuracy, reliability, and ethical responsibilities of the models carries risks that may have negative impacts on society (Fui-Hoon Nah et al., 2023). For example, fake content (deepfake) and misinformation are among the issues that these technologies need to be carefully regulated.

To overcome these limitations, researchers are developing more efficient and energy-efficient algorithms, as well as exploring integrations with innovative technologies such as quantum computing (Manduchi et al., 2024). In the future, AI governance and regulations are expected to gain more importance in order to create more ethical and transparent systems.

10.7.2 Assessing the Technological and Social Impacts of GANs

Generative Adversarial Networks (GANs) offer revolutionary innovations in various sectors as a groundbreaking technology in content generation. In particular, their ability to produce high quality and original content in areas such as medical imaging, game development, art, and design has attracted attention (Carnevale et al., 2023). For example, GANs are being used to enhance low-resolution images of medical imaging devices, paving the way for more accurate diagnoses (Al-Khazraji et al., 2023). They also play an important role in the game and movie industries, creating realistic visuals and characters (Vinothkumar & Karunamurthy, 2022).

The technological impacts of GANs are also prominent in terms of data privacy and data generation. These models offer the opportunity to protect data privacy and accelerate educational processes through synthetic data generation (Sengar et al., 2024). However, the development of this technology also faces technical challenges such as energy consumption and the high cost of training processes (Zhao et al., 2017).

The societal impacts of GANs are evaluated on a broad spectrum, with both positive and negative aspects. Positive impacts include contributions such as enhancing human creativity in creative industries and improving user experiences in the entertainment industry (Fui-Hoon Nah et al., 2023). On the other hand, the proliferation of deepfake technologies leads to negative social consequences such as information pollution and the production of fake content (Al-Khazraji et al., 2023). Misinformation, especially on social media platforms, has the potential to undermine public trust.

GANs also have ethically controversial aspects. For example, it is stated that these models may cause legal problems in copyright violations or intellectual property issues (Carnevale et al., 2023). It is also emphasised that social impacts should be continuously monitored and regulatory frameworks should be established to better understand the impacts of GANs on society (Vinothkumar & Karunamurthy, 2022).

While GANs offer both productivity and creative potential as a leading vehicle for technological innovation, they also pose significant social and ethical challenges. Developing more sustainable and ethical solutions is critical to maximising the benefits and minimising the risks of this technology.

10.7.3 Recommendations for Productive Artificial Intelligence Research

Emerging generative AI models create environmental impacts such as high energy consumption and carbon footprint. Future research should focus on the development of more energy efficient algorithms (Zhao et al., 2017). In particular, the implementation of hybrid models based on Energy-Based GANs (EBGANs) and quantum computing can play a critical role in reducing the environmental impact of these models (Kasgari et al., 2021).

The importance of ethical and societal responsibilities is increasing with the expansion of the use of generative artificial intelligence. Bias problems and lack of transparency are key challenges limiting the acceptability of these technologies (Holmes et al., 2023). Research should focus on developing ethical frameworks and regulatory policies. These frameworks can ensure responsible application of the technology while protecting the rights of users.

Developing effective models in areas where data scarcity is prevalent is a critical priority for future research. By improving the performance of methods such as Few-Shot GANs and Zero-Shot GANs, high accuracy rates can be achieved with less data (Abdollahzadeh et al., 2023). Especially in biomedical fields, such methods have great potential in the diagnosis of rare diseases.

Increasing the multimodal data processing capacity of generative AI is an important opportunity for future research. Developing models that combine image, text, and audio data will enable more complex applications (Cao et al., 2023). This could offer innovative solutions, especially in areas such as virtual reality, gaming, and education.

Generative Adversarial Networks (GANs) have revolutionised generative AI by enabling the creation of highly realistic synthetic data, such as images, text, and audio. However, their inherent "black box" nature raises significant concerns regarding interpretability and trustworthiness, especially in high-stakes applications like healthcare, finance, and autonomous systems. This opacity can lead to ethical dilemmas, such as unintended biases or unexplainable outputs, which limit the broader acceptance of GAN-based technologies (Goodfellow et al., 2014). Explainable artificial intelligence (XAI) is emerging as a critical area of research to address these challenges by developing methods that elucidate the inner workings of AI models. Integrating XAI techniques with GANs can provide insights into both the generator and discriminator components, allowing stakeholders to understand and evaluate the rationale behind the generated outputs (Arrieta et al., 2020). For example, in medical imaging, XAI-enhanced GANs could enable practitioners to validate the authenticity and diagnostic relevance of synthesised images, ensuring that models are both accurate and transparent (Noroozi et al., 2024). Furthermore, XAI could play a pivotal role in mitigating biases by revealing the decision-making pathways within GANs, thereby ensuring fairness and accountability. Future research should prioritise the development of hybrid frameworks that combine the generative power of GANs with the interpretability of XAI, fostering trust and ethical responsibility in the deployment of these models across diverse fields (Schneider, 2024).

REFERENCES

Abdollahzadeh, M., Malekzadeh, T., Teo, C. T. H., Chandrasegaran, K., Liu, G., & Cheung, N.-M. (2023). *A Survey on Generative Modeling with Limited Data, Few Shots, and Zero Shot*. https://arxiv.org/abs/2307.14397

Abunaseer, H. (2023). The Use of Generative AI in Education: Applications, and Impact. *Technology and the Curriculum: Summer 2023*, 1–228.

Achicanoy, H., Chaves, D., & Trujillo, M. (2021). StyleGANs and Transfer Learning for Generating Synthetic Images in Industrial Applications. *Symmetry, 13*(8), 1497. https://doi.org/10.3390/SYM13081497

Ahmadova, S. (2024). A Comparative Quality Assessment of ChatGPT-4 and Human Translation of Scientific Texts. (Master's thesis), Khazar University (Azerbaijan). ProQuest.

Ahmed, S. (2023). Machine Learning for Quantum Information and Computing. *Chalmers University of Technology*. https://research.chalmers.se/publication/539445

Al-kfairy, M., Mustafa, D., Kshetri, N., Insiew, M., & Alfandi, O. (2024). Ethical Challenges and Solutions of Generative AI: An Interdisciplinary Perspective. *Informatics, 11*(3). https://doi.org/10.3390/informatics11030058

Al-Khazraji, S. H., Saleh, H. H., KHALID, A. I., & MISHKHAL, I. A. (2023). Impact of Deepfake Technology on Social Media: Detection, Misinformation and Societal Implications. *The Eurasia Proceedings of Science Technology Engineering and Mathematics, 23*, 429–441.

Alabi, M. (2024). Generative AI and its Applications in Creative Industries. (Thesis), Ladoke Akintola University of Technology.

Alanazi, S., Asif, S., & Moulitsas, I. (2024). Examining the Societal Impact and Legislative Requirements of Deepfake Technology: A Comprehensive Study. *International Journal of Social Science and Humanity, 14*(2), 58–64. https://doi.org/https://doi.org/10.18178/ijssh.2024.14.2.1194

Alasadi, E. A., & Baiz, C. R. (2023). Generative AI in Education and Research: Opportunities, Concerns, and Solutions. *Journal of Chemical Education*. https://doi.org/10.1021/acs.jchemed.3c00323

Arjovsky, M., Chintala, S., & Bottou, L. (2017). {W}asserstein Generative Adversarial Networks. In D. Precup & Y. W. Teh (Eds.), *Proceedings of the 34th International Conference on Machine Learning* (Vol. 70, pp. 214–223). PMLR. https://proceedings.mlr.press/v70/arjovsky17a.html

Arrieta, A. B., Díaz-Rodríguez, N., Del Ser, J., Bennetot, A., Tabik, S., Barbado, A., Garcia, S., Gil-López, S., Molina, D., Benjamins, R., & others. (2020). Explainable Artificial Intelligence (XAI): Concepts, taxonomies, opportunities and challenges toward responsible AI. *Information Fusion, 58*, 82–115.

Ashraf, M. (2024). Generative AI: Challenges and the Road Ahead. *International Journal of Science and Research (IJSR), 13*, 716–725. https://doi.org/10.21275/SR241009154508

Balasubramaniam, S., Chirchi, V., Kadry, S., Agoramoorthy, M., Gururama, S. P., Satheesh, K. K., & Sivakumar, T. A. (2024). The Road Ahead: Emerging Trends, Unresolved Issues, and Concluding Remarks in Generative AI—A Comprehensive Review. *International Journal of Intelligent Systems, 2024*, 7.

Bengesi, S., El-Sayed, H., Sarker, M. D. K., Houkpati, Y., Irungu, J., & Oladunni, T. (2024). Advancements in Generative AI: A Comprehensive Review of GANs, GPT, Autoencoders, Diffusion Model, and Transformers. *IEEE Access*, *12*, 69812–69837. https://doi.org/10.1109/ACCESS.2024.3397775

Bergamin, F. (2024). *Advances in Deep Generative Models, Approximate Inference, and their Applications*. Technical University of Denmark.

Böhm, V., & Seljak, U. (2020).*Probabilistic Autoencoder*. https://arxiv.org/abs/2006.05479v4

Boscardin, C. K., Gin, B., Golde, P. B., & Hauer, K. E. (2024). ChatGPT and Generative Artificial Intelligence for Medical Education: Potential Impact and Opportunity. *Academic Medicine*, *99*(1), 22–27.

Brock, A., Donahue, J., & Simonyan, K. (2018). Large Scale GAN Training for High Fidelity Natural Image Synthesis. *arXiv:1809.11096*.

Cao, Y., Sheng, Q. Z., McAuley, J., & Yao, L. (2023). *Reinforcement Learning for Generative AI: A Survey*. https://arxiv.org/abs/2308.14328

Carbone, D. (2024). Generative Models as Out-of-equilibrium Particle Systems: The Case of Energy-Based Models (Ph.D Thesis), Università degli Studi di Torino.

Carnevale, A., Delgado, C. F., & Bisconti, P. (2023). Hybrid ethics for generative AI: Philosophical inquiries on GANs. *Humana.Mente Journal*, *44*, 33–56.

Celik, A., & Eltawil, A. M. (2024). At the Dawn of Generative AI Era: A Tutorial-cum-Survey on New Frontiers in 6G Wireless Intelligence. *IEEE Open Journal of the Communications Society*, *5*, 2433–2489. https://doi.org/10.1109/OJCOMS.2024.3362271

Chen, A., Liu, L., & Zhu, T. (2024). Advancing the Democratization of Generative Artificial Intelligence in Healthcare: A Narrative Review. *Journal of Hospital Management and Health Policy*, *8*. https://jhmhp.amegroups.org/article/view/8842

Chen, C., Zhao, Q., Zhou, M., He, Z., Sun, Z., & Situ, H. (2024). *Quantum Generative Diffusion Model: A Fully Quantum-Mechanical Model for Generating Quantum State Ensemble*. https://arxiv.org/abs/2401.07039

Choi, H. (2015). *Generative AI Art Exploration and Image Generation Fine Tuning Techniques*. California Institute of the Arts.

Creely, E. (2023). *The Possibilities, Limitations, and Dangers of Generative AI in Language Learning and Literacy Practices*. International Graduate Research Symposium 2023. Proceedings, pp. 1–14.

Dale, M. (2022). Advancement of Generative Adversarial Model for Image Synthesis with Human Language Description. Technical Report.

Das, S. (2019). Generating Synthetic Images from Textual Description Using GANs. Medium. Retrieved from https://towardsdatascience.com/generating-synthetic-images-from-textual-description-using-gans-e5963bae0df4

Dasgupta, D., Venugopal, D., & Gupta, K. D. (2023). *A Review of Generative AI from Historical Perspectives*. https://doi.org/10.36227/techrxiv.22097942.v1

Durall, R., Chatzimichailidis, A., Labus, P., & Keuper, J. (2020). *Combating Mode Collapse in GAN Training: An Empirical Analysis Using Hessian Eigenvalues*. https://doi.org/10.48550/arxiv.2012.09673

Ehrhardt, J., & Wilms, M. (2022). Chapter 8 - Autoencoders and Variational Autoencoders in Medical Image Analysis. In N. Burgos & D. Svoboda (Eds.), *Biomedical Image Synthesis and Simulation* (pp. 129–162). Academic Press. https://doi.org/https://doi.org/10.1016/B978-0-12-824349-7.00015-3

Fui-Hoon Nah, F., Zheng, R., Cai, J., Siau, K., & Chen, L. (2023). Generative AI and ChatGPT: Applications, Challenges, and AI-human Collaboration. *Journal of Information Technology Case and Application Research*, *25*(3), 277–304).

Gangwal, A., Ansari, A., Ahmad, I., Azad, A. K., Kumarasamy, V., Subramaniyan, V., & Wong, L. S. (2024). Generative Artificial Intelligence in Drug Discovery: Basic Framework, Recent Advances, Challenges, and Opportunities. *Frontiers in Pharmacology, 15*, 1331062.

Gangwal, A., & Lavecchia, A. (2024). Unleashing the Power of Generative AI in Drug Discovery. *Drug Discovery Today, 29*(6), 103992. https://doi.org/https://doi.org/10.1016/j.drudis.2024.103992

Gao, X., Deng, F., & Yue, X. (2020). Data Augmentation in Fault Diagnosis Based on the Wasserstein Generative Adversarial Network with Gradient Penalty. *Neurocomputing, 396*, 487–494. https://doi.org/https://doi.org/10.1016/j.neucom.2018.10.109

Gayam, S. R. (2023). Enhancing Creative Industries with Generative AI: Techniques for Music Composition, Art Generation, and Interactive Media. *Journal of Machine Learning in Pharmaceutical Research, 3*(1), 54–88.

Golfe, A., Del Amor, R., Colomer, A., Sales, M. A., Terradez, L., & Naranjo, V. (2023). ProGleason-GAN: Conditional Progressive Growing GAN for Prostatic Cancer Gleason Grade Patch Synthesis. *Computer Methods and Programs in Biomedicine, 240*, 107695.

Goodfellow, I., Pouget-Abadie, J., Mirza, M., Xu, B., Warde-Farley, D., Ozair, S., Courville, A., & Bengio, Y. (2014). Generative Adversarial Nets. *Advances in Neural Information Processing Systems, 27*, 1–9.

Goodfellow, I., Pouget-Abadie, J., Mirza, M., Xu, B., Warde-Farley, D., Ozair, S., Courville, A., & Bengio, Y. (2020). Generative Adversarial Networks. *Communications of the ACM, 63*(11), 139–144. https://doi.org/10.1145/3422622

Gui, J., Sun, Z., Wen, Y., Tao, D., & Ye, J. (2023). A Review on Generative Adversarial Networks: Algorithms, Theory, and Applications. *IEEE Transactions on Knowledge and Data Engineering, 35*(4), 3313–3332. https://doi.org/10.1109/TKDE.2021.3130191

Gulrajani, I., Ahmed, F., Arjovsky, M., Dumoulin, V., & Courville, A. C. (2017). Improved Training of Wasserstein GANs. In I. Guyon, U. Von Luxburg, S. Bengio, H. Wallach, R. Fergus, S. Vishwanathan, & R. Garnett (Eds.), *Advances in Neural Information Processing Systems* (Vol. 30). Curran Associates, Inc.

Gutiérrez, C. (2024). Generative AI and the Arts: An exploration of the Social and Cultural Impact of Generative AI in the Visual Arts (Master Thesis), Linnaeus University.

Harper, C. (2020). Generative Machine Learning. In *Libraries, and Cross-Disciplinary Research: Possibilities and Provocations* (pp. 13–28). https://doi.org/https://doi.org/10.7274/r0-wxg0-pe06

Hicsonmez, S., Samet, N., Akbas, E., & Duygulu, P. (2020). GANILLA: Generative Adversarial Networks for Image to Illustration Translation. *Image and Vision Computing, 95*, 103886. https://doi.org/https://doi.org/10.1016/j.imavis.2020.103886

Ho, J., Jain, A., & Abbeel, P. (2020). Denoising Diffusion Probabilistic Models. *Advances in Neural Information Processing Systems, 33*, 6840–6851.

Holmes, W., Miao, F., & others. (2023). *Guidance for Generative AI in Education and Research.* UNESCO Publishing.

Huang, C.-Z. A., Vaswani, A., Uszkoreit, J., Shazeer, N., Simon, I., Hawthorne, C., Dai, A. M., Hoffman, M. D., Dinculescu, M., & Eck, D. (2018). *Music Transformer.* https://arxiv.org/abs/1809.04281

Hughes, R. T., Zhu, L., & Bednarz, T. (2021). *Generative Adversarial Networks–Enabled Human–Artificial Intelligence Collaborative Applications for Creative and Design Industries: A Systematic Review of Current Approaches and Trends.* https://doi.org/10.3389/frai.2021.604234

Isola, P., Zhu, J.-Y., Zhou, T., & Efros, A. A. (2017). *Image-to-image Translation with Conditional Adversarial Networks*. Proceedings of the IEEE Conference on Computer Vision and Pattern Recognition, pp. 1125–1134.

Jabbar, A., Li, X., & Omar, B. (2021). A Survey on Generative Adversarial Networks: Variants, Applications, and Training. *ACM Computing Surveys*, *54*(8). https://doi.org/10.1145/3463475

Karras, T., Laine, S., & Aila, T. (2019). *A Style-Based Generator Architecture for Generative Adversarial Networks*. Proceedings of the IEEE/CVF Conference on Computer Vision and Pattern Recognition (CVPR).

Karras, T., Laine, S., Aittala, M., Hellsten, J., Lehtinen, J., & Aila, T. (2020). *Analyzing and Improving the Image Quality of StyleGAN*. Proceedings of the IEEE/CVF Conference on Computer Vision and Pattern Recognition (CVPR).

Kasgari, A. T. Z., Saad, W., Mozaffari, M., & Poor, H. V. (2021). Experienced Deep Reinforcement Learning With Generative Adversarial Networks (GANs) for Model-Free Ultra Reliable Low Latency Communication. *IEEE Transactions on Communications*, *69*(2), 884–899. https://doi.org/10.1109/TCOMM.2020.3031930

Kirova, V. D., Ku, C. S., Laracy, J. R., & Marlowe, T. J. (2023). The Ethics of Artificial Intelligence in the Era of Generative AI. *Journal of Systemics, Cybernetics and Informatics*, *21*(4), 42–50.

Kodali, N., Abernethy, J., Hays, J., & Kira, Z. (2017). On Convergence and Stability of Gans. *ArXiv Preprint ArXiv:1705.07215*.

Kumar, B., Kumar, T., & Nadakuditi, S. (2023). Ethical Implications of Generative AI: The Case of Large Language Models. *The Journal of Scientific and Engineering Research*, *7*, 122–127.

Law, L. (2024). Application of Generative Artificial Intelligence (GenAI) in Language Teaching and Learning: A Scoping Literature Review. *Computers and Education Open*, *6*, 100174.

Li, M., Jiang, Y., Zhang, Y., & Zhu, H. (2023). Medical Image Analysis Using Deep Learning Algorithms. *Frontiers in Public Health*, *11*. https://doi.org/10.3389/fpubh.2023.1273253

Luk, C.-Y., Chung, H.-L., Yim, W.-K., & Leung, C.-W. (2024). *Regulating Generative AI: Ethical Considerations and Explainability Benchmarks*. OSF Preprints.

Madaan, G., Asthana, S. K., & Kaur, J. (2024). Generative AI: Applications, Models, Challenges, Opportunities, and Future Directions. In J. Gomathi Sankar & A. David (Eds.), *Generative AI and Implications for Ethics, Security, and Data Management* (pp. 88–121). IGI Global Scientific Publishing. https://doi.org/10.4018/979-8-3693-8557-9.ch004.

Manduchi, L., Pandey, K., Bamler, R., Cotterell, R., Däubener, S., Fellenz, S., Fischer, A., Gärtner, T., Kirchler, M., Kloft, M., Li, Y., Lippert, C., de Melo, G., Nalisnick, E., Ommer, B., Ranganath, R., Rudolph, M., Ullrich, K., den Broeck, G. Van, … Fortuin, V. (2024). *On the Challenges and Opportunities in Generative AI*. https://arxiv.org/abs/2403.00025

Megahed, M., & Mohammed, A. (2024). Collaborative-GAN: An Approach for Stabilizing the Training Process of Generative Adversarial Network. *IEEE Access*, *12*, 138716–138735. https://doi.org/10.1109/ACCESS.2024.3457902

Mirza, M., & Osindero, S. (2014). *Conditional Generative Adversarial Nets*. https://arxiv.org/abs/1411.1784v1

Moreno, F. R. (2024). Generative AI and Deepfakes: A Human Rights Approach to Tackling Harmful Content. *International Review of Law, Computers \& Technology*, *38*(3), 297–326. https://doi.org/10.1080/13600869.2024.2324540

Nikolenko, S. I. (2021). Generative Models in Deep Learning. In *Synthetic Data for Deep Learning* (pp. 97–137). Springer International Publishing. https://doi.org/10.1007/978-3-030-75178-4_4

Noroozi, O., Soleimani, S., Farrokhnia, M., & Banihashem, S. K. (2024). Generative AI in Education: Pedagogical, Theoretical, and Methodological Perspectives. *International Journal of Technology in Education, 7*(3), 373–385.

Novo Diaz, O. (2023). *Exploring the Quantum Frontiers of Generative Adversarial Networks in Chemical Catalysis.* https://oa.upm.es/76810/

Nowozin, S., Cseke, B., & Tomioka, R. (2016). f-GAN: Training Generative Neural Samplers using Variational Divergence Minimization. In D. Lee, M. Sugiyama, U. Luxburg, I. Guyon, & R. Garnett (Eds.), *Advances in Neural Information Processing Systems* (Vol. 29). Curran Associates, Inc.

Pack, A., & Maloney, J. (2023). Using Generative Artificial Intelligence for Language Education Research: Insights from Using OpenAI's ChatGPT. *TESOL Quarterly, 57*(4), 1571–1582. https://doi.org/https://doi.org/10.1002/tesq.3253

Parra Bautista, Y. J., Theran, C., & Aló, R. (2024). Ethical Considerations of Generative AI: A Survey Exploring the Role of Decision Makers in the Loop. *Proceedings of the AAAI Symposium Series, 3*(1 SE-Impact of GenAI on Social and Individual Well-being), 391–398. https://doi.org/10.1609/aaaiss.v3i1.31243

Radford, A., Wu, J., Child, R., Luan, D., Amodei, D., Sutskever, I., & others. (2019). Language Models are Unsupervised Multitask Learners. *OpenAI Blog, 1*(8), 9.

Ramesh, A., Pavlov, M., Goh, G., Gray, S., Voss, C., Radford, A., Chen, M., & Sutskever, I. (2021). Zero-shot text-to-image Generation. *International Conference on Machine Learning, PMLR, 139*, 8821–8831.

Ranjan, R., Mishra, A., Maharana, S. P., & Kumari, S. (2024). AI in Visual Arts: Exploring Generative Algorithm. In R. Kumar, S. Sahu, & S. Bhattacharya (Eds.), *The Pioneering Applications of Generative AI* (pp. 41–60). IGI Global.

Reichwein, F. L. (2024). *Ethical and Societal Implications of Generative AI-Models* [Technische Hochschule Ingolstadt]. https://opus4.kobv.de/opus4-haw/files/4694/I001867595Thesis.pdf

Saxena, D., & Cao, J. (2021). Generative Adversarial Networks (GANs): Challenges, Solutions, and Future Directions. *ACM Computing Surveys, 54*(3). https://doi.org/10.1145/3446374

Saxena, D., Cao, J., Xu, J., & Kulshrestha, T. (2023). *Re-GAN: Data-Efficient GANs Training via Architectural Reconfiguration.* Proceedings of the IEEE/CVF Conference on Computer Vision and Pattern Recognition (CVPR), pp. 16230–16240.

Schneider, J. (2024). Explainable Generative AI (GenXAI): A Survey, Conceptualization, and Research Agenda. *Artificial Intelligence Review, 57*(11), 289. https://doi.org/10.1007/s10462-024-10916-x

Sengar, S. S., Hasan, A. Bin, Kumar, S., & Carroll, F. (2024). Generative Artificial Intelligence: A Systematic Review and Applications. *Multimedia Tools and Applications.* https://doi.org/10.1007/s11042-024-20016-1

Sharma, P., Kumar, M., Sharma, H. K., & Biju, S. M. (2024). Generative Adversarial Networks (GANs): Introduction, Taxonomy, Variants, Limitations, and Applications. *Multimedia Tools and Applications.* https://doi.org/10.1007/s11042-024-18767-y

Shen, D., Wu, G., & Suk, H. Il. (2017). Deep Learning in Medical Image Analysis. *Annual Review of Biomedical Engineering, 19*, 221–248. https://doi.org/10.1146/ANNUREV-BIOENG-071516-044442/CITE/REFWORKS

Shu, R., Xu, X., Yung, M.-H., & Cui, W. (2024). *Variational Quantum Circuits Enhanced Generative Adversarial Network.* https://arxiv.org/abs/2402.01791

Singh, S. K. (2023). Ethical Considerations and Challenges in Generative AI Development. *Advances in Computer Sciences*, *6*(1), 1–9.

Takale, D. G., Mahalle, P. N., & Sule, B. (2024). Advancements and Applications of Generative Artificial Intelligence. *Journal of Information Technology and Sciences*, *10*(1), 20–27.

Thorne, S. L. (2024). Generative Artificial Intelligence, Co-evolution, and Language Education. *Modern Language Journal*, *108*(2), 567–572.

Vaswani, A., Shazeer, N., Parmar, N., Uszkoreit, J., Jones, L., Gomez, A. N., Kaiser, L., & Polosukhin, I. (2017). Attention Is All You Need.(Nips), 2017. *ArXiv Preprint ArXiv:1706.03762*.

Vinothkumar, J., & Karunamurthy, A. (2022). Recent Advancements in Artificial Intelligence Technology: Trends and Implications. *Quing: International Journal of Innovative Research*. *2*(1), 1–11.

Viswa, C. A., Bleys, J., Leydon, E., Shah, B., & Zurkiya, D. (2024). *Generative AI in the Pharmaceutical Industry: Moving from Hype to Reality*. McKinsey & Company.

Wang, Y. (2020). *A Mathematical Introduction to Generative Adversarial Nets (GAN)*. https://arxiv.org/abs/2009.00169v1

Welfert, M., Kurri, G. R., Otstot, K., & Sankar, L. (2024). Addressing GAN Training Instabilities via Tunable Classification Losses. *IEEE Journal on Selected Areas in Information Theory*, *5*, 534–553. https://doi.org/10.1109/JSAIT.2024.3415670

Wiatrak, M., Albrecht, S. V., & Nystrom, A. (2019). Stabilizing Generative Adversarial Networks: A Survey. *ArXiv Preprint ArXiv:1910.00927*.

Ye, Y., Hao, J., Hou, Y., Wang, Z., Xiao, S., Luo, Y., & Zeng, W. (2024). Generative AI for Visualization: State of the Art and Future Directions. *Visual Informatics*, *8*(2), 43–66. https://doi.org/https://doi.org/10.1016/j.visinf.2024.04.003

Zhao, J., Mathieu, M., & LeCun, Y. (2017). *Energy-based Generative Adversarial Network*. https://arxiv.org/abs/1609.03126

Zhu, J.-Y., Park, T., Isola, P., & Efros, A. A. (2017). *Unpaired Image-to-image Translation Using Cycle-consistent Adversarial Networks*. Proceedings of the IEEE International Conference on Computer Vision, pp. 2223–2232.

Zlateva, P., Steshina, L., Petukhov, I., & Velev, D. (2024). A Conceptual Framework for Solving Ethical Issues in Generative Artificial Intelligence. In A. J. Tallón-Ballesteros et al. (Eds.), *Electronics, Communications and Networks* (pp. 110–119). IOS Press.

11 Applications of Big Data Analytics in Healthcare

Insights from Medical Tourism

Zeynep Dereli

11.1 INTRODUCTION

The rapid development of medical tourism has been driven by the growing need for reasonably priced and high-quality healthcare services. Medical tourism is becoming a competitive sector in the global healthcare market as patients travel across borders to receive modern medical procedures, specialty treatments, and reduced wait periods. The rise in international patient mobility leads to the generation of substantial amounts of healthcare-related data, including patient demographics, response to treatment, effectiveness of healthcare services, and market trends. Healthcare providers, legislators, and industry stakeholders will have to analyze and manage extremely large datasets to enhance service quality and optimal operational efficiency and to better understand patient demands.

Digital revolution is playing a massive role in influencing the medical tourism industry. Online patient reviews, social media discussions, and electronic word of mouth (e-WOM) are increasingly influencing patients' choice of where to be treated and by which doctor. This can help healthcare organizations increase quality of service, design data-driven marketing campaigns, and tailor care based on patient needs. In this regard, Big Data Analytics enable researchers to better manage large and complex datasets and consequently improve decision-making and medical tourism service delivery. By employing machine learning, sentiment analysis, and predictive modeling, healthcare professionals can optimize clinical decision-making and enhance patient experience.

The purpose of this chapter is to explore the use of Big Data Analytics in medical tourism with a specific focus on the use of Big Data Analytics in the management and analysis of large-scale healthcare data. It also examines how data analytics approaches can be employed to capture patient preferences, enhance service delivery, and aid healthcare decision-makers in the provision of transnational health services. The chapter introduces the concept of medical tourism, listing its main features and importance. It subsequently delves into Big Data Analytics related to

DOI: 10.1201/9781003605416-11

healthcare, specifically its sources as well as the techniques used for their analyses. Then, the applications of Big Data Analytics concerning medical tourism are addressed, emphasizing the role of data-driven approaches in service optimization and improvement in cross-border healthcare decision-making.

11.2 MEDICAL TOURISM: A GLOBAL HEALTHCARE SERVICE EXPORT

Medical tourism has grown into an important part of international healthcare services exports, enabling individuals to travel abroad for affordable and top-quality medical care. This dynamic industry constitutes a unique mixture of economic, cultural, and social benefits to patients and host countries by combining state-of-the-art medical treatment with tourism opportunities. Travel for healthcare and wellness has been a longstanding practice. In the past, medical tourism primarily consisted of elites from developing and Third World countries traveling to developed nations to access advanced and high-quality medical treatments (Abd Mutalib et al., 2017). However, in recent decades, patients from developed nations have increasingly sought care in less developed countries, driven by cost, access, service, and quality, thereby challenging the traditional territoriality of healthcare (Crooks et al., 2010).

Although often confused with medical tourism, health tourism is a broader concept that encompasses various forms of travel aimed at maintaining, improving, or restoring health (Figure 11.1). It includes medical tourism, wellness tourism, and spa tourism, each serving distinct yet interconnected purposes. While medical tourism primarily focuses on curative treatments, such as surgical procedures, organ

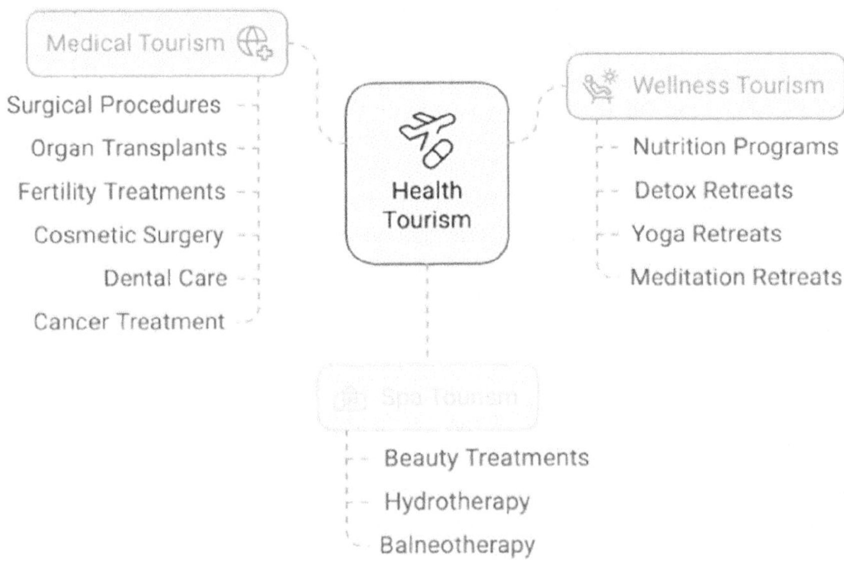

FIGURE 11.1 Health tourism: categories and services.

Source: Adopted from Hall (2012).

transplants, and fertility treatments, wellness tourism promotes preventive health practices, including nutrition programs, detox retreats, and sports activities. Spa tourism, on the other hand, emphasizes relaxation and rejuvenation through beauty treatments and therapeutic recreation (Hall, 2012, p. 12).

In a broader sense, health tourism encompasses all interactions and phenomena that arise when individuals temporarily relocate from their usual place of residence or work to access healthcare services aimed at enhancing, maintaining, or restoring their physical, mental, and social well-being (Hofer et al., 2012; Kaspar, 1996, p. 56). As a subcategory of health tourism, medical tourism specifically refers to individuals traveling to other nations to receive healthcare, often seeking advanced treatments, cost-effective medical procedures, or shorter waiting times (Kundury et al., 2024, p. 2) (Table 11.1).

Medical tourism is a form of service export, as it involves the cross-border provision of healthcare services to international patients who travel for medical treatment. International guidelines for the liberalization of international service trade have been created by the General Agreement on Trade in Services (GATS), which went into effect on January 1, 1995. The goal of this agreement has been to facilitate the international flow of services and lower trade barriers (World Trade Organization, 2022). Global trade in services grew between 2018 and 2019 but declined in 2020 due to the COVID-19 pandemic, which disrupted international travel and service-related sectors. From 2021 onward, service trade gradually recovered, surpassing pre-pandemic levels by 2023 as key industries, including digital trade and medical tourism, resumed activity (Table 11.2).

Medical tourism falls under Mode 2 (Consumption Abroad) of the GATS Modes of Service Supply, as it involves individuals traveling to another country to receive healthcare services. Under this mode, the service provider (hospital, clinic, or healthcare professional) stays in its native nation while the consumer (patient) travels across borders to receive medical treatment. This sets medical tourism apart from other types, such as Mode 3 (Commercial Presence), in which foreign healthcare organizations set up shop overseas, or Mode 4 (Presence of Natural Persons), in which

TABLE 11.1
Definitions of Medical Tourism

Author(s)	Definitions
Connell (2006)	A widely embraced trend in which individuals travel abroad to access healthcare services, including dental and surgical care, while also exploring the tourist attractions of the destination country.
Whittaker (2008)	Medical tourism refers to patients traveling abroad from their country of residence, outside of established cross-border healthcare agreements, primarily to seek medical treatment, often surgical procedures.
Kamassi et al. (2020)	A form of traveling abroad to obtain high-quality treatment at a lower cost, often combined with the opportunity for a pleasant holiday.

TABLE 11.2
Global Trade in Services (Trillion USD)

	2018	2019	2020	2021	2022	2023
Global Service Exports	6.1	6.3	5.2	6.1	7.1	7.8
Global Service Imports	5.8	6.0	4.9	5.6	6.5	7.2

Source: World Trade Organization.

medical personnel relocate abroad to offer services (World Trade Organization, 2022, p. 3).

A number of important locations, such as Costa Rica, India, Israel, Malaysia, Mexico, Singapore, South Korea, Taiwan, Thailand, Turkey, and the United States, are the centers of medical tourism. International patients frequently seek treatments like cosmetic surgery, general and cosmetic dentistry, cardiovascular procedures (CABG, angioplasties, transplants), orthopedic surgeries (joint and spine procedures, sports medicine), cancer treatments, reproductive healthcare (IVF, fertility treatments, women's health), weight loss surgeries (gastric bypass, LAP-BAND), and diagnostic services like scans, health screenings, and second opinions in these countries (Sağ and Zengul, 2019).

Numerous push and pull factors impact medical tourism, influencing people's decisions to seek medical care overseas. Push factors stem from domestic constraints, whereas pull factors are associated with destination-specific benefits that draw medical tourists (John and Larke, 2016). High healthcare costs in countries like the US and Western Europe, coupled with long waiting times in public healthcare systems, limited insurance coverage for specific procedures, and the unavailability of advanced treatments in patients' home countries drive individuals to seek medical care abroad. Additional concerns such as distrust in local healthcare standards, the desire for greater privacy in sensitive treatments, and cultural or religious considerations further push patients toward international medical tourism (John and Larke, 2016; Moghimehfar and Nasr-Esfahani, 2011; Sağ and Zengul, 2019; Henson et al., 2015).

Lower treatment expenses, superior healthcare services, international accreditation of medical institutions, diminished waiting periods, availability of advanced medical technologies and treatments not offered in the home country, skilled and reputable medical practitioners, linguistic proficiency of healthcare providers, and advantageous exchange rates collectively entice medical tourists to particular destinations, enhancing their trust and confidence in pursuing medical care overseas (John and Larke, 2016; Mathijsen, 2019) (Figure 11.2).

Medical tourism is a process consisting of specific stages that enable patients to receive treatment abroad. Initially, patients apply to a medical facilitator who

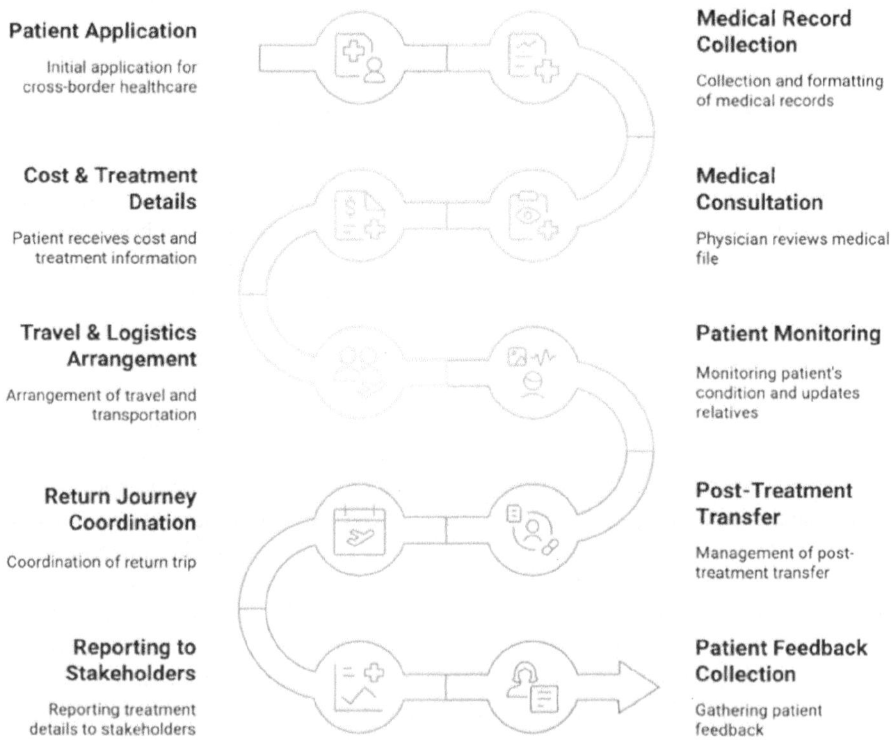

FIGURE 11.2 Medical tourism service stages.

Source: Adapted from SATURK (2020), "Health Tourism Worldwide."

organizes medical records according to the destination's requirements. An affiliated physician reviews the file, provides consultation, and shares details on costs, facilities, and the medical team. After obtaining written consent, a Medical Treatment Travel Form is prepared, along with visa documents if needed. The facilitator coordinates travel and transfers responsibility to a case coordinator in the destination country, who oversees treatment and provides updates to relatives if necessary. Post-treatment, the case coordinator ensures a smooth return journey, while the facilitator reports treatment details to insurers and primary physicians. Finally, patient feedback is collected to assess service quality (Saturk, 2020, p. 6).

11.3 THE ROLE OF BIG DATA IN ENHANCING MEDICAL TOURISM

Large volumes of data are being generated as a result of healthcare systems becoming more digitally integrated, making sophisticated analytical tools necessary to glean valuable insights. Big Data is essential for enhancing healthcare services and has become a key component of medical tourism by enhancing patient experiences and enabling well-informed decision-making. Prior to discussing its particular use cases in medical tourism using real-world examples, this section will first examine the broad uses of Big Data in the healthcare industry.

11.3.1 Big Data Analytics in Healthcare: An Overview

Big Data has emerged as a revolutionary influence in the healthcare sector, significantly impacting medical tourism by facilitating data-driven decision-making, individualized treatment alternatives, and enhanced service efficiency for both providers and patients. Many organizations today are actively collecting, storing, and analyzing extensive datasets, commonly known as "Big Data" due to its *volume*, representing the sheer scale of data generated, its *velocity*, indicating the speed at which it is produced and processed, and its *variety*, reflecting the diverse formats and sources from which it originates (Watson, 2014).

Volume refers to the massive amount of data produced by organizations, with healthcare data already reaching terabytes, petabytes, or exabytes and expected to grow to zettabytes or yottabytes in the future, posing significant challenges in storage and large-scale analysis (Senthilkumar et al., 2018). These datasets are massive not only in terms of size but also in heterogeneity and complexity, encompassing structured, semi-structured, and unstructured data from various sources, including operational, transactional, sales, and marketing records (Vassakis et al., 2018, p. 5). Additionally, velocity plays a crucial role, as Big Data is generated and processed at a substantial speed, requiring advanced real-time analytics and computational capabilities. Thus, the three Vs—volume, variety, and velocity—provide a more comprehensive definition, challenging the misconception that Big Data is only about data volume (Russom, 2011, p. 6) (Figure 11.3).

11.3.1.1 Sources of Big Data in Healthcare

Big Data in healthcare is collected from various sources, encompassing structured, semi-structured, and unstructured data. Structured data in the healthcare sector includes laboratory results, clinical records, sensor-generated data, and information from relational databases, while semi-structured data consists of information stored in formats such as Extensible Markup Language (XML) (Senthilkumar et al., 2018). On the other hand, unstructured data originates from web clickstreams, social media platforms, video recordings from healthcare facilities, call center logs, real-time sensor data, RFID systems, GPS tracking devices, mobile phones, and other monitoring technologies that continuously generate and store healthcare-related information (Batko and Ślęzak, 2022, p. 4). These data have led to a vast influx of information that healthcare organizations must efficiently manage (Manogaran et al., 2018).

Dash et al. (2019) have provided a detailed explanation of the sources of Big Data in healthcare, identifying various systems and technologies that generate, store, and process large volumes of health-related information:

- **Electronic Health Records (EHRs)**: These encompass extensive patient information, comprising medical history, diagnosis, medications, test findings, and demographic details.

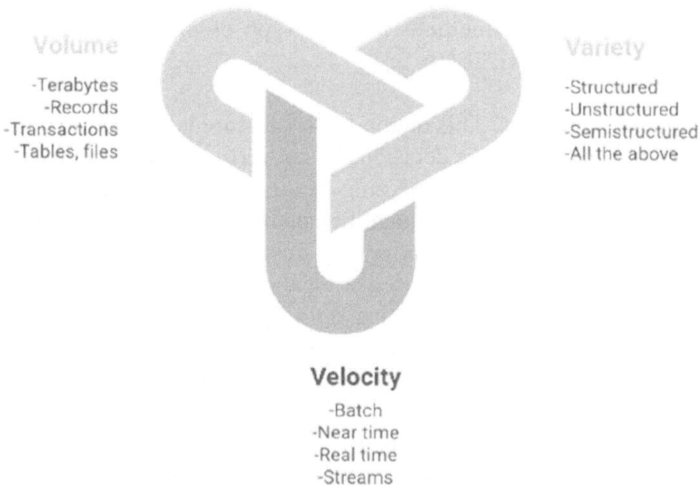

FIGURE 11.3 The three Vs of Big Data.

Source: Adopted from Russom (2011).

- **Medical Imaging Data**: This includes technologies such as MRI, CT scans, X-rays, ultrasound, and PET, which generate vast amounts of data used for disease diagnosis and monitoring.
- **Genomic Sequencing and Biomedical Research**: These generate large volumes of high-resolution biological data, especially through next-generation sequencing (NGS) and genome-wide association studies (GWAS).
- **Internet-Based Health Data (IoT and Mobile Devices)**: Internet-based health data produced by smartphones, smartwatches, fitness trackers, mobile health applications, and wearable sensors for monitoring health metrics generates vast amounts of real-time data.

11.3.1.2 Analysis of Big Data in Healthcare

Considering the vast amount, diversity, and speed of data produced in the healthcare industry, using efficient analytical techniques is crucial to turning these intricate datasets into insightful knowledge. The field of Big Data Analytics is expanding and holds significant potential to enhance healthcare services (Kumar and Singh, 2018). It specifically benefits healthcare by boosting data security, enabling efficient strategic planning, identifying fraud, increasing predictive diagnoses, facilitating thorough patient involvement, and streamlining telemedicine procedures. Additionally, it can predict epidemics, help treat illnesses, improve quality of life, and drastically lower the number of avoidable fatalities (Kankanhalli et al., 2016).

The primary analytical approaches used in Big Data Analytics within the healthcare context can be classified into three main categories: descriptive analytics, predictive analytics, and prescriptive analytics. This taxonomy is based on the characteristics of analytical methods and the type of information obtained from them (Galetsi and Katsaliaki, 2020).

- **Descriptive Analytics**: This method in healthcare is utilized to understand past and current healthcare decisions by converting patient-related data into actionable information for analyzing healthcare decisions, outcomes, and quality (Islam et al., 2018). It identifies patterns of patient care, unnoticed patient trends, and imbalances among cost, capacity, and patient needs, thereby supporting evidence-based clinical practices (Rehman et al., 2022). Additionally, it facilitates reporting on hospitalizations, physician performance, and resource allocation, while supporting visualization, customized reports, drill-down tables, and historical data queries (Batko and Ślęzak, 2022).
- **Predictive Analytics**: This method is utilized to forecast future outcomes by applying various statistical methods, including modeling, machine learning, and data mining, to analyze current and historical data for forecasting future outcomes (Kankanhalli et al., 2016). The concept of machine learning is closely related to data mining, as both analyze data to identify patterns. However, unlike data mining, which extracts data based on human-defined parameters, machine learning utilizes this data to enhance the system's autonomous learning and understanding (Kumar and Singh, 2018). The clinical applications of predictive analytics are extensive and impactful, enabling highly individualized forecasts of patient outcomes. For instance, it can predict whether a patient is at high risk of a heart attack, identify those likely to be readmitted post-surgery, or estimate whether a patient's hospital stay will exceed the average duration (Alharthi, 2018).
- **Prescriptive Analytics**: This method builds upon predictive analytics by not only forecasting outcomes but also guiding decision-making and recommending actionable solutions. In healthcare organizations, it is utilized to evaluate available and feasible alternatives to support informed decision-making (Rehman et al., 2022). As a less mature yet more advanced approach, prescriptive analytics leverages the insights derived from descriptive and predictive analytics to determine and implement the most effective course of action. It focuses on addressing key questions such as "what should we do?" to enhance decision-making processes in clinical settings (Mosavi and Santos, 2020; Delen, 2019). Prescriptive analytics is widely applied in healthcare, particularly in medication prescriptions and treatment selection, supporting both personalized and evidence-based medicine by optimizing medical decision-making (Batko and Ślęzak, 2022).

11.3.2 Applications of Big Data Analytics in Medical Tourism

The analysis of extensive healthcare data has become crucial as the number of patients traveling internationally for medical treatments keeps increasing. Healthcare providers may maintain patient information, forecast treatment results, allocate resources optimally, and improve service efficiency with the use of Big Data Analytics. Furthermore, it helps healthcare businesses better control costs and comprehend consumer preferences. To gain deeper insight into the role of Big Data Analytics in medical tourism, it is important to explore its main applications, such as recommendation systems and sentiment analysis for patient satisfaction.

11.3.2.1 Recommendation Systems in Medical Tourism

Medical tourism recommendation systems employ data-driven methods and machine learning to offer consumers tailored suggestions for hospitals, physicians, treatment alternatives, and destinations based on their medical needs, interests, and past experiences. Studies have looked into the use of these systems in medical tourism, with an emphasis on helping patients make decisions and offering more individualized medical care. For example, Harinivas et al. (2023) reported a knowledge-based medical tourism recommender system that collects hospital data via automated web scraping and subsequently ranks the facilities by google ratings, treatment costs, accreditation status, hospital ranking and score, and review quantity.

Panteli et al. (2021) developed a recommender system for medical tourism based on facility location to achieve optimal diversity in recommendations. The system retrieves matching records from its database of medical, wellness, and tourism providers considering attributes like service category, service cost, infrastructure, and accreditations. Initially, it sorts these cases against those scores for an ideal case with regard to the best ratings, subsequently employing a facility location approach to both relevance and diversity to guarantee the ultimate recommendations.

11.3.2.2 Sentiment Analysis for Patient Satisfaction

Online medical services have gained widespread popularity, and patient feedback plays a crucial role in shaping the medical decisions of other patients. As these platforms continue to expand rapidly, they generate a vast amount of user-generated content. Consequently, the large-scale patient feedback available on these platforms requires in-depth analysis to extract meaningful insights (Zhao et al., 2023). Sentiment analysis or opinion mining is the computational procedure of articulating people's opinions, sentiments, evaluations, attitudes, and emotions for entities, individual, issues, events, topics, and their attributes (Lestari and Anugrahni, 2021). A provider can predict usage behavior by understanding customer sentiment toward its products or services and their intent to transact with the organization, allowing for targeted marketing and advertising strategies (George and Ramos, 2024).

Among others, the electronic word of mouth (e-WOM) is one of the main aspects impacting patients' choices regarding medical tourism. International patients searching for health service options in overseas countries generate a lot of online reviews, ratings, and testimonials that are invaluable knowledge resources for consumers contemplating cross-border healthcare services. This means medical tourism platforms can leverage sentiment analysis, which is a method of measuring patient feedback in a systematic manner to gain clarity as to the level satisfaction, the quality of the treatment, and the overall service experience. By assessing this feedback in detail, healthcare providers can enhance the quality of the service they offer and successfully meet medical tourists' expectations.

Aspect-Based Sentiment Analysis (ABSA) is a kind of sentiment analysis method, which not only recognizes the sentiment but also detects the specific aspects in texts and analyzes the sentiment of individual aspects separately. While traditional sentiment analysis determines document or sentence-level sentiment, ABSA offers further insights by associating opinions with specific aspects of an entity, yielding a more fine-grained and structured view of user opinions (Nazir et al., 2020). Zhao et al. (2023) suggest an Aspect-Level Sentiment Analysis (ALSA) model that classifies patient reviews based on a number of medical service elements, such as hospital amenities, medical ethics, cost, and doctor–patient interactions. By improving the assessment of patient satisfaction, the ALSA model can be used to evaluate medical tourism locations and healthcare professionals.

11.3.2.3 Other Potential Applications of Big Data Analytics in Medical Tourism

In addition to its main applications, Big Data Analytics can be implemented in other areas of medical tourism. One such area is AI-driven chatbots that aid international patients by offering real-time data regarding treatments and healthcare solutions across borders. Powered by Big Data Analytics, such AI-based chatbots generate tailored responses according to patient queries, past correspondences, and health records. Moreover, social media sites produce a wealth of user-generated content that can be analyzed through Big Data methods to detect rising trends within medical tourism sectors. Studying online conversations, patient feedback, and search patterns enables healthcare providers and medical tourism agencies to recognize growing trends in treatments and destinations; adjusting marketing efforts and service offerings accordingly.

AI-Powered Predictive Analytics: Another use of Big Data Analytics can help identify patients more likely to develop complications or adversity after a particular medical procedure. It allows the physicians to take precautions and enhances the safety of patients (Sharma et al., 2023). In addition, patient health records, demographic information, and previous treatment histories can be analyzed to formulate personalized treatment plans. Utilizing Big Data knowledge enables medical practitioners to create treatment plans more specific to the individual patient, which not only results in better health services but adds to the patient's experience.

11.4 CONCLUSIONS

The use of Big Data Analytics in medical tourism has been explored in this chapter, with a focus on how it can be used to improve patient care, manage healthcare data, and aid in decision-making. The conversation looked at how particular analytical techniques, such sentiment analysis and predictive modeling, can evaluate patient input, enhance service quality, and support data-driven tactics in international healthcare.

Due to the growing need for reasonably priced, high-quality medical care, medical tourism has become a vibrant segment of the global healthcare market. Along with wellness and spa tourism, it is frequently included in the more general category of health tourism, which serves different but related objectives. Affordability, shorter wait times, access to cutting-edge medical technologies, and internationally recognized healthcare facilities draw medical tourists to particular locations, while obstacles like exorbitant treatment costs, protracted waiting times, and a lack of medical options in home countries push patients to seek treatment overseas.

In the healthcare industry, Big Data Analytics makes it easier to process large datasets from genomic research, medical imaging, electronic health records, and Internet of Things devices in order to produce insightful information. Healthcare professionals can support evidence-based medical practices, spot patient trends, and improve overall healthcare management by using descriptive, predictive, and prescriptive analytics. In addition to enhancing patient care, these analytical techniques increase operational effectiveness in the medical tourism industry.

Big Data Analytics's incorporation into medical tourism has reinforced data-driven decision-making even further, allowing for better service delivery and more individualized patient experiences. Recommendation systems evaluate hospital ratings, treatment prices, and accreditation status to help patients select healthcare providers. Sentiment analysis uses online patient reviews and electronic word of mouth (e-WOM) to gauge satisfaction and identify new trends in medical travel. Furthermore, using patient health records and demographic information, AI-driven predictive analytics helps medical personnel anticipate problems and personalize treatment regimens.

As technological advancements continue, the role of Big Data Analytics in medical tourism is expected to expand, offering more refined patient profiling, enhanced predictive models, and optimized healthcare services. Future developments in data-driven methodologies may lead to increasingly personalized treatment options, improved patient satisfaction, and greater efficiency in managing cross-border healthcare, reinforcing the strategic importance of Big Data in shaping the future of medical tourism.

REFERENCES

Abd Mutalib, N. S., Soh, Y. C., Wong, T. W., Yee, S. M., Yang, Q., Murugiah, M. K., & Ming, L. C. (2017). Online narratives about medical tourism in Malaysia and Thailand: A qualitative content analysis. *Journal of Travel & Tourism Marketing*, 34(6), 821–832.

Alharthi, H. (2018). Healthcare predictive analytics: An overview with a focus on Saudi Arabia. *Journal of Infection and Public Health*, 11(6), 749–756.

Batko, K., & Ślęzak, A. (2022). The use of big data analytics in healthcare. *Journal of Big Data*, 9(1), 3.

Connell, J. (2006). Medical tourism: Sea, sun, sand and… surgery. *Tourism Management*, 27(6), 1093–1100.

Crooks, V. A., Kingsbury, P., Snyder, J., & Johnston, R. (2010). What is known about the patient's experience of medical tourism? A scoping review. *BMC Health Services Research*, *10*, 1–12.

Dash, S., Shakyawar, S. K., Sharma, M., & Kaushik, S. (2019). Big data in healthcare: Management, analysis and future prospects. *Journal of Big Data*, 6(1), 1–25.

Delen, D. (2019). *Prescriptive analytics: The final frontier for evidence-based management and optimal decision making*. FT Press.

Galetsi, P., & Katsaliaki, K. (2020). A review of the literature on big data analytics in healthcare. *Journal of the Operational Research Society*, 71(10), 1511–1529.

George, O. A., & Ramos, C. M. (2024). Sentiment analysis applied to tourism: Exploring tourist-generated content in the case of a wellness tourism destination. *International Journal of Spa and Wellness*, 7(2), 139–161.

Hall, C. M. (2012). Medical and health tourism: The development and implications of medical mobility. In *Medical tourism* (pp. 3–27). Routledge.

Harinivas, A., Bharathi, R., Gowda, C. A., Mohata, P., & Sharmila, R. (2023, April). Knowledge-based medical tourism recommender system. In *2023 IEEE 8th international conference for convergence in technology (I2CT)* (pp. 1–7). IEEE.

Henson, J. N., Guy, B. S., & Dotson, M. J. (2015). Should I stay or should I go?: Motivators, decision factors, and information sources influencing those predisposed to medical tourism. *International Journal of Healthcare Management*, 8(1), 4–14. https://doi.org/10.1179/2047971914Y.0000000083.

Hofer, S., Honegger, F., & Hubeli, J. (2012). Health tourism: Definition focused on the Swiss market and conceptualisation of health (i) ness. *Journal of Health Organization and Management*, 26(1), 60–80.

Islam, M. S., Hasan, M. M., Wang, X., Germack, H. D., & Noor-E-Alam, M. (2018, May). A systematic review on healthcare analytics: application and theoretical perspective of data mining. In *Healthcare* (Vol. 6, No. 2, p. 54). MDPI.

John, S. P., & Larke, R. (2016). An analysis of push and pull motivators investigated in medical tourism research published from 2000 to 2016. *Tourism Review International, 20*, 73–90. https://doi.org/10.3727/154427216X14713104855810.

Kamassi, A., Abd Manaf, N. H., & Omar, A. (2020). The identity and role of stakeholders in the medical tourism industry: State of the art. *Tourism Review, 75*(3), 559–574.

Kankanhalli, A., Hahn, J., Tan, S., & Gao, G. (2016). Big data and analytics in healthcare: Introduction to the special section. *Information Systems Frontiers, 18*, 233–235.

Kaspar, C. (1996). Gesundheitstourismus im Trend. In Institut für Tourismus und Verkehrswirtschaft (Ed.), *Jahrbuch der Schweizer Tourismuswirtschaft 1995/1996* (pp. 53–61). Eigenverlag.

Kumar, S., & Singh, M. (2018). Big data analytics for healthcare industry: Impact, applications, and tools. *Big Data Mining and Analytics*, *2*(1), 48–57.

Kundury, K. K., Shylaja, K. C., Namitha & Gowdappa, H. B. (2024). Medical tourism: An overview on the cross-border care. *Medical Tourism in Developing Countries: A Contemporary Approach*, 1–27.

Lestari, U., & Anugrahni, D. (2021). Sentiment analysis of performance effectiveness of malioboro pedestrian using sentistrength method on twitter. *Jurnal Tam (Technology Acceptance Model), 12*(1), 75–79. https://doi.org/10.56327/jurnaltam.v12i1.1044

Manogaran, G., Varatharajan, R., Lopez, D., Kumar, P. M., Sundarasekar, R., & Thota, C. (2018). A new architecture of Internet of Things and big data ecosystem for secured smart healthcare monitoring and alerting system. *Future Generation Computer Systems*, *82*, 375–387.

Mathijsen, A. (2019). Home, sweet home? Understanding diasporic medical tourism behaviour. Exploratory research of Polish immigrants in Belgium. *Tourism Management*, *72*, 373–385.

Moghimehfar, F., & Nasr-Esfahani, M. H. (2011). Decisive factors in medical tourism destination choice: A case study of Isfahan, Iran and fertility treatments. *Tourism Management, 32*(6), 1431–1434. https://doi.org/10.1016/j.tourman.2011.01.005.

Mosavi, N. S., & Santos, M. F. (2020). How prescriptive analytics influences decision making in precision medicine. *Procedia Computer Science, 177*, 528–533.

Nazir, A., Rao, Y., Wu, L., & Sun, L. (2020). Issues and challenges of aspect-based sentiment analysis: A comprehensive survey. *IEEE Transactions on Affective Computing, 13*(2), 845–863.

Panteli, A., Kompothrekas, A., Halkiopoulos, C., & Boutsinas, B. (2021, June). An innovative recommender system for health tourism. In *Culture and tourism in a smart, globalized, and sustainable world: 7th international conference of IACuDiT, Hydra, Greece, 2020* (pp. 649–658). Springer International Publishing.

Rehman, A., Naz, S., & Razzak, I. (2022). Leveraging big data analytics in healthcare enhancement: Trends, challenges and opportunities. *Multimedia Systems, 28*(4), 1339–1371.

Russom, P. (2011). Big data analytics. *TDWI Best Practices Report, Fourth Quarter, 19*(4), 1–34.

Sağ, I., & Zengul, F. D. (2019). Why medical tourists choose Turkey as a medical tourism destination? *Journal of Hospitality and Tourism Insights, 2*(3), 296–306. https://doi.org/10.1108/JHTI-05-2018-0031.

SATURK. (2020). *Health tourism worldwide.* Retrieved December 6, 2024, from http://saturk.gov.tr/images/pdf/tyst/03.pdf.

Senthilkumar, S. A., Rai, B. K., Meshram, A. A., Gunasekaran, A., & Chandrakumarmangalam, S. (2018). Big data in healthcare management: A review of literature. *American Journal of Theoretical and Applied Business, 4*(2), 57–69.

Sharma, S., Chauhan, Y., & Tyagi, R. (2023, July). Artificial intelligence based applications in medical tourism. In *2023 14th International Conference on Computing Communication and Networking Technologies (ICCCNT)* (pp. 1–6). IEEE.

Vassakis, K., Petrakis, E., & Kopanakis, I. (2018). Big data analytics: Applications, prospects and challenges. *Mobile Big Data: A Roadmap from Models to Technologies, 10*, 3–20.

Watson, H. J. (2014). Tutorial: Big data analytics: Concepts, technologies, and applications. *Communications of the Association for Information Systems, 34*(1), 65.

Whittaker, A. (2008). Pleasure and pain: Medical travel in Asia. *Global Public Health, 3*(3), 271–290.

World Trade Organization. (2022). *The general agreement on trade in services: An introduction.* Trade in Services and Investment Division. Retrieved from https://www.wto.org/english/tratop_e/serv_e/gsintr_e.pdf.

Zhao, Y., Zhang, L., Zeng, C., Lu, W., Chen, Y., & Fan, T. (2023). Construction of an aspect-level sentiment analysis model for online medical reviews. *Information Processing & Management, 60*(6), 103513.

12 Data Management and Integration

José Antonio Marmolejo Saucedo, Utku Kose, Jafar Ahmad Abed Alzubi, Ilhan Uysal, and Gamze Kose

12.1 INTRODUCTION

Managing data in healthcare remains a major challenge today. The rapid development and adoption of AI systems, paired with an increasing focus on precision medicine and tailored patient management approaches based on individual needs, have transformed data into a core element guiding progress in biomedical research, clinical practice, and diagnostics. The shift from paper-based records to electronic health records (EHRs) creates additional challenges related to data integration and governance (Kruse et al., 2016; Muhunzi et al., 2024; Raghupathi and Raghupathi, 2014).

Interoperability is an essential part of the process of digital transformation, meaning how different healthcare systems interact and intelligibly convey their data. Achieving interoperability is difficult owing to the existence of legacy IT systems, varying levels of data filing and data storage architectures, and the absence of uniform data structures. Some organizations, such as HL7 and FHIR, have created information technology frameworks to organize medical record systems; however, there has been inadequate progress in data formatting, dependency relations, and compliance (Kruse et al., 2016; Kim and Park, 2016). The application of big data analytics intensifies other kinds of regulation, in particular, relating to HIPAA and GDPR because they can impede open data sharing and integration (Song and Ryu, 2015; Hassan et al., 2021).

Moreover, the efficacy of AI applications in healthcare highly depends on the precision and completeness of the data. Using datasets that are incomplete, unrepresentative, or incorrectly curated leads to flawed AI predictions, which can cause critical misdiagnoses and worsen the existing inequalities in the quality of care provided to patients (Yelne et al., 2023; Tsopra et al., 2021). Thus, the application of AI in clinical practice increases the requirement for data management sophistication to safeguard the ethical validity of the conclusions derived from AI systems. This pressure grows with the expansion of big data and predictive analytics, which improve clinical decision-making but increase the risk of breaching patient privacy and data confidentiality (Thopate et al., 2023; Alowais et al., 2023).

Integrated artificial intelligence that carries out explainable artificial intelligence (XAI) is rapidly growing as a significant tool that increases trust and transparency

DOI: 10.1201/9781003605416-12

in AI systems used in healthcare. The so-called black box nature of AI models makes it difficult for healthcare professionals to trust or validate their suggestions. Techniques that fall under the umbrella of XAI, like SHAP and LIME, work on providing insights into how AI makes its decisions to ensure adherence to best clinical practices and accountability for medical applications of AI systems (Uysal, 2023). In addition, XAI augments the ability to uncover gaps within datasets situated on different databases that improve comprehensive data validation, compliance with regulations, and data inconsistency, promoting effective data integration (Allen, 2024).

It is increasingly evident as AI propels international collaborations into medical research that there is a need to adopt the principles of XAI. While the use of AI technologies across diverse healthcare systems makes huge strides to enhance service delivery, it raises ethical, legal, and clinical questions vis-a-vis the protection of sensitive patient information. These challenges are central in maintaining the integrity of patient data as well as optimizing healthcare outcomes (Palaniappan et al., 2024). The big data analytics, AI, and XAI convergence is no doubt a revolution to modern healthcare as it guarantees enhanced quality of care through better decision-making while solving the multifaceted issues of data privacy, security, and interoperability.

This chapter will analyze considerations surrounding the management and integration of data in healthcare systems with an emphasis on the following issues, and the section framework is given in Figure 12.1:

- The method of merging various types of data, ranging from structured (EHRs and lab results) to unstructured datasets (clinical notes and imaging data).
- The issues surrounding healthcare data management, including the management of data privacy, system interoperability, security risks, and adherence to compliance frameworks.

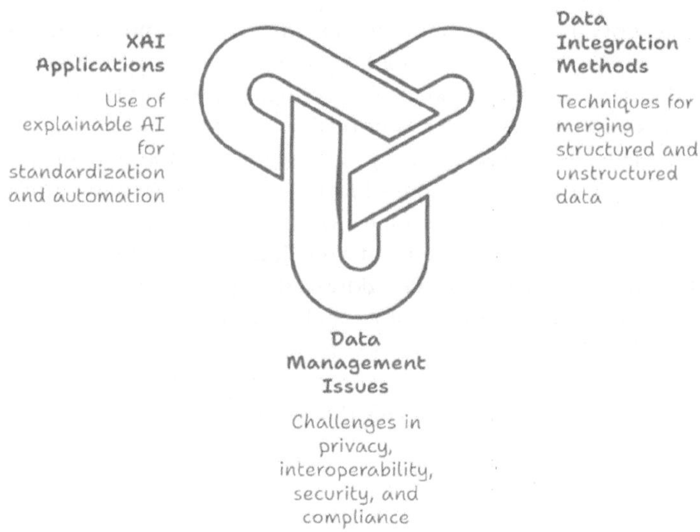

FIGURE 12.1 Healthcare data management overview.

- The use of XAI in supporting the standardization, governance, and automation of workflows within AI systems in healthcare decision-making processes.

12.2 DATA INTEGRATION TECHNIQUES FROM VARIOUS SOURCES IN HEALTHCARE

The rapid digitization of the healthcare sector is associated with the creation of enormous datasets from different origins, including EHR, medical imaging equipment, and even wearable gadgets. This variation highlights the need for data integration that accomplishes all-encompassing patient care, precision approaches, and AI-enhanced decision support systems. However, the complexities associated with healthcare data (mainly its distributed nature and absence of uniformity) are deeply problematic with regard to interoperability, security, and privacy (Denhere et al., 2024; Sony et al., 2024).

Data integration in healthcare entails synthesizing both structured and unstructured medical data to aid in clinical decision-making and artificial intelligence use. Integration processes can be classified into three categories: syntactic, semantic, and technical integration. Syntactic integration concerns itself with the uniformity of data structures across various systems. For example, standards like HL7 and FHIR (Fast Healthcare Interoperability Resources) have been designed to promote data exchange and interoperability between healthcare applications (Ndlovu et al., 2021; Lekkala, 2023). Information interchange semantics is a step deeper in integration; it considers how data is encoded and exchanged while preserving its meaning across different settings. This is difficult because different healthcare institutions tend to use different formats and terminologies (Sony et al., 2024; Denhere et al., 2023).

In the context of data sharing, the technical integration approach focuses on constructing necessary systems and protocols, even though it often requires complex technological infrastructure and extensive development work (Durneva et al., 2020). Moreover, the significance of XAI is critical with respect to enabling integration system transparency as well as ensuring the accuracy of the integrated data. XAI facilitates grasping the inner workings of artificial intelligence algorithms and their rationale, which is necessary for clinicians who must have faith and validate the reliability of the systems' outputs (Kwon and Yoo, 2021; Pine, 2019).

Data integration issues need to be addressed in parallel with advancements in healthcare systems if the advantages of AI and effective care delivery are to be realized. Bridging the gaps in interoperability not only advances quality in patient care but also strengthens adherence to the very important legislative frameworks on privacy and data protection, which are critical to modern healthcare systems (Denhere et al., 2024; Tsinale et al., 2023a; Naveed, 2020). Visualization of data integration techniques in healthcare is given in Figure 12.2.

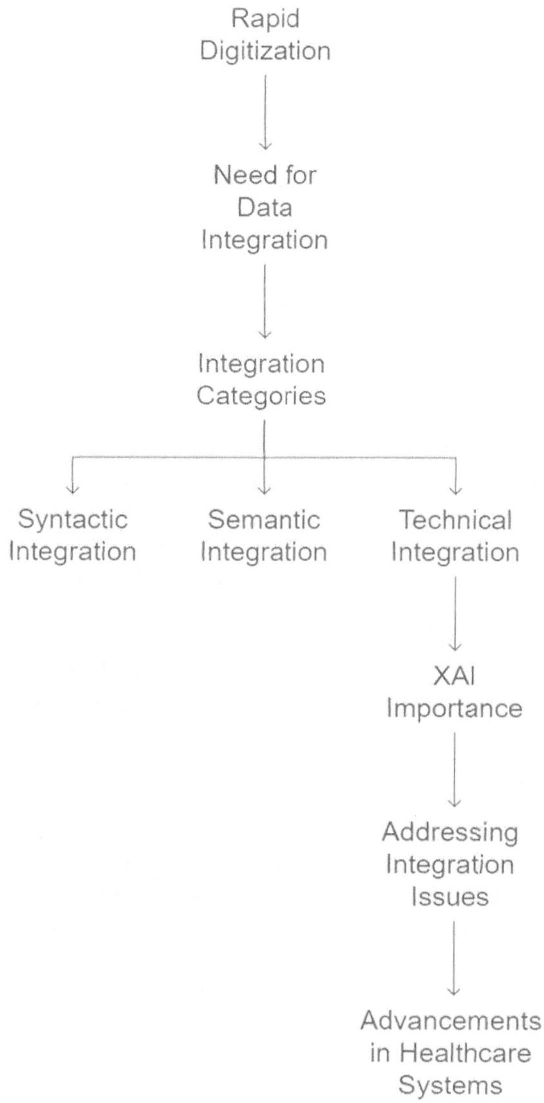

FIGURE 12.2 Data integration techniques in healthcare.

12.2.1 Syntactic Data Integration: Standardizing Data Formats and Structures

In the healthcare sector, the integration of disparate systems requires a high degree of syntactic data integration; this becomes even more complex given the JSON- and XML-type data producers as well as HL7 and FHIR interfaces. The absence of a universal architecture for healthcare data results in an intricate web of healthcare information systems, presenting problems for integration and information sharing. To mitigate these issues, several standards have been created, including HL7 and FHIR.

- *HL7* (Health Level Seven) is one of the most used implemented standards in healthcare, providing a model for the integration of EHRs, Laboratory Data, and Billing information, so that these repositories may work with each other, which serves as the basis for integrating and exchanging data (Rho et al 2015, Reps et al, 2018).
- *FHIR* (Fast Healthcare Interoperability Resources) builds on this further by providing the easier use of RESTful APIs for conveying both clinical and administrative data to older systems powered by the cloud and even non-cloud-based systems (Reinecke, Zoch, Reich et al., 2021; Shin et al 2019). This helps augment the interoperability levels in the growing and digitalized healthcare system region (Garza et al 2016), marking the growing importance of digital platforms in healthcare systems.
- *DICOM* (Digital Imaging and Communications in Medicine) proves to be important in the integration of imaging data like CT scans and MRIs across healthcare departments for a more efficient workflow and diagnostics automation (Park et al., 2022).
- Similarly, *LOINC* (Logical Observation Identifiers Names and Codes) ensures uniformity in coding laboratory tests and clinical observations by providing a standardized representation of the results, which is critical for AI-supported clinical decision-making systems (Khalid et al., 2021; Abhyankar et al., 2012).
- With regard to observatory health data, the *OMOP* (Observational Medical Outcomes Partnership) Common Data Model enhances data integration for large-scale clinical studies and AI analytics through its standardized structure (Burkard et al., 2024; Ji et al., 2024). This model enables the integration of disparate data while ensuring the privacy of patient information. A unified approach to data analysis improves the capability of healthcare organizations to conduct consistent multicontext research, thus improving interoperability between institutions (Belenkaya et al., 2021; Reinecke, Zoch, Wilhelm et al., 2021).

In conclusion, the integration of these standards regarding data syntax improves data sharing among disparate healthcare systems and enables meaningful examinations and applications of healthcare data, which are vital for advancing the quality of patient care and sophisticated research efforts (Jin et al., 2020; Finster et al., 2025).

12.2.2 Semantic Data Integration: Harmonizing Meaning Across Datasets

While syntactic integration standardizes data formats, semantic integration ensures that data from different sources carry the same meaning, enabling accurate AI-driven predictions and clinical interpretations. Semantic heterogeneity arises due to variability in terminologies, coding systems, and domain-specific knowledge representations. Some of the key approaches for achieving semantic data interoperability include the following:

Ontology-Based Data Integration: Medical ontologies such as SNOMED-CT, ICD-10, and RxNorm offer semi-structured ontological frameworks to facilitate the mapping of medical concepts and diagnoses to various datasets. These ontological frameworks also assist in resolving gaps in the multidimensional vocabularies prevalent in medical data and maintain understanding across different frameworks (Ghosh et al., 2024; Mello et al., 2022). AI-powered NLP models with more stable area under the curve (AUC) values align stratified clinical text data with standard ontologies. This alignment, even without cross-referencing, improves harmonization and aids integration processes. Such frameworks have successfully automated the conversion of elaborate clinical narratives into coded, structured formats, enhancing the applicability of simplified analysis and interpretation (Pacaci et al., 2018; Miranda et al., 2024).

Knowledge Graphs and Linked Data Approaches: With the integration of AI technologies, knowledge graphs allow for the interrelation of clinical concepts such as symptoms, treatments, and drug interactions. Hence, it offers a strong basis for data interlinking across countless systems. This approach allows for the better integration of EHRs, biomedical research, and even the pharmaceutical industry databases (Zhang et al., 2019). Also, applying Linked Data and RDF (Resource Description Framework) principles enhances the healthcare data domain by enriching it to become more interpretable and readable for AI and automated machine processes (Jozashoori et al., 2018). Knowledge graphs, by organizing facts about relationships and properties into a semantic network, improve the contextual understanding of medical data and the quality of insights yielded by AI systems (Nath et al., 2020).

Interoperability Frameworks for Multisource Data Alignment: The models by OHDSI (Observational Health Data Sciences and Informatics) and CDISC (Clinical Data Interchange Standards Consortium) contribute toward capturing and maintaining uniform semantic models for disparate data streams from multiple research institutions. These frameworks promote cooperation and collective analytics and data sharing during clinical and observational studies with clinical trials (Ali and Chong, 2019; Yadav, 2023). By these standards, a higher level of semantic interoperability may be achieved by healthcare institutions, which positively influences patient care and research (Alamri, 2018).

In closing, the accomplishment of semantic interoperability in healthcare is critical for enhancing the integration of data and the functioning of AI insights and applications powered by AI. Healthcare systems can solve the semantic issues through the application of ontological frameworks, knowledge graphs, adherence to interoperability policies, and improvement of the reliability of clinical interpretation and prediction. This leads to better data sharing, as well as safer and more efficient care processes for the patients (Tsinale et al., 2023b; Peng and Goswami, 2019; Zhang et al., 2018).

12.2.3 Technical Data Integration: ETL Pipelines, Data Lakes, and Federated Learning

The technical integration approaches in healthcare are particularly important in the aggregation, storage, and processing of heterogeneous datasets since they safeguard security and compliance with applicable laws and standards. One of the common methods employed is the use of ETL pipelines for data integration, which is the crux of most healthcare data system processing.

ETL (Extract, Transform, Load) Pipelines: The standard workflow of ETL details the extraction of raw data from a plethora of sources like EHRs, reporting systems, and imaging systems, while the actual inclusion of clinical data includes the addition of laboratory reports, radiology, and other document repositories. After this data is truly formatted, it is then organized into systems like FHIR and HL7, which aid in offloading processed data into central databases or AI-powered decision support systems (Budrionis et al., 2021). Enhanced ETL processes powered by AI have demonstrated improvement on data accuracy and quality through the use of automated validation, abnormality detection, missing value correction, and explainable transformation XAI techniques (Sim et al., 2019; Gachabayov et al., 2016). These automation techniques guarantee essential integrity and reliability of the data, which is a prerequisite for efficacious clinical decision-making.

Cloud-Based Healthcare Data Lakes: Major healthcare companies and many AI development centers have incorporated cloud-based data lakes like AWS HealthLake, Google Cloud Healthcare API, and Microsoft Azure for Health that hold enormous volumes of both structured and unstructured healthcare data. These platforms support numerous datasets' collaboration that enables real-time analysis and AI modeling training tasks for predictive analytics. Prediction-based data lakes are equipped with AI-powered data harmonization engines that provide advanced integration and analysis that enhances AI deployment in healthcare (Çabuk et al., 2018; Demir, 2017; F. et al., 2020).

Federated Learning for Decentralized AI Training: As a newer approach, federated learning attempts to mitigate privacy concerns by training AI models at different institutions without having to collect sensitive patient data into a single repository. Such an approach not only minimizes legal compliance concerns but also allows models to be trained across different populations and datasets to enhance their generalizability (Křepelka et al., 2017; Johnson et al., 2015). XAI can provide additional benefit to federated learning by clarifying the manner in which data from various regions affect different AI predictions, thereby improving trust from healthcare practitioners and regulatory authorities (Blom, 2016; Hirai et al., 2019). Hybrid analytics work as such enables patient privacy through federated learning while allowing substantive model development for healthcare analytics, making it an integral approach in the contemporary healthcare environment (Kitajima et al., 2023; Marya et al., 2024).

12.2.4 The Role of XAI in Enhancing Data Integration Transparency and Trust

The application of XAI improves the transparency, equity, and auditability of data harmonization, transformation, and analytics powered by AI in healthcare data management systems. There are several significant contributions of XAI to data integration that try to resolve existing challenges related to data accuracy, biases, and the trust in AI applications in healthcare.

Explainable Data Quality Assessment: The majority of AI systems use automated techniques for data cleaning and anomaly detection. This leads to hiding underlying structures that are not interpretable (Linardatos et al., 2020). XAI certainly lifts some aspect of the "black box" problem with some methods like LIME and SHAP, explaining which data sources are responsible for inconsistencies within the datasets and detailing the alterations provided. This ultimately provides better data quality assessments, which leads to enhanced clinical decision-making (Tsopra et al., 2021).

Bias Detection in Integrated Datasets: The absence of equity frameworks in healthcare datasets can exacerbate biases across demographic, clinical, and socioeconomic lines, which can be very damaging to the performance of AI models (Lee and Park, 2022). Real-time bias detection is possible through XAI-enabled frameworks, which ensures that the development of AI models happens in a just and equitable manner. This fairness is accomplished because XAI allows analysis of dataset use to attend to biases, foster critical examination of model outputs, and promote fairness in healthcare (Vaira et al., 2024).

Interpretable Data Harmonization Algorithms: XAI enhances data harmonization that provides a record of data changes across several origins while enabling healthcare organizations to preserve system-wide records of data (Linardatos et al., 2020). XAI allows stakeholders to trace data ownership that permits smooth governance as well as compliance with established policies throughout the life cycle of the data. This is paramount for the General Data Protection Regulation and the Health Insurance Portability and Accountability Act that require powers of robust purview over stored sensitive private information and data (Makubhai et al., 2023).

12.3 CHALLENGES AND SOLUTIONS IN HEALTH DATA MANAGEMENT

The management of healthcare data poses a variety of problems, including fragmentation, interoperability, security, and compliance with legal obligations. Despite these hurdles, enhanced healthcare data management is key to the functionality and effectiveness of contemporary healthcare systems. The storage of medical data in disparate systems that do not communicate with each other leads to healthcare data fragmentation. This fragmentation is problematic for the exchange of real-time data essential for effective clinical workflows and the full functionality of AI-based analytics power (Adeghe et al., 2024).

The fragmentation of healthcare data remains a main hurdle, as entire EHRs, alongside laboratory and imaging databases, are often siloed and utilize proprietary data formats. This lack of standardization makes comprehensive data aggregation and analysis nearly impossible. In an attempt to improve interoperability and standardize data within healthcare, standards like HL7 FHIR have been proposed; however, significant gaps remain (Bennacer et al., 2023). Fortunately, blockchain has emerged as an alternative to traditional security frameworks. It not only increases a system's security and interoperability but also provides reliable audit trails that ease data sharing among healthcare institutions (Ojo and Kiobel, 2024; Quazi et al., 2024).

Data security and privacy are critical factors of concern with the increased use of cloud-based IT solutions in healthcare and AI-centric models. Legal frameworks such as GDPR and HIPAA have strict regulations with respect to data sharing, anonymization, and encryption, making compliance cumbersome due to ever-changing laws and different regions' peculiarities (Ranjan et al., 2023). Moreover, cyber risks like ransomware and data breaches pose serious threats to the confidentiality of patients and trust in the institutions (Agbo et al., 2019). With regard to these issues, blockchain is increasingly seen as a suitable technology in healthcare due to its capability to provide safe and decentralized data management (Ali et al., 2023).

Another crucial challenge is associated with the quality and completeness of health data such as missing values, duplicate records, and inconsistent use of medical terminology. These discrepancies can bias AI-enabled clinical decision support systems, resulting in inaccuracy and worsening the existing health inequities (Rao and Manvi, 2023). The unrepresentativeness of the training data given to AI models intensifies these disparities, increasing the need for strong data validation systems and fairness frameworks. In the realm of healthcare analytics, improved data quality and reduced biases can be achieved through AI-powered automated data cleansing and anomaly detection algorithms (Rajput et al., 2021).

To address these multifaceted issues, innovative approaches such as blockchain, federated learning, and AI-based data management systems are being adopted. These technologies present new options for security enhancement, privacy preservation, and cross-system cooperation improvement or interoperability (Gandhi et al., 2024). With such technological advances, healthcare organizations can strive toward developing a comprehensive, effective health data management system that optimally serves the patients (Bodemer, 2023). A diagram showing innovative solutions for effective health data management systems is given in Figure 12.3.

12.4 CONTRIBUTIONS OF XAI SYSTEMS TO HEALTHCARE DATA MANAGEMENT STRATEGIES

XAI is working toward the improvement of the management of data in the healthcare sector. This improvement is carried out through AI systems that enhance trust and its usage in the healthcare sector via better explainability and strengthened trust frameworks. Unlike many AI models termed "black boxes," predictive AI is one

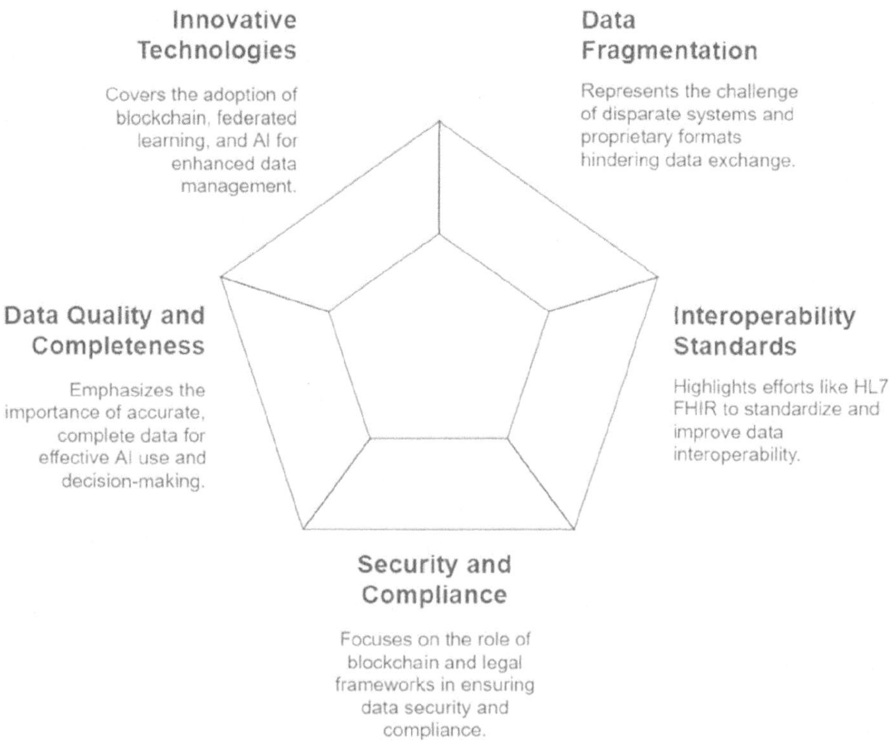

FIGURE 12.3 Innovative solutions for effective health data management systems.

of the few exceptions to this rule. Predictive analytics AI provides an output, but a clear and rational explanation does not accompany the output. Therefore, the within model predictors do not allow a clinician or administrator to appreciate the insight offered or perform data cleansing and ensure integrity without bias ascertainment. Regarding the above problems, XAI provides solutions with interpretable models that can explain algorithmic steps in the computation of health data, tell patient-relative important factors, and argue rational understanding (Mienye et al., 2024; Labkoff et al., 2024).

XAI's contribution to validation and quality assessment has proven to be the most significant. With SHAP and LIME, XAI equips healthcare practitioners with sophisticated methods to document errors, discrepancies, or absent values in integrated datasets (SHAP and LIME, respectively). These refined datasets ensure that AI models function with appropriate and non-biased inputs, which is critical in multinational healthcare partnerships where diverse datasets undergo merging and regulatory compliance (Lauritsen et al., 2020).

Moreover, XAI is crucial in bias and fairness analysis for AI-enabled healthcare systems. XAI's explainable approaches help identify and mitigate inequities stemming from demographic, socioeconomic, or genetic factors that may inform model discrimination during patient stratification, risk of malignancy prediction, or treatment recommendations. Such steps are important toward the responsible use of AI to counteract biases that weaken equity in population health (Ferrara, 2023; Kerasidou, 2021). In the context of underdiagnosis bias, XAI may also demonstrate how inequitable assumptions regarding lower-than-expected AI performance across varying populations can drive inequity in care delivery (Seyyed-Kalantari et al., 2021).

XAI-assisted approaches to data integration ensure that disparate data systems can interact meaningfully, thus providing a seamless fusion of both quantitative (EHRs and Lab Results) and qualitative (clinical notes, imaging, as well as video reports) data, which are unstructured. Given the rapid rise in data protection laws, integrating XAI into AI-powered data integration systems enables healthcare institutions to enhance the use of cross-border data within the limits of privacy laws while fostering the development of explainable AI systems for timely clinical interventions (Mienye et al., 2024); Arrieta et al., 2020).

With the advancement of XAI-driven healthcare systems, the application of explainable AI-based data management techniques will be critical for developing trust, transparency, and efficacy in medical AI solutions. Such developments enhance data governance and security compliance but also create gaps for AI systems that contradict medical norms and ethics (Ali et al., 2024; Kerasidou, 2021). These milestones remain prerequisites for optimizing AI technologies aimed at improving patient care and achieving fairness in healthcare systems (Ejjami, 2024; Zhang et al., 2023).

REFERENCES

Abhyankar, S., Demner-Fushman, D., and McDonald, C. (2012). Standardizing clinical laboratory data for secondary use. *Journal of Biomedical Informatics*, 45(4), 642–650. https://doi.org/10.1016/j.jbi.2012.04.012

Adeghe, E., Okolo, C., and Ojeyinka, O. (2024). Evaluating the impact of blockchain technology in healthcare data management: a review of security, privacy, and patient outcomes. *Open Access Research Journal of Science and Technology*, 10(2), 013–020. https://doi.org/10.53022/oarjst.2024.10.2.0044

Agbo, C., Mahmoud, Q., and Eklund, J. (2019). Blockchain technology in healthcare: a systematic review. *Healthcare*, 7(2), 56. https://doi.org/10.3390/healthcare7020056

Alamri, A. (2018). Ontology middleware for integration of IoT healthcare information systems in EHR systems. *Computers*, 7(4), 51. https://doi.org/10.3390/computers7040051

Ali, A., Ali, H., Saeed, A., Ahmed, A., Tin, T., Assam, M., and Mohamed, H. (2023). Blockchain-powered healthcare systems: enhancing scalability and security with hybrid deep learning. *Sensors*, 23(18), 7740. https://doi.org/10.3390/s23187740

Ali, K., Garcia, A., and Vadsariya, A. (2024). Impact of the AI dependency revolution on both physical and mental health. *Journal of Strategic Innovation and Sustainability*, 19(2). https://doi.org/10.33423/jsis.v19i2.7006

Ali, S. and Chong, I. (2019). Semantic mediation model to promote improved data sharing using representation learning in heterogeneous healthcare service environments. *Applied Sciences*, 9(19), 4175. https://doi.org/10.3390/app9194175

Allen, B. (2024). The promise of explainable AI in digital health for precision medicine: a systematic review. *Journal of Personalized Medicine*, 14(3), 277. https://doi.org/10.3390/jpm14030277

Alowais, S., Alghamdi, S., Alsuhebany, N., Alqahtani, T., Alshaya, A., Almohareb, S., ... Albekairy, A. (2023). Revolutionizing healthcare: the role of artificial intelligence in clinical practice. *BMC Medical Education*, 23(1), 689. https://doi.org/10.1186/s12909-023-04698-z

Arrieta, A., Díaz-Rodríguez, N., Ser, J., Bennetot, A., Tabik, S., Barbado, A., and Herrera, F. (2020). Explainable Artificial Intelligence (XAI): concepts, taxonomies, opportunities and challenges toward responsible ai. *Information Fusion*, 58, 82–115. https://doi.org/10.1016/j.inffus.2019.12.012

Belenkaya, R., Gurley, M., Golozar, A., Dymshyts, D., Miller, R., Williams, A., and Reich, C. (2021). Extending the omop common data model and standardized vocabularies to support observational cancer research. *JCO Clinical Cancer Informatics*, 5, 12–20. https://doi.org/10.1200/cci.20.00079

Bennacer, S., Sabiri, K., Aaroud, A., Akodadi, K., and Cherradi, B. (2023). A comprehensive survey on blockchain-based healthcare industry: applications and challenges. *Indonesian Journal of Electrical Engineering and Computer Science*, 30(3), 1558. https://doi.org/10.11591/ijeecs.v30.i3.pp1558-1571

Blom, J. (2016). Alice in wonderland syndrome. *Neurology Clinical Practice*, 6(3), 259–270. https://doi.org/10.1212/cpj.0000000000000251

Bodemer, O. (2023, October 12). When javabeans meet blockchain: brewing a robust healthcare data management system. *TechRxiv*. https://doi.org/10.36227/techrxiv.24258688.v1

Budrionis, A., Miara, M., Miara, P., Wilk, S., and Bellika, J. (2021). Benchmarking PySyft federated learning framework on mimic-iii dataset. *IEEE Access*, 9, 116869–116878. https://doi.org/10.1109/access.2021.3105929

Burkard, T., López-Güell, K., Gorbachev, A., Bellas, L., Jödicke, A., Burn, E., and Català, M. (2024). Calculating daily dose in the observational medical outcomes partnership common data model. *Pharmacoepidemiology and Drug Safety*, 33(6). https://doi.org/10.1002/pds.5809

Çabuk, F., Aktepe, F., Kusku, E., Çoban, İ., and Doğusoy, G. (2018). Histological features in abdominal wall endometriosis. *Medicine Science | International Medical Journal*, 398. https://doi.org/10.5455/medscience.2018.07.8788

Demir, Y. (2017). A rare cause of shoulder pain: axillary web syndrome. *Turkish Journal of Physical Medicine and Rehabilitation*, 63(2), 178–180. https://doi.org/10.5606/tftrd.2017.21855

Denhere, P., Matanana, N., Zhou, M., Manjeese, C., and Mawere, T. (2024). Evaluating and addressing interoperability constraints in health information systems for enhanced healthcare delivery in Zimbabwe. *Journal of Computer and Communications*, 12(07), 133–154. https://doi.org/10.4236/jcc.2024.127010

Denhere, P., Ruhode, E., and Zhou, M. (2023). A togaf based interoperable health information system needs assessment for practitioner–patient interaction. *The Electronic Journal of Information Systems in Developing Countries*, 89(6). https://doi.org/10.1002/isd2.12284

Durneva, P., Cousins, K., and Chen, M. (2020). The current state of research, challenges, and future research directions of blockchain technology in patient care: systematic review. *Journal of Medical Internet Research*, 22(7), e18619. https://doi.org/10.2196/18619

Ejjami, R. (2024). The ethical artificial intelligence framework theory (EAIFT): a new paradigm for embedding ethical reasoning in AI systems. *International Journal for Multidisciplinary Research (IJFMR)*, 6(5).

Ferrara, E. (2023). *Fairness and bias in artificial intelligence: a brief survey of sources, impacts, and mitigation strategies* (preprint). https://doi.org/10.2196/preprints.48399

Finster, M., Moinat, M., and Taghizadeh, E. (2025). Etl: from the german health data lab data formats to the omop common data model. *PLoS One*, 20(1), e0311511. https://doi.org/10.1371/journal.pone.0311511

Gachabayov, M., Horta, R., Afanasyev, D., and Gilyazov, T. (2016). Abdominal wall endometrioma: our experience in Vladimir, Russia. *Nigerian Medical Journal*, 57(6), 329. https://doi.org/10.4103/0300–1652.193858

Gandhi, J., Maurya, K., Panwar, V., Patel, U., Bhattacharjee, S., and Patel, M. (2024). Leveraging blockchain and IPFS for secure and privacy-preserving patient medical record management: a government-controlled approach. *International Journal for Research in Applied Science and Engineering Technology*, 12(3), 2138–2144. https://doi.org/10.22214/ijraset.2024.59289

Garza, M., Fiol, G., Tenenbaum, J., Walden, A., and Zozus, M. (2016). Evaluating common data models for use with a longitudinal community registry. *Journal of Biomedical Informatics*, 64, 333–341. https://doi.org/10.1016/j.jbi.2016.10.016

Ghosh, M., Kalokyri, V., Sambres, M., Vaterkowski, M., Duclos, C., Tannier, X., and Dhombres, F. (2024). *From syntactic to semantic interoperability using a hyperontology in the oncology domain*. https://doi.org/10.3233/shti240670

Hassan, S., Dhali, M., Zaman, F., and Tanveer, M. (2021). Big data and predictive analytics in healthcare in Bangladesh: regulatory challenges. *Heliyon*, 7(6), e07179. https://doi.org/10.1016/j.heliyon.2021.e07179

Hirai, T., Taniyama, T., Yoshii, T., Mizuno, K., Okamoto, M., Inose, H., and Okawa, A. (2019). Clinical outcomes of surgical treatment for arachnoid web: a case series. *Spine Surgery and Related Research*, 3(1), 43–48. https://doi.org/10.22603/ssrr.2018-0027

Ji, H., Kim, S., Sunwoo, L., Jang, S., Lee, H., and Yoo, S. (2024). Integrating clinical data and medical imaging in lung cancer: feasibility study using the observational medical outcomes partnership common data model extension. *JMIR Medical Informatics*, 12, e59187. https://doi.org/10.2196/59187

Jin, S., Kostka, K., Posada, J., Kim, Y., Seo, S., Lee, D., and You, S. (2020). Prediction of major depressive disorder following beta-blocker therapy in patients with cardiovascular diseases. *Journal of Personalized Medicine*, 10(4), 288. https://doi.org/10.3390/jpm10040288

Johnson, J., Collins, T., Degeling, C., Fawcett, A., Fisher, A., Freire, R., and McGreevy, P. (2015). The first shared online curriculum resources for veterinary undergraduate learning and teaching in animal welfare and ethics in australia and new zealand. *Animals*, 5(2), 395–406. https://doi.org/10.3390/ani5020362

Jozashoori, S., Novikova, T., and Vidal, M. (2018). *Data integration for supporting biomedical knowledge graph creation at large-scale*. https://doi.org/10.48550/arxiv.1811.01660

Kerasidou, A. (2021). Ethics of artificial intelligence in global health: explainability, algorithmic bias and trust. *Journal of Oral Biology and Craniofacial Research*, 11(4), 612–614. https://doi.org/10.1016/j.jobcr.2021.09.004

Khalid, S., Yang, C., Blacketer, C., Duarte-Salles, T., Fernández-Bertolín, S., Kim, C., and Reps, J. (2021). A standardized analytics pipeline for reliable and rapid development and validation of prediction models using observational health data. *Computer Methods and Programs in Biomedicine*, 211, 106394. https://doi.org/10.1016/j.cmpb.2021.106394

Kim, M. and Park, J. (2016). Identifying and prioritizing critical factors for promoting the implementation and usage of big data in healthcare. *Information Development*, 33(3), 257–269. https://doi.org/10.1177/0266666916652671

Kitajima, H., Ichiseki, T., Kaneuji, A., and Kawahara, N. (2023). A case of axillary web syndrome caused by venous blood sampling. *Healthcare*, 11(17), 2390. https://doi.org/10.3390/healthcare11172390

Křepelka, P., Velebil, P., Feyereisl, J., and Krofta, L. (2017). A retrospective study of 17 patients who had excision of abdominal wall endometriosis after caesarean section over an 11-year period. *Journal of Endometriosis and Pelvic Pain Disorders*, 9(4), 293–296. https://doi.org/10.5301/jeppd.5000300

Kruse, C., Goswamy, R., Raval, Y., and Marawi, S. (2016). Challenges and opportunities of big data in health care: a systematic review. *JMIR Medical Informatics*, 4(4), e38. https://doi.org/10.2196/medinform.5359

Kwon, O. and Yoo, S. (2021). Interoperability reference models for applications of artificial intelligence in medical imaging. *Applied Sciences*, 11(6), 2704. https://doi.org/10.3390/app11062704

Labkoff, S., Oladimeji, B., Kannry, J., Solomonides, A., Leftwich, R., Koski, E., and Quintana, Y. (2024). Toward a responsible future: recommendations for AI-enabled clinical decision support. *Journal of the American Medical Informatics Association*, 31(11), 2730–2739. https://doi.org/10.1093/jamia/ocae209

Laura, F. R., Laier, F., Fonseca, V., Juliana, L., and Luz, C. (2020). Chronic axillary web syndrome: 83 months post lumpectomy-a case report. *Journal of Novel Physiotherapy and Physical Rehabilitation*, 7(1), 13–14. https://doi.org/10.17352/2455-5487.000069

Lauritsen, S., Kristensen, M., Olsen, M., Larsen, M., Lauritsen, K., Jørgensen, M., and Thiesson, B. (2020). Explainable artificial intelligence model to predict acute critical illness from electronic health records. *Nature Communications*, 11(1). https://doi.org/10.1038/s41467-020-17431-x

Lee, M. and Park, J. (2022). Do parasocial relationships and the quality of communication with AI shopping chatbots determine middle-aged women consumers' continuance usage intentions?. *Journal of Consumer Behaviour*, 21(4), 842–854. https://doi.org/10.1002/cb.2043

Lekkala, L. (2023). How AI analytical models can use fhir (fast healthcare interoperability resources) data. *Voice of the Publisher*, 09(04), 197–206. https://doi.org/10.4236/vp.2023.94016

Linardatos, P., Papastefanopoulos, V., and Kotsiantis, S. (2020). Explainable AI: a review of machine learning interpretability methods. *Entropy*, 23(1), 18. https://doi.org/10.3390/e23010018

Makubhai, S., Pathak, G., and Chandre, P. (2023). Prevention in healthcare: an explainable AI approach. *International Journal on Recent and Innovation Trends in Computing and Communication*, 11(5), 92–100. https://doi.org/10.17762/ijritcc.v11i5.6582

Marya, K., Iqbal, S., and Marya, A. (2024). An unusual cause of shoulder pain: a case report and review of the literature. *Cureus*. https://doi.org/10.7759/cureus.70488

Mello, B., Rigo, S., Costa, C., Righi, R., Donida, B., Bez, M., and Schunke, L. (2022). Semantic interoperability in health records standards: a systematic literature review. *Health and Technology*, 12(2), 255–272. https://doi.org/10.1007/s12553-022-00639-w

Mienye, I., Obaido, G., Jere, N., Mienye, E., Aruleba, K., Emmanuel, I., and Ogbuokiri, B. (2024). *A survey of explainable artificial intelligence in healthcare: concepts, applications, and challenges*. https://doi.org/10.20944/preprints202408.1702.v1

Miranda, N., Machado, M., and Moreira, D. (2024). Semantic web technologies in healthcare: a scoping review. In *Anais estendidos* (pp. 171–184). SBC. https://doi.org/10.5753/webmedia_estendido.2024.244455

Muhunzi, D., Kitambala, L., and Mashauri, H. (2024). Big data analytics in the healthcare sector: opportunities and challenges in developing countries. a literature review. *Health Informatics Journal*, 30(4). https://doi.org/10.1177/14604582241294217

Nath, R., Hose, K., Pedersen, T., Romero, O., and Bhattacharjee, A. (2020). Setlbi: an integrated platform for semantic business intelligence. In *Companion proceedings of the web conference* (pp. 167–171). ACM. https://doi.org/10.1145/3366424.3383533

Naveed, T. (2020). Addressing semantic interoperability, privacy and security concerns in electronic health records. *Journal of Engineering and Scientific Research*, 2(1). https://doi.org/10.23960/jesr.v2i1.40

Ndlovu, K., Scott, R., and Mars, M. (2021). Interoperability opportunities and challenges in linking mhealth applications and erecord systems: botswana as an exemplar. *BMC Medical Informatics and Decision Making*, 21(1). https://doi.org/10.1186/s12911-021-01606-7

Ojo, O. and Kiobel, B. (2024). Optimizing data management in healthcare: lessons from clinical trials and beyond. *World Journal of Biology Pharmacy and Health Sciences*, 19(3), 218–231. https://doi.org/10.30574/wjbphs.2024.19.3.0626

Pacaci, A., Gönül, S., Sınacı, A., Yüksel, M., and Ertürkmen, G. (2018). A semantic transformation methodology for the secondary use of observational healthcare data in postmarketing safety studies. *Frontiers in Pharmacology*, 9. https://doi.org/10.3389/fphar.2018.00435

Palaniappan, K., Lin, E., and Vogel, S. (2024). Global regulatory frameworks for the use of artificial intelligence (AI) in the healthcare services sector. *Healthcare*, 12(5), 562. https://doi.org/10.3390/healthcare12050562

Park, C., You, S., Jeon, H., Jeong, C., Choi, J., and Park, R. (2022). Development and validation of the radiology common data model (R-CDM) for the international standardization of medical imaging data. *Yonsei Medical Journal*, 63(Suppl), S74. https://doi.org/10.3349/ymj.2022.63.s74

Peng, C. and Goswami, P. (2019). Meaningful integration of data from heterogeneous health services and home environment based on ontology. *Sensors*, 19(8), 1747. https://doi.org/10.3390/s19081747

Pine, K. (2019). The qualculative dimension of healthcare data interoperability. *Health Informatics Journal*, 25(3), 536–548. https://doi.org/10.1177/1460458219833095

Quazi, F., Raju, N., Gorrepati, N., and Kareem, S. (2024). *Blockchain applications in electronic health records* (EHRS). https://doi.org/10.21428/e90189c8.5043b7de

Raghupathi, W. and Raghupathi, V. (2014). Big data analytics in healthcare: promise and potential. *Health Information Science and Systems*, 2(1). https://doi.org/10.1186/2047-2501-2-3

Rajput, A., Li, Q., and Ahvanooey, M. (2021). A blockchain-based secret-data sharing framework for personal health records in emergency condition. *Healthcare*, 9(2), 206. https://doi.org/10.3390/healthcare9020206

Ranjan, P., Yadav, A., Verma, A., Patil, A., and Gupta, D. (2023). Healthcare data management system using blockchain. *International Journal of Scientific Research in Computer Science Engineering and Information Technology*, 382–387. https://doi.org/10.32628/cseit2390250

Rao, K. and Manvi, S. (2023). Survey on electronic health record management using amalgamation of artificial intelligence and blockchain technologies. *Acta Informatica Pragensia*, 12(1), 179–199. https://doi.org/10.18267/j.aip.194

Reinecke, I., Zoch, M., Reich, C., Sedlmayr, M., and Bathelt, F. (2021). *The usage of OHDSI OMOP – a scoping review.* https://doi.org/10.3233/shti210546

Reinecke, I., Zoch, M., Wilhelm, M., Sedlmayr, M., and Bathelt, F. (2021). *Transfer of clinical drug data to a research infrastructure on omop – a fair concept.* https://doi.org/10.3233/shti210815

Reps, J., Schuemie, M., Suchard, M., Ryan, P., and Rijnbeek, P. (2018). Design and implementation of a standardized framework to generate and evaluate patient-level prediction models using observational healthcare data. *Journal of the American Medical Informatics Association*, 25(8), 969–975. https://doi.org/10.1093/jamia/ocy032

Rho, M., Kim, S., Park, S., Jang, K., Park, B., Hong, J., and Choi, I. (2015). Common data model for decision support system of adverse drug reaction to extract knowledge from multi-center database. *Information Technology and Management*, 17(1), 57–66. https://doi.org/10.1007/s10799-015-0240-6

Seyyed-Kalantari, L., Zhang, H., McDermott, M., Chen, I., and Ghassemi, M. (2021). Underdiagnosis bias of artificial intelligence algorithms applied to chest radiographs in under-served patient populations. *Nature Medicine*, 27(12), 2176–2182. https://doi.org/10.1038/s41591-021-01595-0

Shin, S., You, S., Park, Y., Roh, J., Kim, J., Haam, S., and Park, R. (2019). Genomic common data model for seamless interoperation of biomedical data in clinical practice: retrospective study. *Journal of Medical Internet Research*, 21(3), e13249. https://doi.org/10.2196/13249

Sim, K., Zadrazil, P., and Beaufays, F. (2019). *An investigation into on-device personalization of end-to-end automatic speech recognition models*. https://doi.org/10.21437/interspeech.2019-1752

Song, T. and Ryu, S. (2015). Big data analysis framework for healthcare and social sectors in Korea. *Healthcare Informatics Research*, 21(1), 3. https://doi.org/10.4258/hir.2015.21.1.3

Sony, P., Shanmugam, S., and Nagarajan, S. (2024). Enhancement of semantic interoperability in healthcare systems using ifciot architecture. *KSII Transactions on Internet and Information Systems*, 18(4). https://doi.org/10.3837/tiis.2024.04.004

Thopate, S., Dhamdhere, K., Nagarkar, R., Vishwakarma, A., and Somvanshi, R. (2023). Clinical data management in the era of artificial intelligence: a review of challenges and opportunities. *International Research Journal of Modernization in Engineering Technology and Science*, 5(6), 4382–4895. https://doi.org/10.56726/irjmets42732

Tsinale, H., Mbugua, S., and Luvanda, A. (2023a). Architectural health data standards and semantic interoperability: a comprehensive review in the context of integrating medical data into big data analytics. *IJEAST*, 8(4), 17–30. https://doi.org/10.33564/ijeast.2023.v08i04.002

Tsinale, H., Mbugua, S., and Luvanda, A. (2023b). Effective approaches for enhancing data management and semantic interoperability within the healthcare sector. *International Journal of Applied Research*, 9(9). https://doi.org/10.22271/allresearch.2023.v9.i9a.11225

Tsopra, R., Fernández, X., Luchinat, C., Alberghina, L., Lehrach, H., Vanoni, M., and Burgun, A. (2021). A framework for validating AI in precision medicine: considerations from the European ITFOC consortium. *BMC Medical Informatics and Decision Making*, 21(1), 1–14. https://doi.org/10.1186/s12911-021-01634-3

Uysal, I. (2023). Interpretable diabetes prediction using XAI in healthcare application. *Journal of Multidisciplinary Developments*, 8(1), 20–38.

Vaira, L., Lechien, J., Abbate, V., Allevi, F., Audino, G., Beltramini, G., and Riu, G. (2024). *Validation of the QAMAI tool to assess the quality of health information provided by AI*. https://doi.org/10.1101/2024.01.25.24301774

Yadav, R. (2023). *A research review on semantic interoperable archetype models, approaches & methods implemented for electronic health record systems in medical healthcare*. https://doi.org/10.20944/preprints202311.0011.v1

Yelne, S., Chaudhary, M., Dod, K., Sayyad, A., and Sharma, R. (2023). Harnessing the power of AI: a comprehensive review of its impact and challenges in nursing science and healthcare. *Cureus*, 15(11). https://doi.org/10.7759/cureus.49252

Zhang, H., Guo, Y., Li, Q., George, T., Shenkman, E., Modave, F., and Bian, J. (2018). An ontology-guided semantic data integration framework to support integrative data analysis of cancer survival. *BMC Medical Informatics and Decision Making*, 18(S2). https://doi.org/10.1186/s12911-018-0636-4

Zhang, R., Zhang, Z., Wang, D., and Liu, Z. (2023). Editorial: responsible ai in healthcare: opportunities, challenges, and best practices. *Frontiers in Computer Science*, 5. https://doi.org/10.3389/fcomp.2023.1265902

Zhang, X., Yates, A., Vasilevsky, N., Gourdine, J., Carmody, L., Daniš, D., and Robinson, P. (2019). *Semantic integration of clinical laboratory tests from electronic health records for deep phenotyping and biomarker discovery*. https://doi.org/10.1101/519231

13 Revolutionizing Medical Care

The Role of Metaverse and NFTs in Modern Healthcare

V. S. Devi Priya, Sumathi Doraikannan, Vinitha V., Ranjima P., and Mehmet Bilen

13.1 INTRODUCTION

Healthcare professionals find that reviewing the vast amounts of medical data from the electronic medical record (EMR) system takes more and more time. Physicians have to carefully review the data, which in turn increases the time they spend on each patient. This could reflect on the precision and quality of the treatment strategy that should be applied to the patients. If the time required for consulting a single patient increases, the doctor can attend only a few patients in a day. The medical management authority has to deal with it by assigning more physicians and additional funding. In the healthcare sector, the term "innovation," which is widely used in marketing and economic circles, is becoming more widely recognized as a measurable phenomenon. Innovation can be divided into four primary categories: disruptive, architectural, radical, and routine/incremental (Sounderajah et al., 2021). Instead of describing how a product or service has changed over time, the term "disruptive innovation" is used to describe it at a single, fixed point in time. In its most basic definition, "disruption" is the process through which a smaller company with fewer resources can successfully compete with established incumbent businesses (Sounderajah et al., 2021). Several significant characteristics define disruption, such as (1) new market entrants that target underserved or neglected customer segments; (2) a rise in low-end or emerging markets; (3) incumbents that prioritize improving their current products for their core, mainstream customers, making them slow to respond to these new competitive threats; and (4) entrants that establish a strong position by meeting rising demand and frequently offering lower-priced alternatives (Figure 13.1).

The recent information technology (IT) innovations for raising standards across a range of industries, including healthcare, are digital disruption and digital transformation. IT has the potential to greatly enhance healthcare quality and safety by

DOI: 10.1201/9781003605416-13

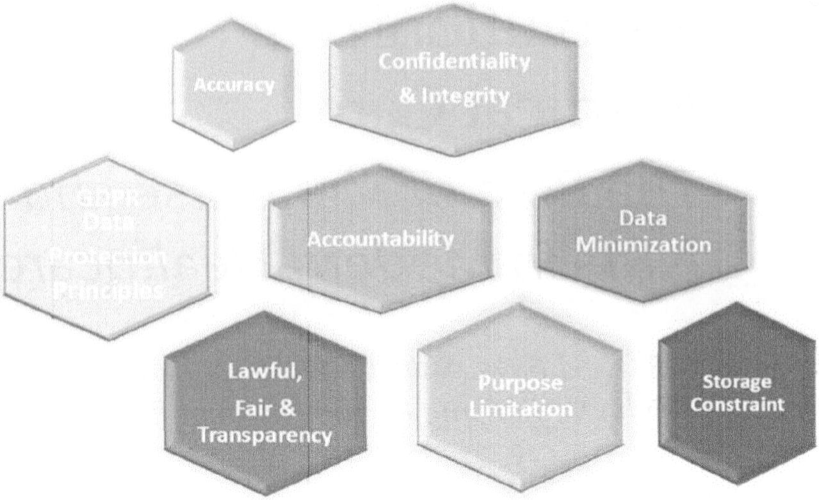

FIGURE 13.1 Innovation landscape map.

facilitating the application of evidence-based practices. Electronic medical records (EMRs), a digital repository for patient data, are considered to be the application with the biggest potential for quality improvement. The outcome of diagnostic and therapeutic interventions, along with the specifics of the prior visit, should be included in the EMRs. In their routine clinical practice, doctors do not have enough time between patient visits to adequately update the incoming patient's record. This time constraint jeopardizes the accuracy and reliability of patient records, which directly affects the quality and safety of patient care. Therefore, it is necessary to analyze large volumes of medical data quickly and accurately to provide high-quality healthcare. The healthcare sector has experienced rapid expansion in recent years, and new technologies have helped them overcome the challenges of analyzing enormous amounts of data. Healthcare providers should ensure that patients' sensitive information is private and secure. They must take privacy precautions into account when storing data on intelligent devices.

Disruptive technologies refer to innovations that significantly alter or transform markets or sectors by replacing established products, services, or practices. When these technologies introduce new ways of doing things that are simpler, less costly, or more efficient than the ones that are currently available, they often result in significant change. Various characteristics of digital disruption include innovation and the development of new markets, as well as efficiency, productivity, scalability, and affordability. The benefits of digital disruption are as follows:

- **Enhanced Productivity**: It facilitates more effective and efficient corporate operations. For instance, companies could manage all of their client data in one location with a customer relationship management (CRM) tool like HubSpot.
- **Increased Interconnections**: Businesses may use technology to establish new connections with their partners and consumers. For instance, social media and internet marketing allow companies to access a worldwide audience.
- **Opportunities and New Markets**: It allows companies to tap into new markets or market niches. The market will require more products as a result of increased digital capabilities.

13.1.1 Disruption Tools

The following tools triggered the advent of digital involvement in healthcare (Pratt, 2019; Albawi et al., 2018; El Khatib et al., 2022) (Figure 13.2).

- **Artificial Intelligence**: The following strategies facilitate the efficient interpretation of enormous amounts of medical data.
  - **Analytics Tools with AI Capabilities**: Descriptive, predictive, and prescriptive analytics are examples of AI-enabled analytic systems that could assist healthcare facilities in analyzing current circumstances, comparing them with records, and providing information on how to prepare better for any impending medical issues.
  - **Neural Networks**: Healthcare institutions find neural networks to be a useful tool in their toolbox. They could greatly assist the Health Information Management (HIM) department and physicians in managing records more effectively, identifying links between cases from the past and present, and even figuring out whether there is a relationship between cases that need to be looked at.

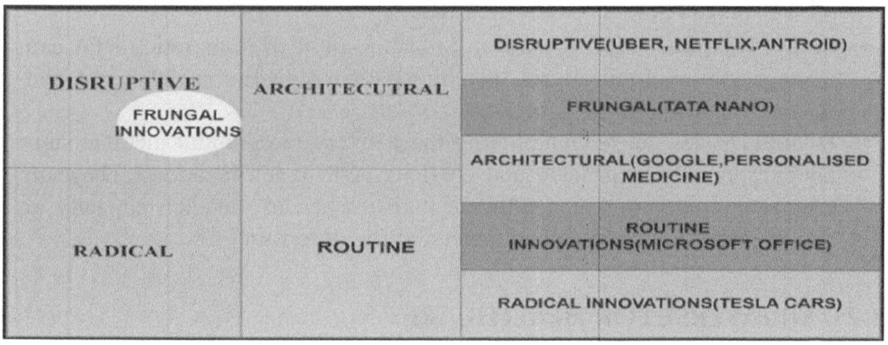

FIGURE 13.2 Disruption tools.

- **System of Double Reading/Entry**: In addition to guaranteeing consistency in the data input, this type of entry system will enable them to store the data in a way that facilitates easy access and analysis when needed in a short time. It can significantly aid in the efficient administration of patient records kept by the HIM department of healthcare institutions. For example, the AI-powered hospital administration system Hivemind-Halemind makes it easier to manage patient registration, appointment scheduling, and electronic health records. It was also possible to download revenue, statistics, trends, average appointment time, and other data with ease.
- **Blockchain**: Doctors could safely record patients' medical histories using blockchain. It is possible to identify fake drugs by looking into the blockchain network's source of purchase for the tablets.
- **IoT**: IoT facilitates remote health monitoring. Under a doctor's supervision, patients could take their heart rates at home, store the data in a central program for real-time analysis, and get the results the same day. An IoT-powered program called Patient Wait Time Prediction keeps track of doctors' availability to efficiently reduce wait times for patients in need of immediate care.
- **Intelligent Pharmacy and Logistics**: The pharmacy ecosystem supports increased operational effectiveness, safe medication distribution, security, and better overall care quality.
- **Robotics and Automation**: By automating the entry of patient data utilizing chatbots and optical character recognition technologies, robotic process automation (RPA) solutions are utilized in hospital process management to give patients prompt service.
- **Virtual Assistance**: Delivers medicine and helps consumers by combining AI and RPA. It also provides alerts and instructional resources.
- **Fraud Detection**: By employing ML and RPA algorithms, it is possible to prevent fraudulent claims and alert the appropriate parties as soon as they are discovered. Data and documentation about a patient's condition help doctors make better data-driven decisions.
- **Smart Hospital Administration**: Smart hospital administration RPA can manage administrative duties, including patient registration, data input, and doctor scheduling for appointment requests.
- **Drone**: Drones are revolutionizing the delivery of essential medical supplies, especially in isolated and challenging-to-reach locations. They are crucial in contemporary healthcare logistics because of their capacity to deliver goods on schedule and traverse difficult terrain.

13.2 METAVERSE FOR HEALTHCARE

Definitions of the Metaverse: "The metaverse is a digital environment that allows people to communicate digitally by fusing elements of social networking, online gaming, augmented reality, virtual reality, and cryptocurrency" (Metaverse, 2022).

"The metaverse is a network of shared, completely immersive virtual environments where people may work, shop, play games, and interact with friends" (Somayaji et al., 2024). "A hypothetical or developing networked online world with digitally permanent surroundings that users occupy as avatars for simultaneous interactions and experiences." Users can access the shared virtual space via smartphone apps, gaming consoles, virtual reality (VR), augmented reality (AR), or conventional PCs.

13.2.1 Core Technologies

- **Sensors**: Human—-machine interface (HMI) devices should be able to perform the following tasks as a link between the real and virtual worlds:

  (1) Gathering data from the actual world to create a virtual environment.
  (2) Data rendering

A large amount of the metaverse's energy usage will come from the electricity used by HMI equipment. HMI devices' sensing technologies form the basis for collecting information from the real world in order to create the metaverse. Wearable sensors are able to project metaverse users' movements, emotions, physiological signals, and interactions with their environment from the real world into the virtual world through the use of VR, AR, and mixed reality (MR). This enables users to manipulate their avatars and produce dynamic, engaging experiences. IoT sensors may be able to provide real-time data to support the metaverse environment by providing environmental data via digital twin technologies (Kaddoura et al., 2021). In IoT-based medical systems, sensors are intentionally incorporated to measure various biological parameters and track real-time patient healthcare data, particularly when connected to remote sensing technologies. Medical systems that use biological sensors are adaptable in their machine-to-machine interactions, saving patients' and healthcare facilities' time while providing treatment options via tele-diagnosis. Aside from blood pressure, accelerometers, and image sensors, temperature and pulse are the widely utilized sensors for assessing physiological conditions.

Enabling Technology—6G:

Hundreds of billion devices and perceptron must be supported by the 6G metaverse in order to offer extensive services, which leads to high demands for spectrum. Furthermore, very high-quality communication is necessary for many metaverse services. A VR application's data traffic must send a 4 × 4-inch full-parallax hologram and an original full-parallax hologram at 30 frames per second (fps), necessitating a 30 Gbps local display rate. To ensure a high-quality user experience and avoid the disorientation that comes with latency, critical real-time metaverse applications demand extremely low latency.

- *BigData*: Formatting, storing, and analyzing massive datasets are all part of the big data idea. Big data is one type of data that is gathered from several sources and includes a variety of data types in different formats. The various dimensions of big data are represented by Vs: Value (in-depth and important information), velocity (data inflow is high and real-time processing), veracity (detailed data accumulation), volume (a significant amount of data), variety (including structured, semi-structured, and unstructured data with various formats), and valence (data interconnection). Big data generation (from various sources, including internal data from hospitals and medical facilities, IoT data, Internet data, and biomedical data), big data acquisition (including data collection, transmission, and pre-processing), big data storage, and big data analysis should be performed effectively (Singh and El-Kassar, 2019; Wu and Gao, 2022).

Enabling Technology—Blockchain: The metaverse platform collects data from a range of IoT devices. A wide variety of hardware, controllers, and tangible objects will be used by the IoT devices to link the metaverse. IoT devices with specialized sensors enable both physical and virtual navigation and connection to the metaverse. The ability of users to function in the metaverse will depend critically on the IoT devices' ability to do so (Zhang et al., 2021). Real-time data storage is made possible in the metaverse via IoT-enabled blockchains. As blockchain transactions are irreversible, all stakeholders can rely on the data and respond quickly and effectively. By enabling stakeholders to monitor their IoT data records in shared blockchain ledgers, blockchain technology will assist in resolving metaverse privacy challenges (Majeed et al., 2021). Further, by decentralizing data storage and verification procedures, the blockchain concept can help protect medical care systems from DDoS attacks, making it more difficult for attackers to interfere with essential healthcare services (Manivannan et al., 2024).

- *Artificial Intelligence*: The use of ML algorithms to simulate human cognition in the presentation, analysis, comprehension, and learning of complex healthcare and medical data is referred to as AI in healthcare (Mughal et al., 2022; Javed et al., 2020). A collection of statistical algorithms use inference to make predictions after learning from data through training. Because machine learning (ML) allows computers to automatically learn patterns from data without explicit and manual programming, it can be used in a wide range of scientific domains, including healthcare and medicine with precision medicine (i.e., analyzing and diagnosing various patient characteristics in order to forecast and suggest the best course of action for a patient's success).

Enabling Technology—Holographic Communication: Cutting-edge technologies are combined on several levels to create holographic communication, which transforms how we interact and perceive digital worlds by enabling immersive, real-time interactions. The Holography Layer captures and reconstructs 3D holographic images and provides realistic visual experiences (Shvetsov and Alsamhi, 2024). The Communication Layer ensures the seamless movement of massive amounts of data while enabling real-time interactions through the use of high-bandwidth channels and low-latency networks. While the Metaverse Layer links the virtual environments to build immersive digital worlds for users to participate in, the Application Layer uses these technologies to provide practical, user-focused applications like remote collaboration, entertainment, and virtual meetings.

- *Wireless Communication Networks*: A proactive examination of the fundamental wireless systems is necessary to manage these intricate computer and wireless resources, particularly in the metaverse, a virtual representation of the real world. The idea of the metaverse is meant to be self-sustaining and enable wireless systems to function smoothly with low operating expenses for effective resource management. The two main elements that make up the metaverse of a wireless system are offline analysis and online control. When it comes to the design and implementation of wireless systems, the former may offer guidance. Numerous simulation tools (such as those for system-level modeling, signal processing, network protocols and routing, and mobility simulations) may be used a priori to carry out this kind of study. It is necessary to create new simulators that can better analyze wireless systems in the meta space to implement a metaverse-based wireless system. Metaverse can be used for run-time control of physical systems in addition to analyzing the virtual wireless world.

Enabling Technology—Quantum Computing: In traditional computing, data is processed sequentially in terms of bits, whereas in quantum computing, qubits are used to represent. This can be done simultaneously and in parallel, a process known as superposition. Entanglement is another feature of quantum computing that allows one qubit's state to be ascertained by the correlation between two or more qubits, which can influence another qubit despite their significant differences.

This feature can readily surpass classical computers because it allows them to perform calculations that are not feasible for a classical computer. A complicated and emerging topic that has the potential to fundamentally alter how we approach restorative research about therapy is the relationship between quantum computing, the metaverse, and healthcare. As quantum computing can efficiently replicate intricate chemical interactions and atomic structures that are difficult or impossible to show with traditional computers, it has the potential to significantly accelerate the development of underutilized medications and therapies. This significantly reduces the time and costs associated with sedate disclosure and enables the development of individualized pharmacological regimens tailored to individual patients. In virtual settings, patients can interact with physicians and therapy professionals to get analysis, treatment recommendations, and even surgery. Additionally, the metaverse can provide a platform for restorative training and education, enabling experts and analysts to work together and exchange knowledge in a virtual setting. Furthermore, by enabling advanced encryption techniques that are impervious to hacking and data breaches, quantum computing can improve the security of confidential information (Bajkoti et al., 2023).

- *Cloud and Edge Computing*: Using shared computing resources instead of local servers or personal devices to manage applications is known as cloud computing. The phrase is typically used to refer to sizable data centers that are accessible to numerous users via a private network (private cloud) or the Internet (public cloud). Enhancing the performance, operational cost, and dependability of applications and services by extending computing capabilities to the logical limits of a network is known as edge computing. By reducing network hops and the distance between devices and the resources that support them, it lessens the latency and bandwidth limitations of the current Internet and opens up new application classes. Massive amounts of unstructured, diversified, and exponentially expanding data acquired from many sources have presented significant issues for many traditional healthcare and medical systems, making it more difficult to store and handle data efficiently and securely. In light of this, the sophisticated methods and large storage capacity of cloud computing enable the analysis of medical and healthcare big data (Rajabion et al., 2019).

Enabling Technology—Computer Vision: In the metaverse universe, computer vision is used to allow users to see the virtual environment. Digital avatars offer an experience that is almost exactly like the real world in computer vision and virtual reality. Computer vision plays an important role in XR applications. Computer vision and visual information are necessary to evaluate and understand visuals, such as digital images or videos, make wise decisions, and act appropriately (Barioni et al., 2018).

- *Immersive Technology*: To give users a realistic and captivating experience in the metaverse, immersive interaction technologies like VR and AR are utilized. VR gaming, 3D films, industrial design, and paramedicine are just a few of the industries that may make extensive use of this technology. Furthermore, developments in cloud computing and 5G networks have enabled the creation of high-fidelity and low-latency virtual environments, enabling real-time interaction between several users in the same virtual world. The following is a quick explanation of the immersive technologies:

VR: This technology makes it possible to create a completely immersive digital environment where the actual world is completely blocked.

AR: This technology allows digital materials to be superimposed over the physical world, creating a composite image of digital and physical elements.

MR: This technology not only makes it possible to superimpose digital components that are being viewed in the actual world, but it also enables interaction between them.

XR: This general phrase refers to any technology that modifies reality, such as incorporating digital or virtual components into the physical world at any scale, essentially eliminating the distinction between the virtual and the real world.

Digital twins: These are virtual versions of real-world projects that are necessary to link actual objects for real-time data processing, reaction, and collecting.

FPV drone flight: This technology allows users to experience the world in the first person by using an unmanned aerial vehicle (UAV) equipped with a camera to transmit high-quality movies to goggles, headphones, mobile devices, or another screen.

Haptics: A technology that interacts with users through tactile (touch) feeling.

Enabling Technology—IoT: IoT is the network of actual items, including buildings, cars, and other vehicles, which are linked to the internet and can gather and exchange data. In contrast, the metaverse is a virtual environment where users may communicate in real time with digital items and one another. The combination of the IoT with the metaverse has garnered a lot of interest in recent years, and studies conducted worldwide indicate that interest in the possible uses of this technology is increasing. IoT can create creative and innovative metaverse user experiences by fusing real-world things with virtual ones (Stasolla et al., 2024; Maier et al., 2019; Wang et al., 2024) (Figure 13.3).

13.2.2 Creating Interoperable Healthcare Ecosystem

Patients, doctors, allied health professionals, state agencies, academic institutions, non-governmental organizations (NGOs), and corporations are just a few of the

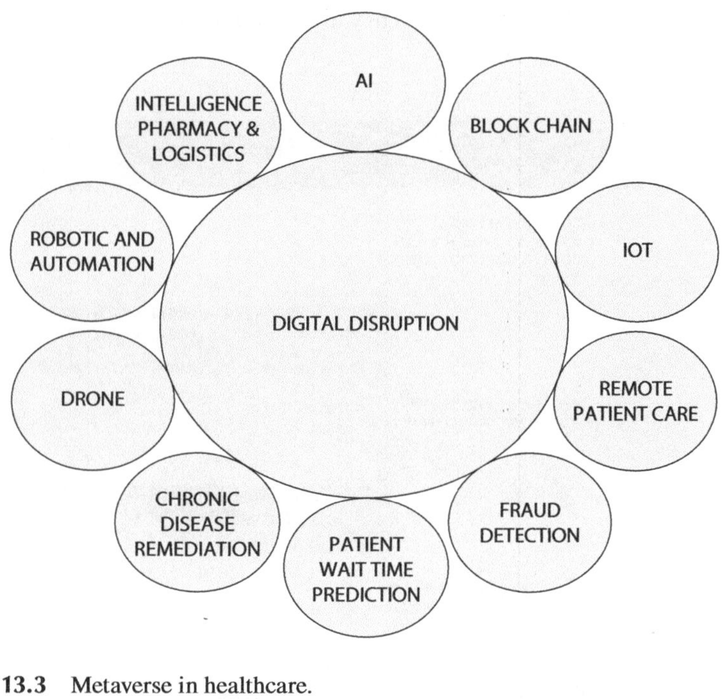

FIGURE 13.3 Metaverse in healthcare.

many entities that make up healthcare ecosystems. To achieve a common objective, they integrate information flows that come from or are co-produced by each of these actors. The many aspects of the metaverse's characteristics include social interactions, immersive simulations, and avatar-based meetups.

Avatar-Based Meetings: The capacity to have meetings using avatars is one of the metaverse's key features. The avatar can serve as the single point of entry and distinct identity where people explore, interact, and engage in the metaverse, which combines many apps and virtual world aspects. Compared to traditional online video meetings, people could engage with each other and the virtual world considerably more when using digital avatars. Using the metaverse, patients can participate in virtual consultations. For real-time contact between patients and medical personnel, traditional online consultations that only allow audio or video chat are frequently ineffective.

Avatars that mimic the behaviors of doctors might provide deeper contact and communication than video or teleconsultation. VR- and AR-based virtual diagnostic and therapeutic tools in avatars are becoming useful (Secundo et al., 2019) (Figure 13.4).

Immersive Simulations: By combining emerging technologies with XR, the metaverse provides more immersive simulation experiences enhancing electronic and digital environments where data is projected and represented.

Social Interactions: The social and gaming sectors currently account for the majority of metaverse apps. In addition to the previously mentioned interactions between patients and healthcare providers, the metaverse offers virtual communities for patients and medical professionals. They are helpful to patients in creating online

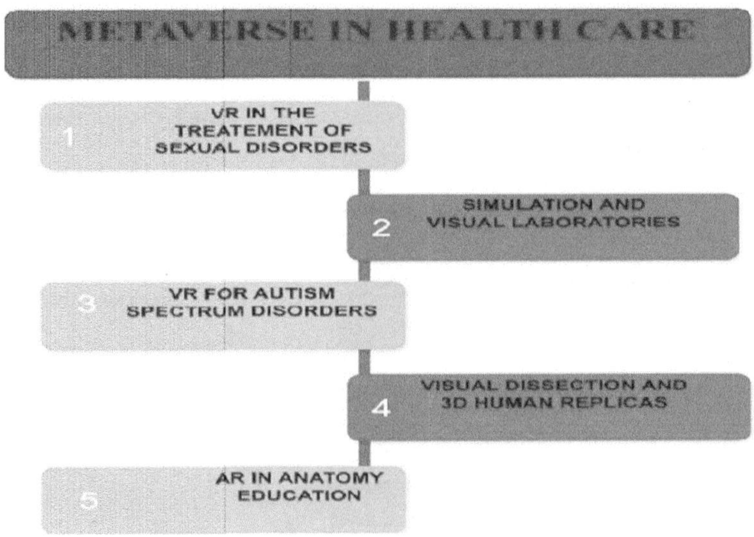

FIGURE 13.4 Creating interoperable healthcare ecosystem.

support groups. Research indicates that participation in organizations that provide patients with emotional support, strength, hope, and confidence improves their quality of life in quantifiable ways (Van Uden-Kraan et al., 2011).

13.3 NON-FUNGIBLE TOKENS (NFTS)

Non-fungible tokens, or NFTs, are digital tokens that are based on blockchain technology and represent exclusive assets, such as artwork, digital content, or media. In essence, an NFT functions as an unalterable digital record of ownership and authenticity for a specific asset, whether it's digital or tangible. The three main goals of NFTs are

- Cryptographic verifiability
- Uniqueness or scarcity
- Ease of transferability

One can quickly ascertain the asset's origin and current owner by utilizing cryptographic signatures that are inherent to the blockchain on which an NFT is issued. NFTs can be made to symbolize almost any kind of asset, be it digital, metaphysical, or physical. Digital artwork, digital collectibles, audio or video content, and event tickets are the most popular NFT assets. Minting is the process by which a creator, artist, or license holder creates a non-fungible token. The process of minting entails signing a blockchain transaction outlining the essential details of the token, which is then sent to the blockchain to initiate a smart contract function that generates the token and allocates it to its owner. NFT is made up of a distinct token ID, or token ID, that is stored inside a smart contract and mapped to an owner identifier. It is simple to confirm ownership and reassign the token to a new owner when the owner of a given token ID wants to give it to another user.

The primary distinction between NFTs and other cryptographic tokens is their non-fungibility, which is how they got their name. An item's fungibility is the quality that establishes whether or not it can be swapped out for other similar items without losing value. Cash is fungible, as evidenced by the fact that one can exchange a 100 Rupee note for five 20 Rupee notes or even another 100 Rupee note. On the other hand, because of its special qualities, a work of art such as the original Mona Lisa cannot be sold like-for-like. The ability to define distinct metadata and a unique token ID allows each NFT to be as unique as its creator desires, providing an entirely open design space that can be tailored to a vast array of applications.

Blockchain currently introduces non-fungibility to the digital realm in the form of NFTs, just as it did fungibility and the ability to exchange value like-for-like in the form of cryptocurrencies. The immutability, dependability, transparency, and decentralization of blockchain technology open up new possibilities for the easy trading, sharing, and exchanging of digital representations of any kind of asset, and this is likely to encourage new blockchain-based innovation for many businesses. The market for NFTs was estimated to be worth USD 36.19 billion in 2023 and is expected to increase at a compound annual growth rate (CAGR) of 34.5 percent from 2024 to 2032, from USD 48.67 billion to USD 521.17 billion. NFTs offer a wide range of market opportunities, and more and more industries are investigating the technology's possible uses. There are several use cases like smart cities and governance, healthcare, gaming, supply chain management, education, and agriculture.

The next section discusses the adoption of NFT in healthcare. The resilience of health systems faces major challenges in the face of new threats to global health, pandemics, armed conflicts, rising service demands, and an aging population (WHO, 2023). The need for continuous innovation and advancement in the health sector is highlighted by the growing demand for healthcare systems to prevent, prepare for, detect, and recover from these challenges (WHO, 2023). As the healthcare industry continues to change and adopt new technologies, the use of NFTs is one innovation that has drawn a lot of interest. NFTs are most frequently linked to the realm of digital art and collectibles, but they are also being investigated as a way to increase the effectiveness and openness of healthcare data management. NFTs have the potential to completely transform the management, sharing, and security of medical records by producing distinct and impenetrable digital records. The use of NFTs in healthcare is a promising development that has the potential to revolutionize the sector, from enhancing patient privacy to enabling more accurate and efficient clinical trials.

13.3.1 Benefits of NFT in Healthcare

There are a number of possible advantages to tokenizing healthcare data on the blockchain with NFTs.

- Enhancing the flow of health information between various healthcare providers can lead to safer care and fewer unnecessary tests or treatments, both of which can have positive financial effects on health.
- In addition to ensuring data authenticity and preventing changes after data has been minted, tokenization of health data can improve clinical decision-making processes and yield more accurate research results.
- By encouraging patient involvement in their care and giving patients control over their data, it can stop businesses from making money off of data gathered by personal health apps or third parties gaining illegal access to institutional databases.
- Businesses can set themselves apart from rivals by providing creative and patient-centered solutions by integrating NFTs into healthcare data management.
- Reliable automation of data exchange is further made possible by smart contracts in NFTs.

Although digital acceleration has not yet reached its full potential, it may become more effective and efficient as blockchain-based solutions that use NFTs proliferate. As a certificate of authenticity, NFTs are used to grant permission to own a portion of a digital representation of a physical asset, in contrast to cryptocurrencies.

i) Combating Counterfeit Pharmaceuticals: By employing this verification process with the aid of a token ID assigned throughout its existence that remains with the NFT leaving a digital footprint, NFT and blockchain play a significant role in the fight against counterfeit medications. The uniqueness of each NFT is defined by the information contained in its metadata, which refers to the priceless digital resources that are updated in real time on the blockchain. To a certain extent, NFTs reduce and even eradicate inconsistencies and fraud by creating an unchangeable ledger record. NFTs protect medications and expedite the tracking process, enabling quick error detection. It is possible to address potential issues like detecting and eliminating prescription drugs obtained illegally from the system considerably faster.
ii) Blood Donation Process: NFTs, in which donors are identified by a unique token that can be tracked through the system, are already encouraged by blood donation organizations. It is possible to register and store blood in a digital "blood bank" using an NFT. The demand for particular blood types can be tracked using blockchain technology, and blood can be effectively delivered to areas with the greatest need. Using NFTs, BloodChain, a blockchain-based biological tracing company, circumvents bottlenecks in the distribution and collection of biological products like blood. With the aid of the BloodChain network, they established an open social blood bank that enables anyone to donate blood. The goal of BloodChain is to provide a safe and secure environment for people to register their blood types while simultaneously meeting supply and demand. Additionally, they employ AI-based applications on blockchain data to compute and comprehend the demand for blood from hospitals and other blood banks in order to promptly supply them with the necessary resources.
iii) Security for Medical Records: Maintaining records, including blood reports and other medical records, and using or sharing the information as needed is one of the difficult tasks in the healthcare industry. This issue is resolved by NFTs, which permit the use of health data across national boundaries and organizational boundaries. It is projected that this interoperability will lower patient costs, eliminate obstacles to care, and create new opportunities for advancement and care.
iv) Healthcare Data Storage: Opportunities for innovation in healthcare are abundant when health data is stored as NFTs. With centralized and easily accessible health data for each patient, better patient outcome monitoring and research may be possible, leading to advancements in care. The development of personalized medicine is one of the most exciting ways that NFTs can spur innovation in the healthcare industry. Researchers can better understand the underlying causes of diseases and create treatments that are suited to each patient's unique needs by safely storing and exchanging genetic data and other health information. The efficacy of these treatments can also be monitored over time with NFTs, enabling ongoing development and innovation. This can help lower healthcare costs and improve patient

outcomes by focusing treatments on the patients who will benefit from them the most. Overall, by making personalized medicine possible, NFTs have the potential to significantly impel innovation in the healthcare sector.

v) Control over the Data: Patients frequently have little or no control over their health information. Since patients own their access key, they have complete control over their data with NFTs. They can decide who can access their data, including researchers, family members, insurance companies, and medical professionals. NFTs also give patients a safe, unchangeable method to store and distribute their health information, which is crucial for private data like genetic information or medical records. Patients can feel more at ease knowing that their personal health information is protected from data breaches and unauthorized access thanks to this. Patients can also take a more active part in their healthcare by tracking treatment results, keeping tabs on their health, and even taking part in medical research when they have control over their data. Overall, by granting patients authority over their health information, NFTs have the potential to empower patients and improve healthcare for all. The next section outlines the use case for patient-centered cardiovascular care that employs NFT.

13.3.2 Case Study: NFT in Cardiovascular Medicine

The storage of EHRs on a blockchain network using NFTs is one of the most exciting uses in the healthcare industry (Teo and Ting, 2023). Compared to centralized hospitals, blockchain is suitable for sharing health information among patients, hospitals, clinics, pharmacies, and research centers, and is virtually immune to violent interventions. NFTs can embed or access text- or image-based data (such as lab results or heart ultrasound scans) and can be published through a blockchain portal. Hanna et al. (2022) discuss the possibility of incorporating ECGs into NFTs and storing patient data on a separate blockchain layer that is only available to patients and healthcare organizations. Historically, doctors and hospitals have been the custodians of important medical information, and patients have had little control over this information. Yet there is a growing recognition that health outcomes improve when patients have access to their own health information, and that they should have greater autonomy and control over their own health information (Figure 13.5).

Cardiovascular care frequently uses mobile health technologies and home medical devices to measure things like blood pressure, glucose, heart rate, electrocardiography, actigraphy, percentage of oxygen-containing hemoglobin in the blood, and body composition. These metrics have a track record of success in managing chronic conditions like heart failure, diabetes, and hypertension and are crucial for self-care and remote patient monitoring. These gadgets connect to vendor-controlled proprietary servers via the Internet of Things (Abdulmalek et al., 2022). These servers have a number of drawbacks, most notably their susceptibility to security breaches and their incapacity to integrate data across platforms. On the other hand, NFTs are extremely secure and vendor-neutral, thus offering a way to integrate data from

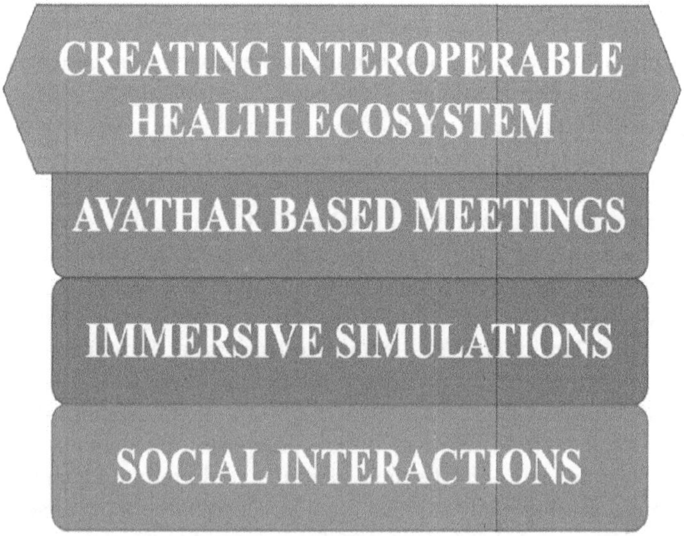

FIGURE 13.5 Updated version of CardioVerse model.

any device, analyze aggregated data from various devices using machine learning, and share patient data with doctors. Additionally, patients maintain ownership of the NFT once it is "minted," and they are free to profit from their anonymized data by sharing it with organizations to which they wish to donate. This incentive may gradually encourage patients to self-measure more health parameters and more frequently, as well as patient-reported outcome measures, in order to increase the data density of their NFTs.

When patients seek medical care or advice outside of their institution's geographic boundaries, NFTs may be able to help. Instead of requesting and sending records between institutions, which would take a lot of time, patients could give doctors instant access to their NFT-based medical records. The doctor would immediately have controlled access to all of their medical records, including diagnoses, prescriptions, tests, inpatient and outpatient visits, and data that they personally gathered. Consequently, the patient would obtain more accurate and prompt medical attention, which is particularly important in cases of acute cardiac events. Following that, hospitalization records would be accessible to the primary care physician or cardiologist who is not part of the hospital ecosystem, and pharmacists from different parts of the town could reconcile prescriptions, guaranteeing continuity of care. Zhang et al. (2023) used an NFT-based blockchain to create a convincing proof-of-concept for patient identification and health information exchange between institutions. The bioinformatic gap between disjointed clinics, pharmacies, test centers, and healthcare facilities is filled by this solution. Opportunities for collaborative care are increased and the likelihood of misunderstandings is reduced by combining all the data into a single NFT-based medical record.

13.3.2.1 CardioVerse

Historically, physical interaction has been the cornerstone of the patient–doctor relationship in cardiovascular medicine. This special relationship between patients and healthcare providers has been called into question by the most recent pandemic, which has resulted in risks to the standard of patient care. The adoption of innovative technologies has shown accelerations in all domains (Wosik et al., 2020; Colbert et al., 2020). Due to the advancements in AR and VR, the health sector shows extensive progress in adopting and extending to the field of the cardiovascular sector. Currently, the metaverse is receiving a lot of attention as a disruptive digital reality that has the potential to change many facets of life, including healthcare. Skalidis et al., envisioned the CardioVerse as a metaverse framework for cardiovascular medicine, introducing immersive approaches to medical pedagogy, telemedicine consultations, patient community forums, patient education, and telehealth (Skalidis et al., 2022, 2023a, 2023b). NFTs serve as digital passports that patients and providers use within the metaverse to verify their identities and credentials and, in the case of patients, to encapsulate their medical records. Despite the metaverse's seemingly vast scope, it is not intended to be separate from current technology or telemedicine services. Compatibility and integration with existing medical devices are two of the most significant and efficient features that will advance the metaverse by leveraging innovations that are already in use. An ideal CardioVerse model (Skalidis et al., 2022) as shown in Figure 13.5 would involve interoperability through the integration of home-based health devices and applications (such as blood pressure-heart frequency monitors, blood glucose calculators, oxygen saturation meters, and distant 12-lead ECGs), the outcomes of which would be directly projected into the metaverse. After conducting a medical analysis and analyzing the data from all health monitoring devices, the doctor will then communicate with the patient via a virtual avatar, arriving at a final diagnosis that the patient can receive. The integration of telemedicine advancements with the metaverse is regarded as a crucial element of a practical, tangible, and developing CardioVerse.

13.3.2.2 Challenges in Implementing the CardioVerse

As expected, we can assume that opportunities will also present numerous challenges as shown in Figure 13.6. The challenges are likely to be found in a variety of areas, including technical, security, legislative, and regulatory. Because breaches and violations could expose or steal sensitive data, patients' data security and privacy are major concerns in the metaverse. Blockchain-powered metaverses' decentralized nature may open up completely new avenues for patient data encryption and ensure that procedures and practices adhere to medical standards.

Key Players in Many Fields: This technology has given rise to businesses and start-ups that have created and marketed blockchain solutions based on NFT for the healthcare sector. Aimedis (2024), a blockchain-based healthcare ecosystem, was established in the Netherlands in 2016 and offers safe, unchangeable NFTs for storing and exchanging electronic medical records with researchers or other healthcare professionals. In order to receive payment in Ethereum cryptocurrency, patients are

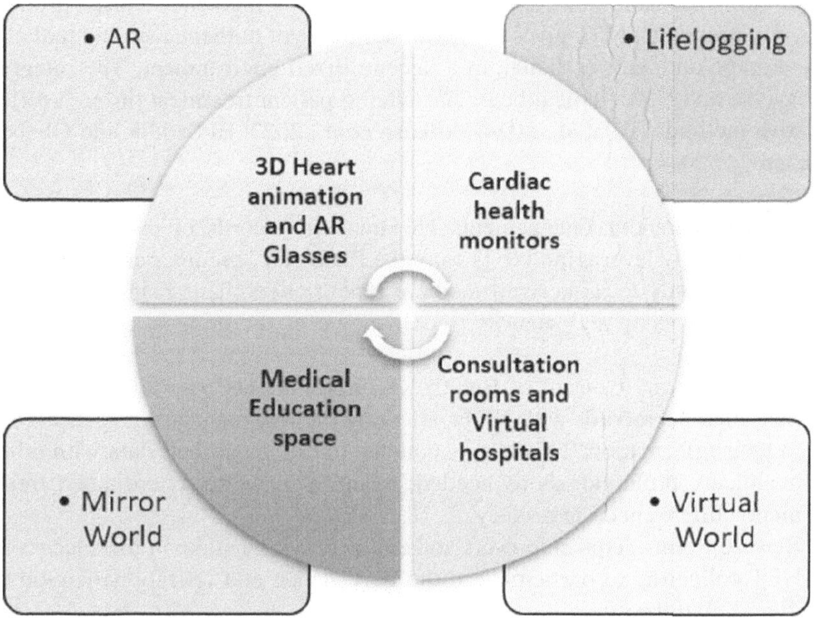

FIGURE 13.6 Challenges in implementation of CardioVerse.

urged to submit depersonalized data, mint their own NFT, peruse the platform for research projects looking for data, and exchange access to their NFT. A variety of services, such as patient-to-patient social networking, digital pharmacy fulfillment, and telemedicine consultations, were recently introduced as part of their metaverse Web3 experience. In 2017, Nebula Genomics (2024) was established in the United States and developed a blockchain-based personal genomics platform and service. In order to mint their own genomic NFT data, patients can either upload their raw DNA or use their kit to perform a home-based genomic sequencing test. They can then choose to share this data with industry or academic researchers in exchange for tokenized rewards. One feature that sets Nebula apart from other personal DNA analysis services is its NFT-based technology, which allows you to submit a sample and get a report without ever revealing your identity. This ensures complete anonymity and allays worries about data leaks.

13.4 INTEGRATION OF METAVERSE AND NFTS IN HEALTHCARE

Metaverse gives better communication, cooperation, and education, hence its use in virtual consultation, remote operation, and medical training. Doctors can use AR, VR, and AI to communicate with patients without meeting them physically. Similarly, NFTs allow users to have genuine and secure ownership of virtual space and create new opportunities for medical records and intellectual property. These technologies—metaverse and NFTs—can be integrated to improve the medical field through online consultations, encrypting the patient's medical records, promoting fitness initiatives, etc. NFT gives a virtual guarantee of authenticity, and that allows secure storage and data exchange in a decentralized environment. The integration of metaverse and NFTs in healthcare has altered patient treatment through different innovative methods (Li et al., 2024; Prakash et al., 2023; El Saddik and Ghaboura, 2023):

1. Enhanced Patient Engagement: The medical records of patients can be tokenized by leveraging NFTs to make them safe, secure, permanent, and available only to authorized medical practitioners. This helps in enhancing data privacy and security, tackling one of the greatest challenges in healthcare.
2. Ownership and Control of Health Records: Patients may take custody of their medical records with NFTs, allowing them to manage who gets access to their information. This allows patients to exchange their data with other healthcare professionals as needed, resulting in better coordinated treatment while respecting privacy.
3. Reward Points: This empowers stakeholders with a stake in the success of NFT collecting to participate in the governance and operationalization of digital platforms.
4. Virtual Health Communities: The metaverse has online forums and groups where users can interact with others having the same interests, share their experiences with others, and help each other. NFTs provide these communities with specific data, tools, or activities that foster a sense of belonging and support.
5. Enhanced Telehealth Services: Healthcare providers can improve telehealth services by utilizing NFTs and the metaverse. For example, patients utilize NFTs to schedule online sessions or access specialized virtual clinic spaces, resulting in a more personalized and engaging experience.
6. Personalized Health Experiences: VR/AR avatars enhance the realism and personalization of remote consultations, minimizing the need for in-person interactions. Avatar-based interactions with physicians can improve patients' understanding of the informed consent procedure.
7. Training and Simulation for Healthcare Professionals: Research has mostly focused on creating healthcare solutions for teaching and training, including metaverse components like AR and VR. VR training was utilized to equip medical staff and rescue workers to tackle bioterrorism threats.
8. Support for Research and Clinical Trials: NFTs can assist patient recruitment for clinical trials by offering a secure and reliable way to handle authorization and involvement. Patients will be rewarded through NFTs to facilitate their involvement, and it acts as a digital record of their involvement in research and trials.
9. Creating Unique Medical Resources: Medical practitioners make use of NFTs to develop unique teaching aids, such as interactive simulations and

e-learning sessions. These resources can be shared or sold, opening up new revenue sources for healthcare professionals (Figure 13.7).

13.4.1 Case Study: Claustrophobia Exposure Therapy

This case study examines the integration and practical uses of NFTs and the metaverse to gain a thorough comprehension of the interaction process between these two technologies. With a focus on ownership, digital assets, and user interactions in the metaverse, this case study will shed light on the application of NFTs in virtual environments. Owing to a phobia of enclosed places like tunnels, elevators, and MRI machines, claustrophobia is an anxiety disorder with a significant impact on a large fraction of the world's population. Conventional treatment methods have significant results but are restricted by their failure to provide a controlled environment for the treatment. NFT was proposed to address the difficulties in the conventional exposure therapy process. An NFT-based approach could break through the barriers of contemporary claustrophobic exposure treatments (Musamih et al., 2024). Also, this approach proposes an innovative approach to cross the boundaries of conventional VR-based therapies. Musamih et al. explained numerous classical techniques used in exposure therapy for claustrophobia.

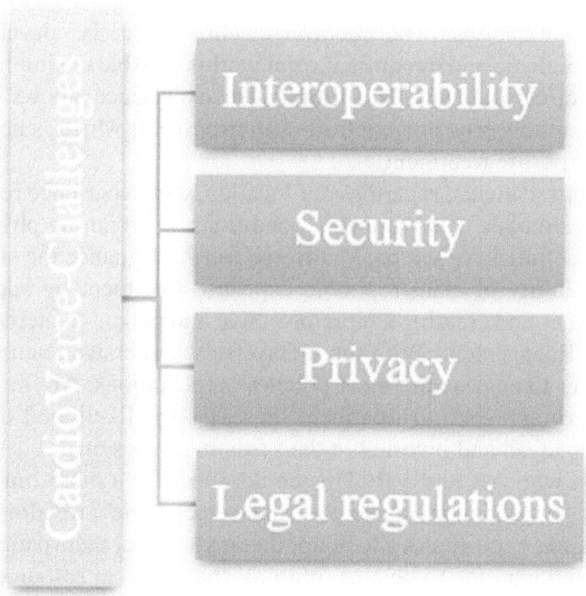

FIGURE 13.7 Advantages of integrating metaverse with NFT.

1. Cognitive Behavioral Therapy (CBT): This therapy includes systematic meetings in which patients discuss their issues through progressive exposure. Traditional CBT has limitations with respect to the necessity for physical presence and may not furnish the deep immersion required for individuals to truly engage with their anxieties.
2. Virtual Reality Exposure Therapy: While VR is beneficial in lowering anxiety and avoidance behaviors, standard VR systems are costly and lack the depth of study required to treat a wide range of illnesses. Conventional VR fails to provide sufficient flexibility based on the patient's demands.
3. Limited Scenarios: Limited exposure to therapy doesn't adequately prepare individuals for real-world situations. The scarcity of variability in therapeutic situations makes it harder to employ treatment in real life.
4. Monitoring and Feedback: Traditional approaches may have limitations in terms of real-time patient development and feedback. This makes it difficult for therapists to adapt treatment programs depending on individual reactions during therapy sessions.
5. Accessibility Issues: Many traditional approaches need physical presence in a professional environment, which can be challenging for certain individuals, like those with mobility challenges or who live in distant places. This may limit the scope and efficacy of exposure treatment.

According to Musamih et al., the metaverse facilitates an immersive setting for therapy in several ways:

- Realistic Simulations: The metaverse allows for the development of extremely realistic and dynamic virtual worlds capable of simulating claustrophobic circumstances. This immersive experience allows patients to address their concerns in a controlled environment, which is necessary for effective exposure treatment.
- Accessibility: Patients, regardless of location, can experience realistic situations that simulate claustrophobic conditions, overcoming physical limits and resource-intensive setups. Metaverse and XR enhance the effectiveness and accessibility of claustrophobic exposure treatment by addressing its specific issues and creating a more inventive and patient-centered approach.
- Enhanced Engagement: With the metaverse's immersive features, patients find it easier to engage and meet policies' expectations. An immersive and participatory approach to treatment increases the likelihood that patients will stay engaged and invested in their treatment sessions.
- Integration with AR and VR: This could allow for a more immersive and interactive environment inside the metaverse while providing therapists with real-time opportunities to adapt therapy to meet their patients' needs.
- Safe Environment for Exposure: With all the different resources available in the metaverse, patients can achieve effective treatment of their psychological problems as they can tackle their fears more safely and protectively.

The architecture proposed by Musamih et al. for improving claustrophobia exposure therapy consists of several important components and layers that function together to provide an integrated and engaging healing experience, as illustrated in Figure 13.8.

The benefits of combining blockchain and NFTs in exposure treatment for claustrophobia are stated below:

- Data Security and Privacy: Patients could obtain greater control over their health records, which in turn increases their willingness to contribute more data. NFTs incentivize persons to proactively involve themselves in therapy by delivering valuable benefits within the healthcare ecosystem.
- Incentivizing Participation: This opens up the door to rewards (NFTs) to motivate individuals to engage more in these therapies. NFTs act as value providers within the healthcare ecosystem, thus generating user engagement and participation. This generates an emotional connection between the platform and its users.
- Transparency and Trust: NFTs allow for transparent ownership and transactions, reducing the need for trusted third parties. Blockchain and NFT-based metaverse systems offer genuine and immersive claustrophobic settings as well as a safe and decentralized platform for exposure therapy.
- Real-Time Monitoring and Insights: Real-time tracking of the patient's status and data-driven insights allow improved therapeutic effectiveness. Traditional approaches frequently lack this capacity, which might negatively impact treatment outcomes (Figure 13.9).

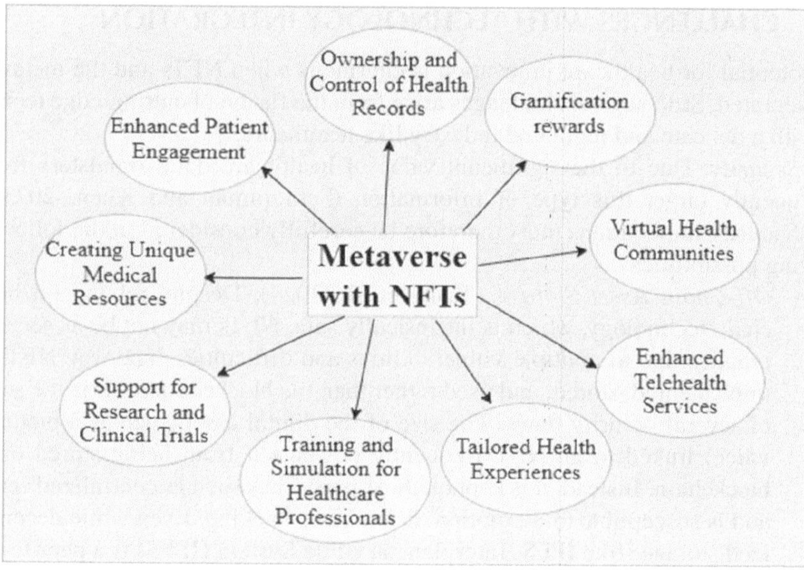

FIGURE 13.8 System architecture of case study.

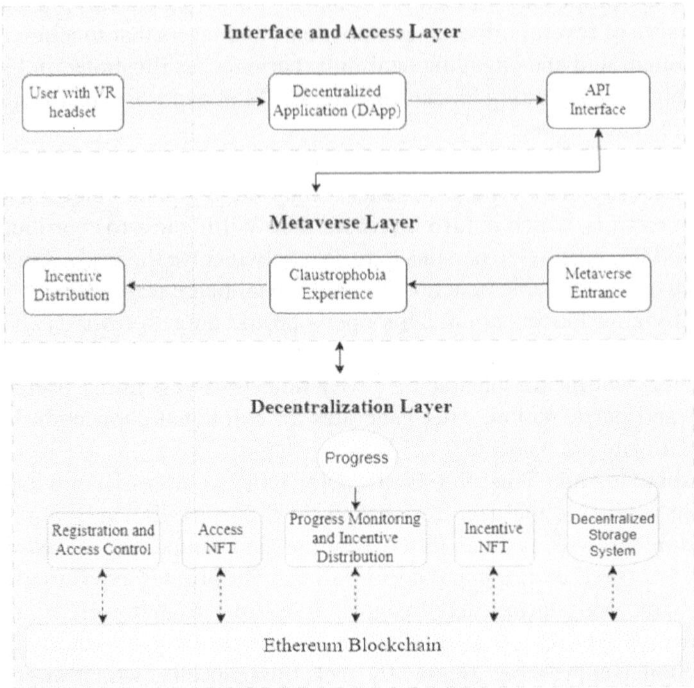

FIGURE 13.9 Challenges of integrating NFT and metaverse.

13.5 CHALLENGES WITH TECHNOLOGY INTEGRATION

The potential for healthcare innovation is enormous when NFTs and the metaverse are integrated. Still, several challenges arise from the fusion of cutting-edge technology with a delicate and regulated industry like healthcare.

- *Security*: Due to the significant value of healthcare data, fraudsters frequently target this type of information (Sethuraman and Khan, 2023). Security implications must therefore be carefully considered in the following possibilities:
  - *Off-Chain Asset Storage* (Tsang et al., 2024): Despite relying on blockchain technology, which is intrinsically safe, NFTs may not be as secure in practice due to multiple vulnerabilities and difficulties. The way NFTs are implemented, stored, and used rather than the blockchain itself is the source of several security flaws. The size of the digital asset (such as a picture or video) linked to an NFT frequently prevents it from being stored on the blockchain. Instead, it is kept on third-party sites such as centralized servers and is susceptible to disruption, deletion, or hacking. Even while decentralized storage (like IPFS: Interplanetary File System (IPFS) is a peer-to-peer (P2P) network and decentralized protocol that is intended for distributed

file and data storage, sharing, and access (Psaras and Dias, 2020) is more secure, files could become unreadable if the nodes that store them go down.

- *Smart Contract Risks* (Mezquita et al., 2019): NFTs are governed by smart contracts, and faults in their coding may result in security vulnerabilities. Forgery or the exposure of sensitive patient information could result from a compromised NFT that represents medical records. Inadequately drafted contracts can be used by hackers to steal NFTs. For instance, NFT project assets have been depleted by vulnerabilities like re-entrancy attacks. In this type of intrusion, an intruder takes advantage of the state of a contract and possibly drains funds or changes data by repeatedly calling it before its first execution is concluded (Moubarak et al., 2018). Due to the immutability of blockchains, smart contract bugs are challenging to resolve.
- *Phishing Attempts*: Phishing attacks use phony websites, emails, or messages that appear to be authentic NFT platforms that deceive users into divulging their private keys or seed phrases (Yang et al., 2024). A hacker can steal NFTs and cryptocurrency if they get access to the user's wallet. Users need to keep the private keys of their wallets safe. Access to NFTs is permanently lost if the private key or seed phrase is lost. Keys are susceptible to theft when they are stored carelessly (for example, by being written down in an unsafe manner). Hacks could result in impersonation, NFT theft, or monetary losses on both the metaverse platforms and blockchain infrastructure.
- *Plagiarism and Counterfeiting*: Anyone can create an NFT, regardless of whether they are the original content owner or not (Garcia et al., 2024). For instance, a digital piece of art could be copied and minted as an NFT without the owner's consent. Unknowingly buying fake NFTs is a possibility for buyers. Having an NFT does not entitle one to the digital asset's copyright or intellectual property. Customers often just own the token associated with a digital asset, even if they may believe they have all rights to it. If the item is used in ways that the creator did not intend, disputes may result. For patients and physicians, the metaverse may employ avatars and virtual profiles, which increases the possibility of impersonation or abuse in the event that authentication procedures are inadequate.

Best Practices for improving NFT security:

To reduce reliance on external storage, keep as much data as you can on the blockchain itself.

Before starting NFT projects, use expert audits to find weaknesses. Hardware wallets are an additional layer of security.

Don't share seed phrases or private keys.

Buy NFTs exclusively from platforms and creators who have been verified.

- Scalability: Metaverse apps demand massive storage capacity, bandwidth, and processing power. It's possible that healthcare organizations, particularly smaller ones, lack the infrastructure necessary for efficient scaling. Healthcare NFT processing could be delayed by the transaction speed and throughput constraints of current blockchains, such as Ethereum. Challenges with interoperability encompass smooth data transfer between NFTs, the metaverse, and state-of-the-art systems like electronic health records (EHRs) (Evans, 2016). Platform incompatibilities, for instance, could result from a lack of standardized data formats (Priya et al., 2023). For quicker and less expensive transactions, employ Layer-2 protocols like Polygon, Optimism, or Arbitrum. By combining several transactions into one, these solutions minimize the overall strain on the primary blockchain network. Transactions involving NFT and medical data tokens can be managed off-chain before being finalized on the main blockchain, which reduces expenses and bottlenecks. Blockchain transactions consume a lot of energy, especially with regard to Proof-of-Work (PoW) (Manivannan et al., 2024; Zhang and Chan, 2020), which raises questions about their effects on the environment and operational expenses. Best practices for improving scalability are as follows:

Leverage Layer-2 scaling solutions (e.g., Polygon, Optimism (Gangwal et al., 2023) for faster and cheaper transactions.
Adopt healthcare interoperability standards (e.g., HL7, FHIR, DICOM) for smooth system integration.
Utilize trusted cloud infrastructure like AWS, Azure, etc. for scalable virtual environments in healthcare.
Implement upgradable smart contracts using proxy patterns for future-proofing.
Leverage high-throughput blockchain networks like Solana, Avalanche, etc. for faster and scalable transactions.

Financial Constraints: Investments in virtual reality (VR)/augmented reality (AR) equipment, integration of blockchain, and medical staff training are necessary to set up a metaverse-based healthcare infrastructure. There may be significant costs associated with blockchain transactions, such as NFT transfers or minting. It may become fiscally unfeasible for standard healthcare operations as a result. The arbitrary charges associated with Ethereum may make minting NFTs for patient data storage unaffordable for a small clinic. Best Practices for reducing cost:

To reduce transaction volume and related expenses, mint NFTs in batches.
Use cloud computing services (AWS, Google Cloud, Azure) to access scalable and adaptable resources, only paying for what is utilized.
For jobs like patient record administration, data verification, and NFT minting, use automated workflows.
Reduce development expenses by integrating with pre-existing healthcare systems (such as EHRs and EMRs) rather than starting from scratch.

- Compatibility with Legacy Systems: For patient management, healthcare institutions frequently rely on legacy systems. It is difficult to integrate these with NFT frameworks or metaverse platforms. For instance, costly and technically complex middleware solutions may be needed to sync NFT-based medical records with conventional EHR systems. Interoperability may be challenging due to the possibility of distinct blockchain networks and metaverse platforms (such as Meta and Decentral) and operating independently. It can be difficult to guarantee that the metaverse experience is consistent across devices with varying capabilities (such as smartphones versus VR headsets).

Best Practices for Ensuring Compatibility:

Utilize healthcare standards like Fast Healthcare Interoperability Resources (FHIR), Digital Imaging and Communications in Medicine (DICOM), and Health Level 7 (HL7) to facilitate data sharing between NFTs, healthcare systems, and the metaverse.

To handle various blockchain ecosystems, employ cross-chain bridges or oracles that facilitate the smooth transfer of NFTs or digital assets between blockchains, improving interoperability.

Employ commonly used metadata platforms (such as ERC-1155 and ERC-721) to guarantee interoperability with different metaverse systems.

Create extendable NFT metadata so that it may be updated and contain a variety of medical information (such as credentials, certificates, and medical records).

- Concerns in Ethics and Regulations: Integrating patient data with NFTs and the metaverse raises concerns regarding adherence to laws such as the General Data Protection Regulation (GDPR) and the Health Insurance Portability and Accountability Act (HIPAA). For instance, HIPAA's stringent patient data security regulations or the GDPR's "right to be forgotten" could conflict with the decentralized storage of NFTs. Ownership concerns are raised by NFTs that depict medical imagery or health data. The ramifications of allowing access or transferring ownership through NFTs may not be completely understood by patients. Disparities in access or results could result from the unintentional introduction of biases in healthcare delivery via virtual platforms and blockchain technologies. Best Practices for Avoiding Concerns in Ethics and Regulations

Employ cryptographic methods (such as encryption and zero-knowledge proofs) to protect private medical information kept in NFTs and the metaverse.

Guarantee that consent is expressly given by patients and healthcare professionals for the metaverse and NFT platforms to gather, store, and share data.

To ensure accountability, implement audit trails that offer verifiable evidence of data access, sharing, and modification.

Follow established moral standards for blockchain and AI in healthcare, guaranteeing equity, justice, and openness.

Implement universal design principles to guarantee that everyone has fair access to online healthcare services.

Keep patients and healthcare professionals informed about regulatory framework changes and their effects on the usage of NFTs and the metaverse on a regular basis.

13.6 DATA PROTECTION LAWS

Although integrating NFTs and the metaverse in the healthcare industry has enormous promise for innovation, data security and adherence to pertinent data protection regulations must be maintained. Healthcare data is sensitive, thus patient information, medical records, and private data should be handled per existing privacy laws and ethical norms. Data protection regulations govern the gathering, processing, sharing, and storing of personal information. Since the metaverse and NFTs are new technologies that include digital data transfers, these regulations guarantee that private and sensitive health data is shielded from breaches, misuse, and illegal access. A thorough overview of data protection laws that must be considered when integrating NFTs and the metaverse into medical treatment is discussed below.

13.6.1 Health Insurance Portability and Accountability Act (HIPAA)

The United States passed the Health Insurance Portability and Accountability Act of 1996 (HIPAA), which restricts how healthcare organizations—referred to as covered entities—may utilize protected health information (PHI). HIPAA, officially known as Public Law 104–191, aims to lower healthcare costs by standardizing the electronic transmission of financial and administrative transactions. It also provides ongoing health insurance coverage for employees who lose or change jobs. Additional objectives include enhancing access to long-term care services and health insurance, as well as preventing fraud, misuse, and waste in healthcare delivery and health insurance (Figure 13.10).

Any of the following could be a covered entity:

- Health plans: This category includes business health plans, health insurance firms, etc.
- Clearing houses for healthcare: Any organization that converts nonstandard health data from another organization into a standard format. Clinics, pharmacies, dentists, doctors, and other medical professionals are included in this category.

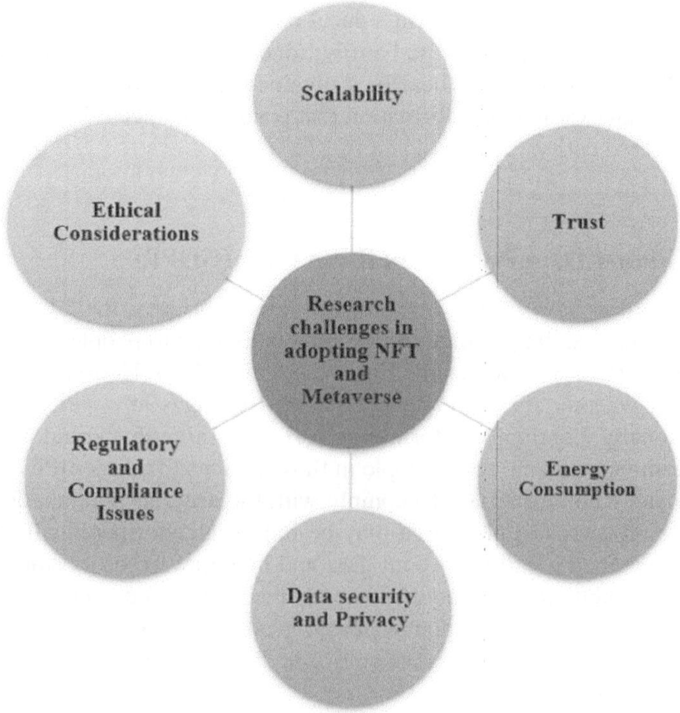

FIGURE 13.10 HIPAA principles of data protection.

The Office for Civil Rights (OCR) enforces HIPAA as it lacks a formal certification or certifying organization. The Transactions and Code Sets (TCS), Security as well as Privacy Rule, Breach Notification, Unique Identifiers, and Omnibus Final are the several rule sections of the HIPAA Regulation. Implementing technical, physical, and administrative safeguards is demanded under the HIPAA Rule of Security. It also requires documentation of procedures similar to those of the HIPAA Privacy Rule, along with other organizational requirements.

13.6.1.1 Which Information Is Covered under HIPAA?

All PHI that is stored or sent by a covered business is protected under the HIPAA Privacy Rule. PHI comprises the following, albeit it is not exclusive to—an individual's name, Social Security number (SSN), location, date of birth (DOB), biometric data identifiers, or other personally identifiable information (PII); their physical or mental health condition, past, present, or future; any care they have received; and details about previous, current, or forthcoming payments for the treatment that can be used to recognize the patient. Medical bills and consultation reports, laboratory reports, etc., are specific instances of PHI. The following are excluded from PHI:

Employment documents, including educational records, and other documents covered by or specified by the Family Educational Rights and Privacy Act (FERPA). Blood pressure/heartbeat obtained from a consumer smart care device is an example of information that is not PHI since it is not disclosed to a covered entity.

13.6.2 General Data Protection Regulation (GDPR)

Among the hardest laws in the world regarding data privacy, the GDPR applies to all businesses that handle personal information belonging to people in the European Economic Area (EEA) as well as the European Union (EU) (Hoofnagle et al., 2019). Regardless of whether they operate (EU/UK), it engages any entity that aims or gathers personally identifiable information (PII—anything that could be utilized to readily determine a person) from people in those nations (Tikkinen-Piri et al.,. 2018; Chellappan and Kannan, 2021). To comply with the criteria, organizations need to have specific processes in place that may be implemented. Specifically, exercising greater caution when handling patient data and being aware of its storage location and processing method. This holds for both the public and commercial sectors, including clinics and hospitals, dental offices, pharmacies, assisted living facilities, diagnostic labs, online pharmacies, and any other business or institution that handles health-related data.

13.6.2.1 Concept of Sensitive Data and Criteria for Processing

The GDPR classifies "sensitive data" as personal information handled in the healthcare industry. Consequently, there are even stricter requirements for its protection, and GDPR specifically refers to three types of health data (Brasher, 2018):

1) Health Information: Specific information on a person's physical or mental well-being, such as the usage of health cards or services, which provide details about their current state of health.
2) Inherited Data: Information about inherited or accumulated genetic traits of an individual that supply particular information about that person's physique or health and which result, specifically, from an examination of the biological specimen taken from the individual.
3) Biometrics: Personal information obtained through specific technical analysis related to an individual's biological, physiological, or mental traits, such as face or dactyloscopic photographs.

Data subjects have additional rights under the GDPR. The most significant one for the healthcare industry is the right to access, which enables individuals to obtain their processed health data, also referred to as subject access requests.

Organizations must protect PII and give documentation of the procedures they use to do so under the GDPR. The following should be covered in the documented steps:

- Consent: Organizations must issue a fresh request for consent to individuals if their data is used for a new purpose. When it comes to consent, the GDPR forbids the use of ambiguous terms and conditions and mandates that the procedure for withdrawing consent be as simple as that for giving it.
- Notifications of Security Breaches: Companies have 72 hours to inform all data subjects of a security breach via phone, email, or public notice.
- Right to Be Forgotten: Organizations are required to immediately delete PII at an individual's request and stop further distribution of that data unless there is a legitimate cause to keep it.
- Right to Access: Businesses have to inform citizens how their PII is used.
- Privacy by Architecture: Businesses are only permitted to process data that is necessary to run their operations.
- Data Protection Officer (DPO): To supervise the GDPR's implementation, organizations are required to designate a DPO. This person guards against abuse, illegal access, and other security lapses involving personal information.

A DPO must be appointed by any organization, regardless of size (Cliza, 2018)—It is a public entity or authority.

- Its primary functions include data processing processes that necessitate extensive, consistent, and methodical data subject monitoring.
- Processing unique data classifications and/or personal information of convictions for crimes and offenses on a very big scale are its main functions (Figure 13.11).

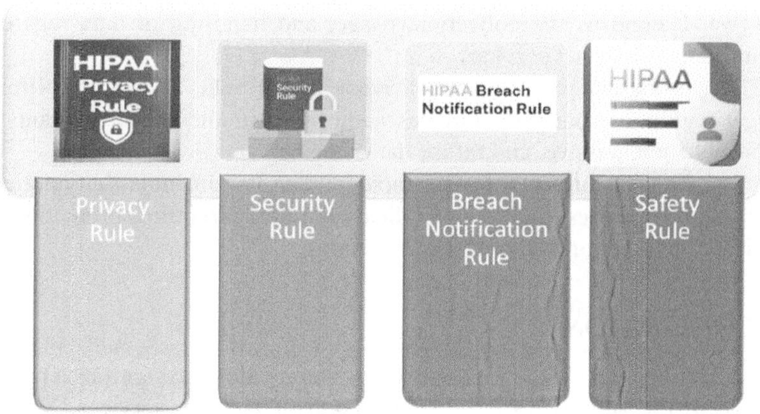

FIGURE 13.11 GDPR principles of data protection.

13.6.3 Comparison between GDPR and HIPAA Compliance

Which sector and jurisdiction each regulation pertains to is the most obvious distinction among these laws (Tovino, 2016; Oakley, 2023). The following are three further distinctions between GDPR and HIPAA:

- Consent: Under HIPAA, PHI could be shared to a specific extent without a patient's permission. For instance, physicians might disclose PHI to another practitioner for therapeutic purposes. However, consent is perpetually appropriate, particularly while treating individuals.
- Data Breaches: According to the HIPAA notification rule, insured companies and business collaborators must inform affected parties of breaches. If the incident affects more than 500 individuals, the firm has 60 days from the date to report it to the OCR and any affected parties. The magnitude of a breach is irrelevant under the GDPR. Article 33 of the GDPR necessitates firms to inform breaches to the appropriate managerial levels within the first 72 hours of the occurrence.
- Right to Exclude: HIPAA prohibits the alteration or deletion of medical records and other personal data. The right to be excluded, which is granted by the GDPR, enables individuals to ask an employer to remove the PHI.

13.6.4 Other Relevant Laws

Other data protection rules and regulations in place globally to protect private information include:

- Gramm–Leach–Bliley (GLBA) Act: The United States (US) law safeguards private financial information and mandates that organizations maintain strong security measures and reveal their data-sharing policies.
- Children's Online Privacy Protection (COPPA) Act (Stoilova et al., 2021): A regulation in the US that protects the information of children less than twelve. It controls the collection, usage, and handling of data regarding children via Internet services.
- CCPA, or California Consumer Privacy Act (Bonta, 2022): A California legal regulation that gives citizens authority over their data. It grants the ability to see, remove, and refuse data sharing.
- Act of 2000 on Information Technology: The law in India that applies to all body corporates, including medical facilities. It requires protections for private information and online transactions.

13.7 CONCLUSION

The incorporation of NFTs and the metaverse into healthcare signifies a revolutionary change in the administration and provision of medical services. These tools promote creative ideas in telemedicine and medical education, improve patient participation, and expedite data administration. However, strong data protection and regulatory compliance are essential for the effective implementation of these digital solutions. Healthcare stakeholders need to keep up with new developments in this field and deal with the challenges brought on by these technological breakthroughs. The healthcare sector could fully realize the potential of these digital advances by investigating practical applications and following best practices.

REFERENCES

Abdulmalek, S., Nasir, A., Jabbar, W.A., Almuhaya, M.A., Bairagi, A.K., Khan, M.A.-M., Kee, S.-H.: Iot-based healthcare-monitoring system towards improving quality of life: A review. *Healthcare* **10**, 1993 (2022). MDPI

Aimedis: Where healthcare meets future. https://aimedis.com/. Accessed on 2024 March 24

Albawi, S., Bayat, O., Al-Azawi, S., Ucan, O.N.: Social touch gesture recognition using convolutional neural network. *Computational Intelligence and Neuroscience* **2018**(1), 6973103 (2018)

Bajkoti, A.S., Tiwari, S., Ranjan, T., Bisht, R.S., Mittal, A.: Role of quantum computing and metaverse in the field of healthcare and medicine. In: *2023 5th International Conference on Inventive Research in Computing Applications (ICIRCA)*, pp. 306–311 (2023). IEEE

Barioni, R.R., Figueiredo, L., Cunha, K., Teichrieb, V.: Human pose tracking from RGB inputs. In: *2018 20th Symposium on Virtual and Augmented Reality (SVR)*, pp. 176–182 (2018). IEEE

Bonta, R.: *California Consumer Privacy Act (CCPA)*. State of California Department of Justice. https://oag. ca. gov/privacy/ccpa (2022)

Brasher, E.A.: Addressing the failure of anonymization: guidance from the European Union's general data protection regulation. *Columbia Business Law Review* 209–253 (2018)

Chellappan, K., Kannan, M.J.: Pii classification and applicability in personal data protection bill 2019. *GIS-Zeitschrift fu¨ Geoinformatik* **1**(8), 1417–1424 (2021)

Cliza, M.-C., Spataru-Negura, L.-C.: The general data protection regulation: what does the public authorities and bodies need to know and to do? the rise of the data protection officer. *Juridical Tribune Journal= Tribuna Juridica* **8**(2), 489–501 (2018)

Colbert, G.B., Venegas-Vera, A.V., Lerma, E.V.: Utility of telemedicine in the covid-19 era. *Reviews in Cardiovascular Medicine* **21**(4), 583–587 (2020)

El Khatib, M., Hamidi, S., Al Ameeri, I., Al Zaabi, H., Al Marqab, R.: Digital disruption and big data in healthcare-opportunities and challenges. *ClinicoEconomics and Outcomes Research*, **14**, 563–574 (2022)

El Saddik, A., Ghaboura, S.: The integration of ChatGPT with the metaverse for medical consultations. *IEEE Consumer Electronics Magazine* (3), 6–15 (2023)

Evans, R.S.: Electronic health records: then, now, and in the future. *Yearbook of Medical Informatics* **25**(S 01), 48–61 (2016)

Gangwal, A., Gangavalli, H.R., Thirupathi, A.: A survey of layer-two blockchain protocols. *Journal of Network and Computer Applications* **209**, 103539 (2023)

Garcıa, R., Cediel, A., Teixid´o, M., Gil, R.: Semantics and non-fungible tokens for copyright management on the metaverse and beyond. *ACM Transactions on Multimedia Computing, Communications and Applications* **20**(7), 1–20 (2024)

Hanna, B., Chatterjee, N.A., Akoum, N.: Ekg as a Non-fungible Token (NFT): a schema for storing healthcare data on the public blockchain. *Cardiovascular Digital Health Journal* **3**(4), 13–14 (2022)

Hoofnagle, C.J., Van Der Sloot, B., Borgesius, F.Z.: The European Union general data protection regulation: what it is and what it means. *Information & Communications Technology Law* **28**(1), 65–98 (2019)

Javed, A.R., Sarwar, M.U., Beg, M.O., Asim, M., Baker, T., Tawfik, H.: A collaborative healthcare framework for shared healthcare plan with ambient intelligence. *Human-centric Computing and Information Sciences* **10**(1), 40 (2020)

Kaddoura, S., Haraty, R.A., Al Kontar, K., Alfandi, O.: A parallelized database damage assessment approach after cyberattack for healthcare systems. *Future Internet* **13**(4), 90 (2021)

Li, Y., Gunasekeran, D.V., RaviChandran, N., Tan, T.F., Ong, J.C.L., Thirunavukarasu, A.J., Polascik, B.W., Habash, R., Khaderi, K., Ting, D.S.: The next generation of healthcare ecosystem in the metaverse. *Biomedical Journal* **47**(3), 100679 (2024)

Maier, J., Weiherer, M., Huber, M., Palm, C.: Imitating human soft tissue on basis of a dual-material 3d print using a support-filled metamaterial to provide bimanual haptic for a hand surgery training system. *Quantitative Imaging in Medicine and Surgery* **9**(1), 30 (2019)

Majeed, U., Khan, L.U., Yaqoob, I., Kazmi, S.A., Salah, K., Hong, C.S.: Blockchain for iot-based smart cities: Recent advances, requirements, and future challenges. *Journal of Network and Computer Applications* **181**, 103007 (2021)

Manivannan, A., Sethuraman, S.C., Vimala Sudhakaran, D.P.: Mcaptcha: Replacing captchas with rate limiters to improve security and accessibility. *Communications of the ACM* **67**(10), 70–80 (2024)

Metaverse: Defining The Metaverse Today. https://www.forbes.com/sites/ cathy-hackl/2021/05/02. Accessed on 2021 May 2

Mezquita, Y., Valdeolmillos, D., Gonz´alez-Briones, A., Prieto, J., Corchado, J.M.: Legal aspects and emerging risks in the use of smart contracts based on blockchain. Knowledge Management in Organizations: 14th International Conference, KMO 2019, Zamora, Spain, July 15–18, 2019, Proceedings 14, pp. 525–535 (2019). Springer

Moubarak, J., Filiol, E., Chamoun, M.: On blockchain security and relevant attacks. In: *2018 IEEE Middle East and North Africa Communications Conference (MENACOMM)*, pp. 1–6 (2018). IEEE

Mughal, H., Javed, A.R., Rizwan, M., Almadhor, A.S., Kryvinska, N.: Parkinson's disease management via wearable sensors: a systematic review. *IEEE Access* **10**, 35219–35237 (2022)

Musamih, A., Salah, K., Jayaraman, R., Seghier, M., Hamdan, H., Ellaham, S., Omar, M.: Enhancing claustrophobia exposure therapy: A blockchain and NFT-enabled metaverse approach. *Computers in Human Behavior* **160**, 108364 (2024)

Nebula Genomics: Health and Ancestry? https://nebula.org/. Accessed on 2024 March 24

Oakley, A.: HIPAA, HIPPA, or HIPPO: What really is the health insurance portability and accountability act? *Biotechnology Law Report* **42**(6), 306–318 (2023)

Prakash, R., Nayar, G.R., Thomas, T.: Security risk assessment of metaverse based health-care systems based on common vulnerabilities and exposures (CVE). In: *2023 IEEE International Conference on Recent Advances in Systems Science and Engineering (RASSE)*, pp. 1–10 (2023). IEEE

Prat, N.: Augmented analytics. *Business & Information Systems Engineering* **61**, 375–380 (2019)

Priya, V.D., Chakkaravarthy, S.S., Chekuri, A.K., Johnson, S.: *Knowledge-twin: Addressing the Current Challenges of Knowledge Management in Industry 4.0 Using Digital Twins* (2023). Nova Science Publishers, Inc

Psaras, Y., Dias, D.: The interplanetary file system and the filecoin network. In: *2020 50th Annual IEEE-IFIP International Conference on Dependable Systems and Networks-Supplemental Volume (DSN-S)*, pp. 80–80 (2020). IEEE

Rajabion, L., Shaltooki, A.A., Taghikhah, M., Ghasemi, A., Badfar, A.: Healthcare big data processing mechanisms: The role of cloud computing. *International Journal of Information Management* **49**, 271–289 (2019)

Secundo, G., Toma, A., Schiuma, G., Passiante, G.: Knowledge transfer in open innovation: a classification framework for healthcare ecosystems. *Business Process Management Journal* **25**(1), 144–163 (2019)

Shvetsov, A.V., Alsamhi, S.H.: When holographic communication meets metaverse: Applications, challenges and future trends. *IEEE Access* **12**, 197488–197515 (2024)

Singh, S.K., El-Kassar, A.-N.: Role of big data analytics in developing sustainable capabilities. *Journal of Cleaner Production* **213**, 1264–1273 (2019)

Skalidis, I., Fournier, S., Hammilos, M., Kaldasch, M., Idrissi, B.E., Kirsch, M., Muller, O., Skalidis, E., Maurizi, N.: Feasibility of using the metaverse as telecardiology platform: remote follow-up of a patient with vasospastic angina. *Canadian Journal of Cardiology* **38**(11), 1768–1769 (2022)

Skalidis, I., Fournier, S., Skalidis, E., Maurizi, N.: *Virtual Hospitals and Digital Doctors: How Far Are We from the CardioVerse?* (2023b). Oxford University Press

Skalidis, I., Muller, O., Fournier, S.: Cardioverse: the cardiovascular medicine in the era of metaverse. *Trends in Cardiovascular Medicine* **33**(8), 471–476 (2023a)

Somayaji, S.R.K.: The metaverse and its related technologies in telesurgery in healthcare 5.0: A case study. In: *The Metaverse for the Healthcare Industry*, pp. 257–274 (2024). Springer

Sounderajah, V., Patel, V., Varatharajan, L., Harling, L., Normahani, P., Symons, J., Barlow, J., Darzi, A., Ashrafian, H.: Are disruptive innovations recognised in the healthcare literature? a systematic review. *BMJ Innovations* **7**(1), 208–216, (2021)

Stasolla, F., Di Gioia, M., Messina, I., Treglia, F., Passaro, A., Zullo, A., Dragone, M.: Assessing and recovering Alzheimer's disease: a comparative analysis of standard neuropsychological approaches and virtual reality interventions with the use of digital storytelling. *Frontiers in Psychology* **15**, 1406167 (2024)

Stoilova, M., Nandagiri, R., Livingstone, S.: Children's understanding of personal data and privacy online – a systematic evidence mapping. *Information, Communication & Society* **24**(4), 557–575 (2021)

Teo, Z.L., Ting, D.S.W.: Non-fungible tokens for the management of health data. *Nature Medicine* **29**(2), 287–288 (2023)

Tikkinen-Piri, C., Rohunen, A., Markkula, J.: Eu general data protection regulation: changes and implications for personal data collecting companies. *Computer Law & Security Review* **34**(1), 134–153 (2018)

Tovino, S.A.: The HIPAA privacy rule and the EU GDPR: illustrative comparisons. *Seton Hall Law Review* **47**, 973 (2016)

Tsang, Y.P., Lee, C.K.M., Zhang, K., Wu, C.-H., Ip, W.: On-chain and offchain data management for blockchain-internet of things: A multi-agent deep reinforcement learning approach. *Journal of Grid Computing* **22**(1), 16 (2024)

Van Uden-Kraan, C.F., Drossaert, C.H., Taal, E., Smit, W.M., Moens, H.J.B., Laar, M.A.: Determinants of engagement in face-to-face and online patient support groups. *Journal of Medical Internet Research* **13**(4), 1718 (2011)

VS, D.P., Sethuraman, S.C., Khan, M.K.: Container security: precaution levels, mitigation strategies, and research perspectives. *Computers & Security* **135**(3), 103490 (2023)

Wang, Y., Zhu, M., Chen, X., Liu, R., Ge, J., Song, Y., Yu, G.: The application of metaverse in healthcare. *Frontiers in Public Health* **12**, 1420367 (2024)

World Health Organization (WHO): Health Systems Resilience Toolkit: A WHO Global Public Health Good to Support Building and Strengthening of Sustainable Health Systems Resilience in Countries with Various Contexts (2023). https://www.who.int/publications/i/item/9789240048751. Accessed on 2023-1228

Wosik, J., Fudim, M., Cameron, B., Gellad, Z.F., Cho, A., Phinney, D., Curtis, S., Roman, M., Poon, E.G., Ferranti, J., *et al.*: Telehealth transformation: Covid-19 and the rise of virtual care. *Journal of the American Medical Informatics Association* **27**(6), 957–962 (2020)

Wu, J., Gao, G.: Edu-metaverse: Internet education form with fusion of virtual and reality. In: *2022 8th International Conference on Humanities and Social Science Research (ICHSSR 2022)*, pp. 1082–1085 (2022). Atlantis Press

Yang, J., Liu, J., Lin, D., Wu, J., Huang, B., Li, Q., Zheng, Z.: Who stole my NFT? investigating web3 NFT phishing scams on ethereum. *IEEE Transactions on Information Forensics and Security* **19**, 9301–9314 (2024)

Zhang, L., Li, F., Wang, P., Su, R., Chi, Z.: A blockchain-assisted massive IoT data collection intelligent framework. *IEEE Internet of Things Journal* **9**(16), 14708–14722 (2021)

Zhang, R., Chan, W.K.V.: Evaluation of energy consumption in block-chains with proof of work and proof of stake. *Journal of Physics: Conference Series* **1584**, 012023 (2020)

Zhang, Y., Shyu, C.-R., Hong, S., Li, P., Zhang, L.: Self-sovereign identity empowered non-fungible patient tokenization for health information exchange using blockchain technology. *Computers in Biology and Medicine* **157**, 106778 (2023)

14 The Future of XAI and Digital Transformation in Healthcare

Gokhan Turan

14.1 INTRODUCTION

The technology has compelled the healthcare sector to undergo a significant restructuring. Digital transformation refers to deploying artificial intelligence, the Internet of Things, big data, and blockchain technology to improve healthcare processes from a patient-centric perspective. These technologies help improve the quality of healthcare services and strengthen the sector's operational efficiency and financial sustainability (Topol, 2019). In particular, explainable artificial intelligence (XAI) offers a paradigm-shifting opportunity to use AI in healthcare. XAI better addresses the issues of healthcare trust and accountability (Eke & Shuib, 2024). Unlike traditional AI, XAI can be adopted on a larger scale in medicine since it is more of a system of trust than a black box. XAI improves transparency and accountability by adhering to ethical standards. Additionally, XAI is more effective and will make diagnostic and treatment processes more efficient since it can explain clinical reasons for decisions (Amann et al., 2020).

The demographic shifts and pressure on healthcare systems are driving the sector's digital transformation. As the population ages and chronic diseases proliferate, demand for more healthcare services increases, leading to an innovation deficit (WHO, 2020). There is also a shortage of trained professionals and rising costs that limit the functionality of existing systems. This transformation seeks to meet these challenges by enhancing system functioning and benefiting individual patients (Marx & Padmanabhan, 2020). This shift impacts many structural elements of the system. For instance, mobile health devices give patients a more active role in their healthcare management. At the same time, AI-powered medical imaging systems increase the likelihood of early diagnosis by enabling doctors to detect diseases from images more accurately (El-Rashidy et al., 2021). Electronic health record (EHR) systems make it easier for physicians to share health records and save time. Moreover, telemedicine provides patients with access to specialists in remote areas with a shortage of healthcare providers (Hollingsworth, 2018).

Furthermore, ethical and societal issues associated with XAI and digital transformation must also be considered. One of the most controversial aspects of AI is

DOI: 10.1201/9781003605416-14

data privacy, security, and biased algorithms. Similar to other systems where ethical compliance and transparency standards are common practice, artificial intelligence systems within the European Union are also expected to follow these standards (EUR, 2021). That is why XAI is essential for technological innovation and legal and increasing ethical standards.

Research shows that AI-based healthcare solutions in diagnosis and treatment processes can significantly reduce error rates and improve individual patient outcomes. In addition, these predictions show that proactive and predictive healthcare systems for 2030 will be established and supported by technological transformation in healthcare services. The impact of artificial intelligence on data democratization will enable individuals to have more control over their health data, contributing to a more patient-centered structure in healthcare services.

This chapter examines the opportunities and challenges related to digital transformation and explainable artificial intelligence in healthcare systems. Furthermore, developing strategic recommendations for the sustainable implementation of these technologies will provide a deeper analysis of the future of healthcare.

14.2 DIGITAL TRANSFORMATION IN HEALTHCARE

Digital transformation describes strategically adopting digital technologies to increase the efficiency, accessibility, and innovation of businesses and services. In the Regulation of the European Programme on Digital Transformation No. 2021/694 of the European Parliament and of the Council, transformation is defined as making changes with digital technologies in businesses and public service sectors.

Digital transformation is a critical process that helps businesses grow in a competitive environment while maximizing operational performance. This process consists of four main components. The first component is "People and Experiences," which focuses on crafting better experiences for both customers and employees while delivering business processes with a people-centric focus. The second component is "Data and Technology." Technology and data transform a business into a modern entity, allowing information to be used in strategic planning via analytics. The third component is "Governance and Trust." Developing governance models that align with digital solutions, implementing a security policy, and trusting stakeholders are all essential. The fourth and final component is "Partnerships and New Business Models." This component aims to enhance organizations' adaptability and foster sustainable development through partnerships and new ventures. All four components are crucial for effectively implementing digital transformation in a company. The key elements of digital transformation are illustrated in Figure 14.1.

The creative and algorithmic data processing will improve the quality and efficiency of digitally integrated technologies in healthcare delivery. Digital healthcare enables patients to manage their health better and use tailored and easier-to-obtain healthcare services (Stoumpos et al., 2023). The provision of digital tools, such as access to online information sources and mobile applications, now enables patients to participate actively in the healthcare decision-making process. Individual health management is increased, but this transformation also affects the healthcare systems.

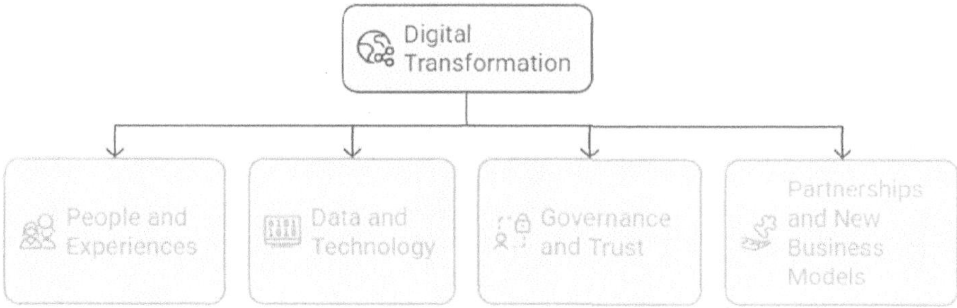

FIGURE 14.1 Foundational elements of digital transformation.

Patient-centered care morphs into a digital practice with the use of modern technologies. In this respect, healthcare mobile applications, remote patient monitoring systems, and telemedical solutions increase healthcare services' availability and contribute to improving their quality (Whitelaw et al., 2020). The implementation of active digital healthcare services enhances individual healthcare experiences and effective healthcare services by increasing the alliances of patient participation in the decision-making process.

14.2.1 Why Is Digital Transformation Needed in Healthcare?

The need for digital transformation in the healthcare sector stems from current challenges and the need to deliver healthcare services more effectively and efficiently. Increasing populations, aging societies, and the prevalence of chronic diseases are increasingly putting pressure on healthcare systems. In addition, increasing healthcare spending and the shortage of qualified healthcare professionals are critical issues that threaten sustainability (WHO, 2020). Current challenges in the health system are given in Figure 14.2.

- **Increasing Number of Patients**: The world's increasing elderly population and scoliosis rate are straining the capacity of health systems and increasing the demand for health services. This situation makes it difficult for existing resources to provide urgent and effective health services (OECD, 2021).
- **Cost Pressures**: The increase in health expenditures continues unabated due to the development of effective new technologies and the rise in drug costs. Traditional management of these expenses will not be sustainable.
- **Human Resource Shortages**: There are difficulties in obtaining sufficient human resources, especially qualified health personnel in special areas such as nursing, surgery, and patient management. This situation causes delays and quality problems in the provision of services (WHO, 2020).

Global digital transformation offers the opportunity to create a more sustainable, efficient, and patient-centered health system by offering innovative solutions to the

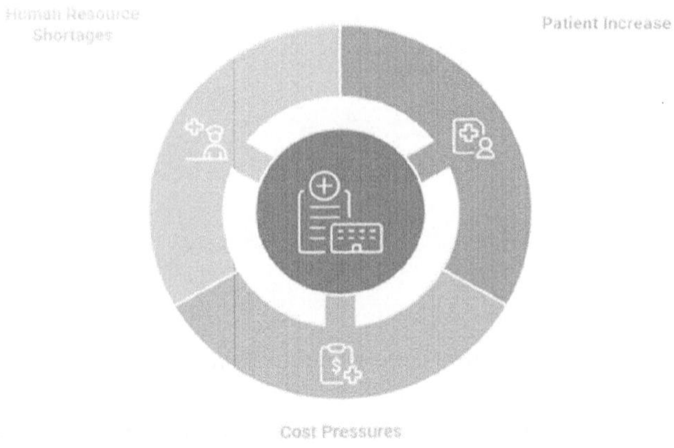

FIGURE 14.2 Challenges facing healthcare systems.

challenges encountered in health service delivery. Effective technology integration will not only alleviate current problems but also determine future health service standards.

14.2.2 Benefits of Digital Transformation in Healthcare

Digital transformation offers excellent opportunities for individuals and organizations in the healthcare sector. Integrating innovative technologies into healthcare delivery makes processes faster, more efficient, and patient-centered. These benefits include patient care, the operational processes of healthcare institutions, and improved performance throughout the healthcare system.

14.2.2.1 Benefits for Patients

- **Faster and More Accurate Diagnosis**: Digital health technologies play an important role in the early and accurate diagnosis of diseases. Artificial intelligence-supported medical imaging enables subtle details that doctors may overlook. For example, algorithms used for chest X-rays can save lives in many cases by early diagnosis of serious diseases such as cancer (Topol, 2019). In addition, technologies such as mobile health devices help monitor symptoms in real-time, accelerating the time to diagnosis.
- **Personalized Treatment**: Digital transformation increases patients' genetic and biomedical data analysis, allowing them to receive customized treatment plans. This development will enable patients to receive more effective treatments with their genetic structures and health history (Reddy et al., 2019).
- **Remote Patient Monitoring**: Remote patient monitoring systems allow patients to access medical services more efficiently. This development provides better access to healthcare for patients in rural areas as it eliminates

geographical limitations. They also help in the early detection of complications through continuous active data monitoring (OECD, 2021).

14.2.2.2 Benefits for Healthcare Institutions Operational Efficiency

Digital transformation helps enhance and refine the operational processes in healthcare institutions, making them more efficient and effective. Systems like electronic health records (EHRs) allow practitioners to obtain patient information within seconds. Thus, the EHR saves valuable time, as its users have reported (Kraus et al., 2021). In addition, the management of patient appointments and even resource allocation is improved with AI-powered scheduling.

- **Cost Reduction**: Avoid dubious medical procedures and redundant tests; one such strategy will invariably benefit healthcare institutions. The use of remote monitoring systems will cut down on other healthcare costs by decreasing the length of hospital stays. For instance, monitoring heart patients remotely can result in quicker treatment when problems are detected. Consequently, the need for intensive nursing will be reduced.
- **Decision Support through Data Analytics**: Artificial intelligence and big data analytics can significantly improve decision-making in healthcare institutions. Data analytics can enhance the allocation of hospital resources, staff scheduling, and patient flow management. This will revolutionize resource allocation and improve the quality of service (Topol, 2019).
- **Public Health and Epidemiological Monitoring**: Digital tools have transformed public health. For instance, during the pandemic, contact tracing applications and epidemiological modeling systems became essential in shaping government interventions. These techniques serve as rapid response devices to effectively reduce the spread of diseases (Whitelaw et al., 2020).
- **Reducing Barriers to Healthcare Access**: Expanding and improving health services through information and communication technologies opens new boundaries to a broader audience regardless of geographical and socio-economic hurdles. Digital health solutions are increasingly deployed in rural regions to bridge the gap in essential healthcare services (OECD, 2021).

Using solutions presented by the multifaceted transformations of the digital world, both patients and healthcare institutions can reap the advantages. One of the greatest strengths of healthcare systems, operational improvement, problem and treatment, cost reduction, and increased patient participation, is these "sustainable" factors that multifaceted transformations bring.

14.2.3 What Is XAI in Healthcare?

Explainable artificial intelligence (XAI) is an approach where the logic behind the operation and decisions of artificial intelligence systems is made understandable to users. XAI enhances the way users interact with even the most complex systems by trying to explain the enigmatic logic behind their workings. This is why models of AI systems – commonly known as "black box" or dependent systems – are the most complex components to break down and understand. These systems are straightforward to construct. However, they provide almost no insight into understanding how the output of a model is produced (Adadi & Berrada, 2018). The key XAI objectives include understanding the output of the resulting reasoning and providing model decision justification and explanation. The main goals of explainable artificial intelligence are given in Figure 14.3.

In healthcare, XAI increases the trust of healthcare professionals and patients in these systems by transparently explaining the role of AI in the diagnosis and treatment processes. Explainable AI is valuable because it explains to the patient the logic behind a diagnosis, what data is used, how it is processed, and what logic is applied to reach the result. XAI enables both healthcare professionals and patients to trust AI-powered decisions (Gunning et al., 2019).

14.2.4 Why Is XAI Needed in Healthcare?

AI systems can improve patient care by streamlining clinical decision-making processes when widely adopted in healthcare. However, uncertainty about how these systems work can result in a lack of trust among healthcare professionals and patients. Explainable artificial intelligence (XAI) offers a critical approach to addressing this trust gap and facilitating broader acceptance of AI applications (Adadi & Berrada, 2018).

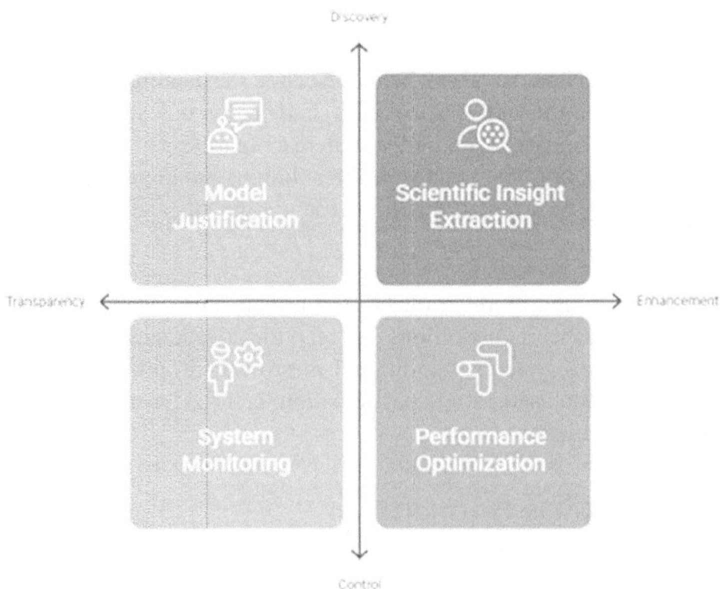

FIGURE 14.3 Explainable AI key objectives and applications.

Trust in healthcare goes beyond having an AI system that can make accurate predictions. It also involves knowing how these predictions were derived. XAI builds trust by explaining how AI systems work for both healthcare professionals and patients. For example, if an AI algorithm explains the biological and clinical parameters on which it diagnoses a disease, doctors can evaluate this decision more consciously (Gunning et al., 2019).

Transparency is essential for AI-powered clinical decisions to be questioned. Understanding how AI systems follow a process, especially in ethically critical situations, will allow healthcare professionals to verify the reliability of these decisions. For example, if the AI model misdiagnoses cancer, if the answer to the question "What did the model miss?" can be found, we will have better answers to correct the errors (Tjoa & Guan, 2020).

14.2.5 Benefits of XAI in Healthcare

Explainable artificial intelligence (XAI) offers many important benefits for both healthcare professionals and patients by enabling the effective and reliable implementation of AI programs in the healthcare field. The healthcare sector is highly sensitive to ethical and legal aspects; therefore, the XAI system's transparency, reliability, and explainability features are important in this area.

- **More Reliable Clinical Decision Systems**: **An** explanation is the most valuable function performed in healthcare using XAI-based systems. It allows physicians to appreciate the clinical decisions that were explained. For example, an XAI model can tell exactly what aspect of data it uses to predict a cancerous risk. This helps practitioners corroborate the predictions made by the models and helps them practice in an augmented clinical environment by coming to conclusions using their clinical experience and the model-made output (Adadi & Berrada, 2018).
- **Increased Patient Confidence**: Patients must trust AI-supported diagnosis and treatment processes. XAI increases patients' sense of trust by explaining the processes behind the AI system's decisions (Gunning et al., 2019).
- **Personalized Medical Applications**: XAI advocates for custom-tailored diagnosis and treatment. Specific approaches to medical concerns can be based on genetic makeup, history of diseases, or even personal habits. This will be of great help, especially in the management of complicated disorders like cancer (Tjoa & Guan, 2020).
- **Ethical and Legal Issues**: Ethical concerns exist in AI uses in medicine, and XAI can aid in these issues remarkably. For instance, the Artificial Intelligence Act of the European Union has provisions that mandate AI systems to be verifiable and justifiable (EUR, 2021). Meeting these standards helps further XAI applications.
- **Wider Acceptance of Technology**: The adoption of AI technologies in the healthcare sector is determined by the level of trust associated with these systems. XAI helps foster this trust by conveying the functionality of AI

models and the rationale behind their results, consequently increasing the acceptance of AI systems in healthcare by physicians and patients (Adadi & Berrada, 2018).

- **Risk Control and Error Reduction**: XAI is much more effective in spotting flaws in AI systems at an earlier stage. For instance, when a model provides an erroneous diagnosis, tracking the data or algorithm steps that led to the incorrect output is straightforward.

14.3 STRATEGIC CHALLENGES FOR XAI AND DIGITAL TRANSFORMATION

A major concern associated with XAI or digital transformation is the security of medical data, coupled with infrastructure gaps, ethical issues, and missing legal frameworks. XAI and digital transformation have led to a revolution in healthcare; however, implementing such technologies is still a work in progress.

14.3.1 Medical Data Security and Privacy

AI applications in the healthcare sector are based on sensitive data sources, which raises the issue of effective and secure data management. This data is critical to protecting patient privacy and complying with legal policies. However, in the long-term digital transformation process, it is becoming increasingly difficult to provide security for sensitive data and reduce unauthorized access (Rieke et al., 2020).

Health data include sensitive personal information such as an individual's medical history, genetic makeup, lifestyle, and previous and existing diseases. Such information is important for building AI models that can improve the healthcare system. Unfortunately, the sensitive nature of such information poses many ethical, legal, and social risks if abused (Davenport & Kalakota, 2019). There is an urgent need for healthcare providers to implement strengthened security protocols to ensure the security of such information.

Patients are increasingly concerned about the privacy of their personal information. In particular, AI-enabled healthcare systems pose a risk of privacy breaches as they collect and process large amounts of data. For example, sharing genetic data without patient consent can lead to ethical and legal issues (EUR, 2021). Therefore, privacy should be protected for the sake of privacy and as an ethical obligation to strengthen trust in healthcare systems.

Healthcare systems are attractive targets for cyberattacks. Data breaches not only compromise the sensitive information of individual patients but can also reduce the reputation and functionality of the healthcare institution. In particular, in an era of accelerating digitalization, it is necessary to provide a strong defense against current cybersecurity threats.

14.3.1.1 Strategic Solution Proposals

- **Federated Learning**: In this process, rather than gathering information on a single server, data is handled on individual devices. As a result, AI models can be developed directly within a device. This approach minimizes the risk of data exposure and ensures that confidentiality policies are implemented (Rieke et al., 2020).

- **AI-Based Security Measures**: The most robust algorithms available should be deployed to protect health information to the utmost. Most importantly, end-to-end encryption during data transfer is extremely efficient for protecting against unwanted intrusion.
- **AI-Supported Security Protocols**: AIC can be applied to ensure the detection of anomalies and also help prevent potential cyber threats. For instance, AIC systems can observe unusual movements in the network and try to block data breaches before they happen.
- **Compliance with Legal Regulations**: In the European Union, GDPR rules, and in the US, HIPAA regulations act as a block to safeguard health data. In the expectation of healthcare institutions, these regulations demand that the regulations be followed, subject to periodic inspections.

The security and privacy of medical data are prerequisites not only for the successful implementation of XAI and digital transformation but also for transforming the healthcare industry. There is an urgent need for healthcare institutions to ensure data security using federated learning, encryption, and AI-powered security protocols. Such strategies ensure patient privacy, build trust in healthcare systems, and accelerate digital transformation processes.

14.3.2 Adapting to Digital Transformation in Healthcare

While digital transformation helps medical services to be more effective, accessible, and patient-centered, the adaptability of healthcare professionals is of great importance in this process. The concept of digital transformation encompasses much more than implementing innovative technologies; it also includes managing human-centered changes. In this context, the challenges faced by healthcare professionals can directly affect the effectiveness of the transformation (Topol, 2019).

Healthcare professionals may resist digital transformation processes for various reasons:

Lack of Knowledge: Insufficient knowledge about digital technologies can make using these systems more complex. In particular, older workers have more difficulty adapting to these new technologies (Davenport & Kalakota, 2019).

Time Constraints: Healthcare professionals often find it challenging to find time to learn and implement new systems due to their busy work schedules.

Distrust of Technology: There may be valid concerns about the reliability of AI and other digital technologies, and this distrust can become a significant barrier preventing healthcare professionals from accepting these systems. For example, anxiety about making mistakes in clinical decision-making with artificial intelligence is quite common.

Fear of Change: The need to change current working methods and adopt new techniques can encourage resistance to change.

To be successful in digital transformation processes, healthcare professionals must first increase their digital literacy levels. Establishing a balance among employees with different levels of knowledge is difficult in this situation.

14.3.2.1 Strategic Solution Proposals

- **Education Programs**: Education programs should be organized to help healthcare professionals adapt to digital transformation. These programs should include basic information about artificial intelligence systems and tools, their use, and data security. Training should not be theoretical, and the practical application part should have a large proportion (Singh et al., 2021).
- **Change Management Strategies**: Change management strategies should be adopted to ensure the successful implementation of digital transformation processes. These strategies include addressing employee concerns, facilitating active participation in the transformation process, and managing the process with free communication.
- **User-Friendly Interfaces**: User-friendly interfaces of digital tools will make it easier for employees to learn and use these systems. The design should focus on increasing the explainability of complex artificial intelligence models and improving healthcare professionals' acceptance of these technologies (Stige et al., 2024).
- **Management Support**: Managers of healthcare organizations should explain the importance of digital transformation to employees and support them throughout the processes. Leadership support increases employee motivation and reduces resistance to change.

Adapting healthcare professionals to digital transformation is about successfully implementing technological solutions and increasing the overall quality of healthcare services. Training programs, change management, and user-friendly devices are some strategic solutions that help effectively manage this process. By doing this, healthcare professionals can be encouraged to participate in digital transformation processes, thus making healthcare systems more sustainable.

14.3.3 Infrastructure Weaknesses and Economic Issues

Digital transformation and explainable artificial intelligence (XAI) offer significant opportunities to the healthcare sector; deficiencies in technology infrastructure, and the associated high costs are some obstacles that prevent the adoption of these processes. This situation can be especially valid in healthcare institutions where legacy systems dominate, and the transition to modern technologies can create financial and operational difficulties.

The healthcare sector still relies on the legacy-based data processing and management systems. Such old systems cannot be easily integrated with the existing AI and XAI utility applications, which leads to poor performance. For instance, the existing electronic health record (EHR) systems and data entry processes are manual and do not support AI-based analytical techniques, severely limiting the application of new technologies. Furthermore, low-capacity operational servers that cannot support sufficient data storage and processing restrict the use of AI-dependent applications that need extensive data computation. Moreover, upgrading old infrastructure or setting up new systems is expensive, so adopting these technologies becomes a costly issue for the healthcare sector.

The perceived expenses associated with digital transformation create serious financial problems in the healthcare industry. Other significant costs include acquiring technology such as advanced equipment, sensors, and servers and paying exorbitant licensing fees for AI systems. Additionally, investment in human capital, such as training programmers to assist healthcare staff in adjusting to advanced technologies, increases healthcare sector expenses. Each of these factors presents a massive hurdle in the financial background. These challenges create a strong barrier to enabling financing from the healthcare sector (Vărzaru, 2022).

14.3.3.1 Strategic Solution Proposals

- **Cloud Computing Solutions**: Implementing cloud computing systems would lower costs while making data management and access easier. Expensive physical servers can be replaced by cost-efficient cloud computing systems. Modern artificial intelligence applications can be efficiently integrated into the healthcare sector by adopting cloud-based storage and analysis solutions.
- **Public–Private Partnerships**: The digital transformation of healthcare systems can be financed through public–private partnerships, which is a valid option. For instance, using public monetary incentives while simultaneously investing in the infrastructure with the support of the private sector makes it feasible to speed up transformation processes (Almosa et al., 2025).
- **Developing Low-Cost Technologies**: Health technology companies can offer more affordable and modular solutions for the needs of developing countries. In addition, open-source software and low-cost hardware can provide solutions for small-scale healthcare institutions.
- **International Funding and Grant Programs**: International organizations like the United Nations, the European Union, and the World Bank provide funds and grants to develop digital health infrastructure. These programs help disseminate technology in low-income regions.

The correct application of digital transformation in healthcare and using other AI relies on strategic methods to address some infrastructural and monetary concerns. Adequate measures, such as cloud computing or public–private collaborations, and the development of new, low-cost technologies can address these obstacles.

14.3.4 Cultural and Social Barriers

While digital techniques and explainable artificial intelligence (XAI) provide a new dimension of opportunities in the healthcare sector, they are met with socio-cultural reluctance within varying geographies. Such reluctance originates from limited access to digital means and is pervasive within societal digital competency and norms. These challenges make it difficult to embrace digital healthcare solutions and hinder the benefits that arise from them (Rane et al., 2024).

The attitudes toward the use of digital technologies differ from culture to culture. Some societies may be more reluctant to use AI-based technologies in healthcare. For example, lacking trust in AI-powered diagnostic systems may negatively impact implementation (Cassidy, 2021). Even in developed countries, the population's digital literacy level varies. Elderly individuals, especially those with low levels of education, may have great difficulty understanding and using digital health solutions. In some societies, concerns about data misuse or exposure of sensitive information may increase skepticism toward digital health technologies. This issue can be addressed with XAI's transparency and explainability features, but cultural factors can limit this trust.

The digital divide refers to differences in digital access between individuals or communities. Again, access to healthcare is one of the effects of the digital divide. Access to healthcare in rural areas is made difficult by inadequate digital infrastructure. For example, telemedical solutions or mobile health applications cannot be used in areas without an internet connection. In addition, high-cost digital devices and internet connections that low-income individuals must purchase will limit access. In order to be effective in using digital technologies, information and education are needed. However, these resources may be limited in developing regions.

14.3.4.1 Strategic Solution Proposals

- **Adaptation to Local Needs**: Digital health solutions should be customized according to each community's cultural and social needs. This can facilitate broader adoption of the technology.
- **Community-Based Approaches**: To increase the acceptance of health technologies, efforts should be made in collaboration with the community and local health workers.
- **Infrastructure Investments**: National and international investments should be encouraged to increase access to internet infrastructure and technological devices, especially in rural areas.
- **Low-Cost Solutions**: Digital health technologies suitable and scalable for developing countries should be developed.
- **Education and Information**: The community should be encouraged to use digital health technologies. Special training courses can target the elderly and those with low digital literacy.
- **Increasing Patient Involvement**: Transparent information should be provided on how digital technologies can improve patient outcomes.

Cultural and social factors are critical barriers to the adoption of digital transformation and the implementation of XAI. Overcoming such barriers is possible only through strategies that increase cultural sensitivity, projects to expand digital access, and awareness campaigns to inform the public.

14.4 MAIN FACTORS SHAPING THE FUTURE OF DIGITAL TRANSFORMATION

Digital transformation is shaping the future by providing more innovative, accessible, and effective services in the healthcare sector. New-generation technologies are optimizing the functioning of healthcare systems and providing a more patient-centered paradigm. Innovations such as blockchain, mobile devices, telemedical solutions, metaverse, and future technologies such as quantum computing and digital copies form the building blocks of digital transformation. In this section, the main factors shaping the future of digital transformation will be discussed.

14.4.1 Blockchain Technology and Healthcare Services

Blockchain technology is considered one of the important digital transformation elements in the healthcare sector. It has a unique potential to ensure health data security, increase processes' transparency, and provide more patient-centered services (Massaro, 2023). The distributed ledger structure of the blockchain allows data to be stored in an encrypted format on a network instead of a centralized system (Figure 14.4). This feature increases protection against unauthorized access, prevents the modification of stored data, and provides full traceability. Protecting health data with this method increases patients' trust in health systems while ensuring that health professionals can access accurate and reliable data easily.

The use of blockchain in healthcare also extends to smart contracts. Processes can be made more efficient and inexpensive with the use of smart contracts. An example is that doctors can utilize a secure environment to share patient records, enabling other healthcare institutions to swiftly and securely access the data. Even insurance transactions can be carried out without manual intervention, permitting

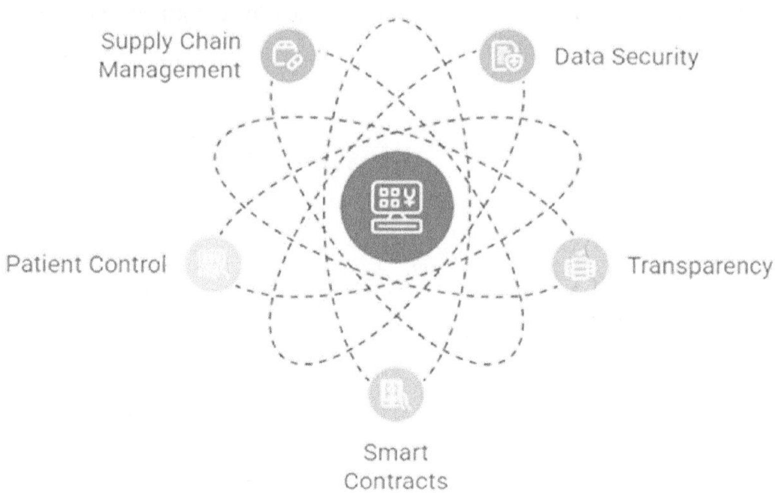

FIGURE 14.4 Blockchain's role in healthcare transformation.

the processes to be done faster and more transparently. Furthermore, treating blockchain technology as an integral part of supply chain management allows for all stages of drug production and delivery to patients to be tracked. This prevents the circulation of counterfeit medicines into the market and enhances the reliability of treatment processes. Blockchain approaches also allow information management to be patient-centric. Patients can, through blockchain, have complete control of their health data and manage who gets to see it and how it will be used. More importantly, sensitive data, which includes genetic information, is more secure with solutions built on blockchain technology. Besides improving patient privacy, this technology promotes greater patient participation in healthcare.

14.4.2 Mobile Medical Devices and Wearable Technologies

The growing population affected by mobile devices and an increasing acceptance of wearable technologies aid patients in monitoring and taking care of their health much better. These smart devices offer accessible data that helps individuals grasp a magnitude of information on their health (Liao, 2019). Smart devices can monitor heart rate, blood pressure, blood glucose level, and sleep patterns, making the diagnosis of illnesses more swift and accurate while improving the management of chronic conditions. For example, a diabetic patient who requires more careful management can significantly benefit from CGM (Continuous Glucose Monitoring) devices, which provide real-time data that makes treatment adjustments easy and helps to avoid complications.

Mobile health applications stimulate patients to monitor and manage their health actively. In addition to using the application to manage one's health, it also makes communication with the doctor efficient, boosting the availability of healthcare services for patients. Essential components of mobile health applications typically include appointment scheduling, prescription tracking, and medication information (Figure 14.5). These applications also allow patients to document and review their

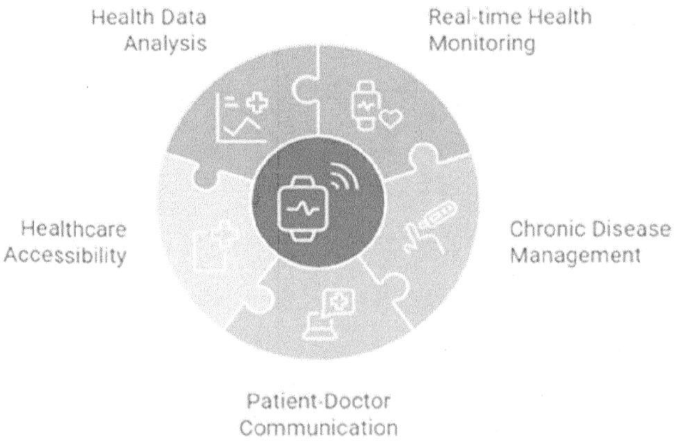

FIGURE 14.5 The impact of mobile health technologies.

health parameters, assisting them to make correct choices concerning their health. With mobile apps, health professionals can manage patients' conditions more effectively and develop better treatment strategies.

Mobile devices and wearable technology are increasing the accessibility of healthcare to a broader population. This implies that people living in rural areas or poor communities will find it easier to receive healthcare. Through a mobile phone, a patient can seek essential medical advice and online consultation while being able to view and even manage their medical records. As a result, personal healthcare management is enhanced, and equity in the supply and distribution of medical services is improved. These mobile devices and other wearable gadgets enable users to interact more dynamically with the healthcare system by allowing access to personal medical records and transforming passive patients into active participants in their healthcare. Such patients can monitor their health more readily and better manage chronic illnesses through personal digital health technologies like mobile phones.

14.4.3 Telemedical Solutions and Remote Healthcare Services

Telemedical solutions can bring specific digital changes to medical services. Especially with the emergence of the COVID-19 pandemic, there has been a shift to online healthcare services. Due to the high pressure on global healthcare systems during the pandemic, people began to turn to telemedicine to maintain social distancing. During this period, online consultation and remote diagnosis and treatment were the best alternatives for patients; they ensured the safety of all participants and, at the same time, allowed healthcare services to function during the global crisis.

Telemedicine is a significant technology for tracking and controlling long-term health ailments (Baker & Stanley, 2018). Complications that could potentially arise may be detected more easily using remote patient monitoring systems, enabling qualitative observation of patients' health (Figure 14.6). For instance, a patient with chronic ailments like hypertension, diabetes, or heart failure can receive regular updates from the physician using remote monitoring mechanisms. This improves the overall health status of individuals while allowing healthcare facilities to allocate resources more intelligently because their workload is reduced. Additionally, telemedical solutions enable healthcare to be more personalized and proactive.

These solutions make the most difference in enhancing the availability of healthcare services in remote locations and areas with poor living conditions. Telemedicine bridges the gap for patients with no local access to doctors by enabling them to consult medical specialists for the required care. This service only requires Internet access and elementary gadgetry, allowing it to bypass physical and financial limitations in numerous situations. For instance, the only requirement for a patient to receive medical guidance and follow-up is a smartphone or a computer. This method frees the need for strict controls concerning the provision of healthcare services, allowing the population to improve their general health. Meeting social needs while providing innovative technology to medicine, telemedicine makes healthcare services more affordable and faster without compromising quality and personalization.

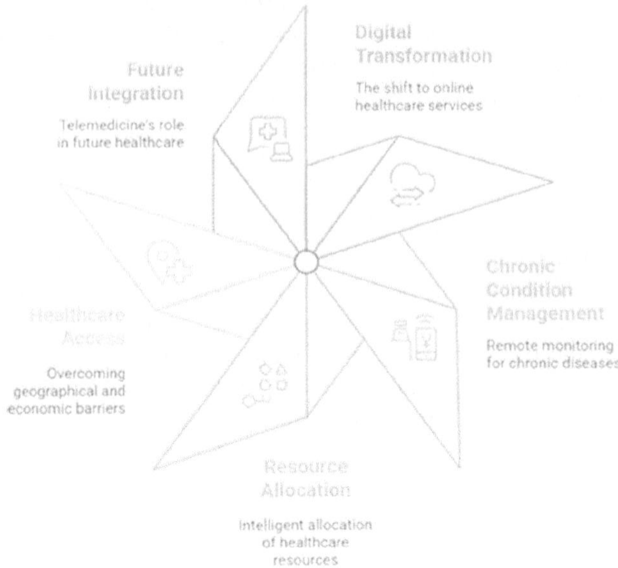

FIGURE 14.6 The impact of telemedicine on healthcare.

The adjustments that the healthcare system was forced to adopt during the pandemic have laid the foundation for the future use of these technologies.

14.4.4 Metaverse and Virtual Healthcare Experience

Metaverse is adding new dimensions to the digital transformation of the healthcare sector by providing advanced virtual clinics. These, along with other sophisticated technologies like VR/AR, are developing and capable of changing treatment and medical educational pedagogy. Vertical clinical processes between patients and physicians and the range of healthcare services can also improve as a result of the virtual healthcare experience (Bansal et al., 2022).

Metaverse is ushering in a new era for patient–doctor relationships. Virtual meetings eliminate physical boundaries and make it possible to meet with doctors from all over the world. The realistic and interactive environments the Metaverse provides allow patients to understand the entire diagnostic and treatment process more deeply. For example, a doctor can explain in detail how they will treat the patient and analyze different processes together with the patient. This helps personalize healthcare and increases the level of patient participation (Figure 14.7).

The development of the metaverse has also led to the creation of virtual hospitals and clinics and the simulation of clinical practice, which demonstrate yet another area of its practicality. Virtual hospitals generally refer to facilities where patients can be diagnosed, treated, and consulted online without face-to-face interaction. Such environments eliminate the waiting times standard in physical hospitals and can reduce costs by optimizing resource allocation. Further, virtual experiences of clinics open new avenues in the field of medical research and drug development. For example,

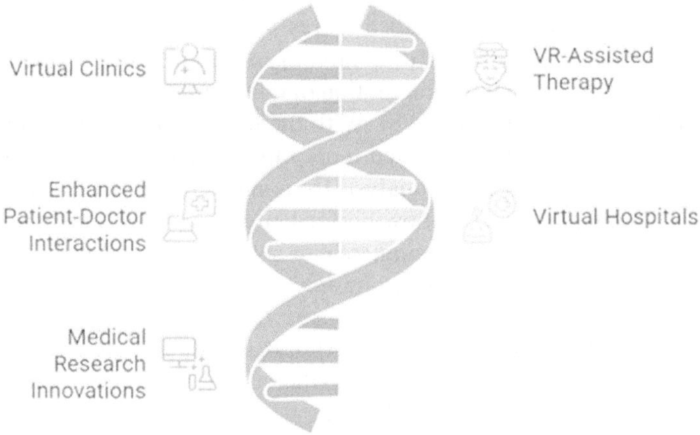
Virtual Clinics
Enhanced Patient-Doctor Interactions
Medical Research Innovations
VR-Assisted Therapy
Virtual Hospitals

FIGURE 14.7 Transforming healthcare with Metaverse and virtual innovations.

a new methodology can be tested on a patient in a simulated clinic to test its safety and efficacy without performing a clinical trial. In general, the metaverse and virtual health experiences can transform how healthcare is provided. Changes in how patients interact with doctors and implementing virtual reality-supported applications like virtual hospitals will make healthcare more affordable, accessible, effective, and inclusive. These technologies are destined to transform the future of healthcare and will undoubtedly be one of the most remarkable aspects of digital transformation.

14.4.5 Quantum Computers: Future Technology in Healthcare

Quantum computers are a next-generation technology that enhances digital transformation opportunities in the healthcare sector. The same has been the case across other industries; the gains in efficiency from the computational power of quantum computers accelerate the solving of problems in the healthcare industry. This technology has tremendous prospects, such as genetic data profiling, speeding up the processes of drug designing, and improving the methods of diagnosis and therapy (Gupta et al., 2023).

For instance, the impact of quantum computing is significant when measuring the performance of large and complex data sets in the analysis field. Processing extremely data-intensive tasks, including genetic data analysis, can be done faster and more efficiently because of quantum computing. Quantum computing is especially beneficial for human genome analysis, identifying genetic disease causes, and individualized treatment development. This leads to the capability of formulating new in-depth genetic analyses, research targets, and advanced treatment methodologies.

According to Kumar et al. (2024), quantum technologies could revolutionize the process of drug development. Unlike classical computers, quantum gains can model drug molecules' chemical interactions and transformations with greater precision and accuracy. This might streamline the entire process, rendering it more efficient and economical. The power of quantum computing might be highly beneficial in researching and developing new medical cures for cancer, Alzheimer's, and other complex health issues stemming from rare diseases. Innovative applications in healthcare are expanding with the integration of quantum technology into diagnostic and therapeutic processes (Figure 14.8). With the help of quantum computing, data from medical imaging can be processed more rapidly and accurately. For instance, quantum technology improves data analysis from magnetic resonance images (MRI) or Computed Tomography (CT), allowing for better diagnosis. Furthermore, algorithms optimized with quantum computers can help the medical team design treatment procedures. As any sector tries to improve productivity, speed, precision, and emphasis, healthcare digitalization must ensure that quantum computing is at the forefront of the most potent technologies within the field. The integration of genetic analysis, drug development, and diagnostic-therapeutic integration will transform the healthcare system while greatly enhancing health outcomes.

14.4.6 Digital Twins: A New Dimension in Healthcare

Digital twins represent a paradigm shift in the patient-specific treatment of pathology, the training of surgeons, and even the management of healthcare systems. They facilitate a type of modeling and simulation through the use of digital replicas of physical entities, systems, or people, which can enable the emergence of new analytical capabilities that add value to the healthcare sector (Sun et al., 2023).

A patient's digital twin makes it possible to create a digital mirror of their health status (Sahal et al., 2022). By utilizing complex algorithms, the model can capture real-time data like genetic markers, a patient's prior medical events, and even specific activities to inform the real-time prognostications of illness progression through innovative health management. One of the well-studied applications of digital twins is in patients suffering from chronic diseases, where treatment plans can be optimized virtually to minimize side effects and improve the effectiveness of therapies.

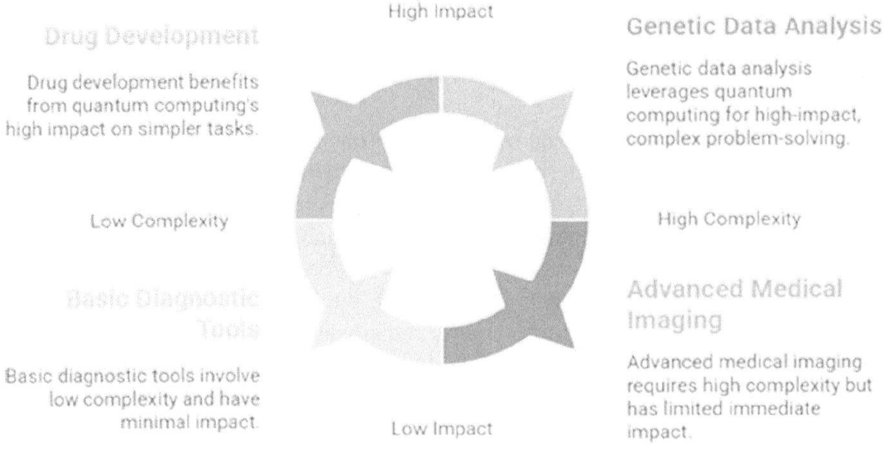

FIGURE 14.8 Quantum computing applications in healthcare.

Digital twin technology has many benefits for health professionals, including the possibility of performing surgical simulations and training. Surgeons can perform such actions in a computerized environment before operating on a patient, which allows them to gauge the patient's risk and develop the most appropriate operational tactics. This improves the maneuvers of the surgeons and decreases surgical blunders, thereby enhancing the safety of patients. Digital twins also assist every medical learner and resident in gaining clinical experience by practicing on lifelike models.

Digital twins of health systems are implemented to improve operational performance and effective resource distribution in hospital governance. The twin of a hospital's digital system enables decision-makers to gain insights by simulating patient traffic, equipment consumption, and employee attendance. Modeling the patient influx helps in the use of emergency departments' digital twin, which aids in efficiency in resource distribution and the reduction of wait time.

Digital twins enhance innovation in services, education, and healthcare management from a personalized perspective. This technology is significantly helping to advance the efficiency and sustainability of healthcare systems while attaining better results for every patient. Digital twins will undoubtedly be a revolutionary tool in the healthcare sector.

14.5 CONCLUSION

Explainable artificial intelligence (XAI) and digital transformation are the most powerful drivers of change in healthcare delivery. These technologies have the potential to improve patients' quality of life by making healthcare systems more accessible, efficient, and tailored to their individual needs. Most importantly, the rapid spread of AI-based solutions in the healthcare industry encourages the sector to take a more proactive and predictive stance.

A recent Research and Markets report suggests that the global market for explainable AI is expected to expand from $3.5 billion in 2020 to $21 billion in 2030. This increase indicates that medical software and AI technology are in high demand. While the magnitude of data increases constantly, the significance of AI technologies increases just as fast. Hence, the issues revolving around data protection and privacy become crucial challenges that must be dealt with carefully. In the near future, governments and the business sector are expected to likely reach an understanding that will allow the potential benefits of AI to be maximally harnessed.

According to the World Economic Forum, 2030 will be a revolutionary year for healthcare systems that employ AI technology. It will introduce many new use cases to make healthcare systems more proactive and predictive. AI will give individuals more control over their data and determine how it is used, paving the way for democratic data use in healthcare. This will contribute to healthcare being more transparent and patient-centered. In particular, setting international standards, establishing regulations, and ensuring ethical and legal compliance are crucial to achieving these goals. Education and awareness-raising efforts should support public adoption of XAI and other digital health technologies. Table 14.1 details the emerging trends and potential impacts of AI in healthcare.

TABLE 14.1
Future Perspectives and Strategic Development for AI in Healthcare

Key Innovations	Transformative Benefits	Obstacles to Overcome	Vision for Progress
Personalized medicine	Revolutionizing care through targeted treatments and genetic insights.	Data security concerns, implementation in clinical workflows, and equitable access.	Expanding into mental health and dynamic care models using real-time monitoring data.
AI-driven predictive analytics	Optimizing preventive care through early diagnosis and risk identification.	Bias in data representation, ensuring inclusivity in predictive models.	Strengthening inter-institutional collaborations and refining bias-free AI algorithms.
Robotic surgery innovations	Enhancing precision and reducing recovery times in surgical procedures.	High cost, training complexities, and ethical implications of autonomous systems.	Developing advanced robotics with sensory feedback for minimally invasive procedures.
Explainable artificial intelligence (XAI)	Fostering trust by making AI decision-making comprehensible for end users.	Bridging the gap between technical complexities and user understanding.	Creating global standards for XAI and implementing explainability into clinical tools.
Wearable health monitoring	Enabling proactive health management through continuous, real-time tracking.	Interoperability and data security across diverse healthcare platforms.	Building IoT-integrated ecosystems for comprehensive patient health management.
AI in drug discovery	Accelerating drug development while reducing costs and enhancing efficacy.	Validation of AI predictions and addressing ethical concerns.	Utilizing advanced analytics to streamline clinical trials and predict drug outcomes.
Healthcare Data Security	Preserving patient privacy while ensuring AI systems' efficiency in data processing.	Balancing data utility and regulatory compliance with technological advancement.	Adopting federated learning and encrypted multi-party computation methods for secure data use.

In conclusion, the role of XAI and the digital transformation of healthcare systems will make the healthcare system structure more inclusive, equitable, and sustainable. A future where information and innovative technology offsets humans to an extent and everyone has access to healthcare facilities is a future that is on the horizon.

REFERENCES

Adadi, A., & Berrada, M. (2018). Peeking inside the black-box: A survey on Explainable Artificial Intelligence (XAI). *IEEE Access*, 6, 52138–52160. https://doi.org/10.1109/ACCESS.2018.2870052

Almosa, N. M., Alonazi, W., & Alonazi, W. B. (2025). Factors influencing patients' choice of public or private hospitals in riyadh city: A cross-sectional study. *Cureus*, 17(2), 1–11. https://doi.org/10.7759/cureus.78756

Amann, J., Blasimme, A., Vayena, E., Frey, D., Madai, V. I., & Precise4Q Consortium. (2020). Explainability for artificial intelligence in healthcare: A multidisciplinary perspective. *BMC Medical Informatics and Decision Making*, 20, 1–9.

Baker, J., & Stanley, A. (2018). Telemedicine technology: A review of services, equipment, and other aspects. *Current Allergy and Asthma Reports*, 18, 1–8.

Bansal, G., Rajgopal, K., Chamola, V., Xiong, Z., & Niyato, D. (2022). Healthcare in metaverse: A survey on current metaverse applications in healthcare. *IEEE Access*, 10, 119914–119946.

Cassidy, R. (2021). Attitudes towards digital health technology: introducing the digital health scale. *medRxiv*, 2021–2009.

Davenport, T., & Kalakota, R. (2019). The potential for artificial intelligence in healthcare. *Future Healthcare Journal*, 6(2), 94–98.

Eke, C. I., & Shuib, L. (2024). The role of explainability and transparency in fostering trust in AI healthcare systems: A systematic literature review, open issues and potential solutions. *Neural Computing and Applications*, 37, 1999–2034.

El-Rashidy, N., El-Sappagh, S., Islam, S. R., M. El-Bakry, H., & Abdelrazek, S. (2021). Mobile health in remote patient monitoring for chronic diseases: Principles, trends, and challenges. *Diagnostics*, 11(4), 607.

European Parliament and Council. (2021). *Digital Europe programme regulation 2021/694.*

Gunning, D., Stefik, M., Choi, J., Miller, T., Stumpf, S., & Yang, G. Z. (2019). XAI – Explainable Artificial Intelligence. *Science Robotics*, 4(37), eaay7120.

Gupta, S., Modgil, S., Bhatt, P. C., Jabbour, C. J. C., & Kamble, S. (2023). Quantum computing led innovation for achieving a more sustainable Covid-19 healthcare industry. *Technovation*, 120, 102544.

Hollingsworth, J. D. (2018). Is there a doctor in the house: How dismantling barriers to telemedicine practice can improve healthcare access for rural residents. *Howard Law Journal*, 62, 653.

Kraus, S., Schiavone, F., Pluzhnikova, A., & Invernizzi, A. C. (2021). Digital transformation in healthcare: Analyzing the current state-of-research. *Journal of Business Research*, 123, 557–567.

Kumar, G., Yadav, S., Mukherjee, A., Hassija, V., & Guizani, M. (2024). Recent advances in quantum computing for drug discovery and development. *IEEE Access,* 12, 64491–64509.

Liao, Y., Thompson, C., Peterson, S., Mandrola, J., & Beg, M. S. (2019, January). The future of wearable technologies and remote monitoring in health care. In *American society of clinical oncology educational book. American society of clinical oncology: Annual meeting* (Vol. 39, p. 115). NIH Public Access.

Marx, E. W., & Padmanabhan, P. (2020). *Healthcare digital transformation: How consumerism, technology and pandemic are accelerating the future.* Productivity Press.

Massaro, M. (2023). Digital transformation in the healthcare sector through blockchain technology: Insights from academic research and business developments. *Technovation*, 120, 102386.

OECD. (2021). *Health at a glance 2021.* https://www.oecd.org/en/publications/health-at-a-glance-2021_ae3016b9-en.html

Rane, N., Choudhary, S. P., & Rane, J. (2024). Acceptance of artificial intelligence: Key factors, challenges, and implementation strategies. *Journal of Applied Artificial Intelligence*, 5(2), 50–70.

Reddy, S., Fox, J., & Purohit, M. P. (2019). Artificial intelligence-enabled healthcare delivery. *Journal of the Royal Society of Medicine*, 112(1), 22–28.

Rieke, N., Hancox, J., Li, W., Milletari, F., Roth, H. R., Albarqouni, S., ... Cardoso, M. J. (2020). The future of digital health with federated learning. *NPJ Digital Medicine*, 3(1), 1–7.

Sahal, R., Alsamhi, S. H., & Brown, K. N. (2022). Personal digital twin: A close look into the present and a step towards the future of personalised healthcare industry. *Sensors*, 22(15), 5918.

Singh, S., Bhatt, P., Sharma, S. K., & Rabiu, S. (2021). Digital transformation in healthcare: Innovation and technologies. In *Blockchain for healthcare systems* (pp. 61–79). CRC Press.

Stige, Å., Zamani, E. D., Mikalef, P., & Zhu, Y. (2024). Artificial Intelligence (AI) for user experience (UX) design: A systematic literature review and future research agenda. *Information Technology & People*, 37(6), 2324–2352.

Stoumpos, A. I., Kitsios, F., & Talias, M. A. (2023). Digital transformation in healthcare: Technology acceptance and its applications. *International Journal of Environmental Research and Public Health*, 20(4), 3407.

Sun, T., He, X., & Li, Z. (2023). Digital twin in healthcare: Recent updates and challenges. *Digital Health*, 9, 20552076221149651.

Tjoa, E., & Guan, C. (2020). A survey on Explainable Artificial Intelligence (XAI): Toward medical XAI. *IEEE Transactions on Neural Networks and Learning Systems*, 32(11), 4793–4813.

Topol, E. (2019). *Deep medicine: How artificial intelligence can make healthcare human again.* Hachette UK.

Vărzaru, A. A. (2022). Assessing digital transformation of cost accounting tools in healthcare. *International Journal of Environmental Research and Public Health*, 19(23), 15572.

Whitelaw, S., Mamas, M. A., Topol, E., & Van Spall, H. G. (2020). Applications of digital technology in COVID-19 pandemic planning and response. *The Lancet Digital Health*, 2(8), e435–e440.

World Health Organization (WHO). (2020). *Global strategy on digital health 2020–20.* World Health Organization.

15 Ensuring Patient Autonomy and Informed Decision-Making in AI-Driven Healthcare

Safa Kaymakci and Bekir Yitik

15.1 THE ROLE OF XAI IN SUPPORTING PATIENT AUTONOMY

The application of artificial intelligence (AI) technology in healthcare is progressively changing the processes of diagnosis, treatment planning, and patient administration. However, with these developments, the sophistication of AI models has brought forth grave issues related to the explainability, transparency, and interpretability of their results (Žlahtič et al., 2024; Amann et al., 2020; Patel et al., 2024). These challenges stem from the fact that there is an inadequate response to requirements related to explainable AI (XAI), which is known to foster trust in automated systems by guaranteeing that the medical conclusions produced by AI are eloquently articulated in a manner that professionals and patients equally understand (Abdullah et al., 2021; Ansari et al., 2024). In tandem with enhanced accessibility, XAI serves an equally important purpose in advancing patient autonomy by providing the capacity to take informed actions regarding one's health, as AI enhancement of health recommendations increases the information transparency (Amann et al., 2020; Mienye et al., 2024).

The application of XAI in the medical field accentuates the need for XAI in terms of boosting confidence and trust toward AI systems, placing it as one of the more important features of AI in medicine. There is an indication that the implementation of XAI contributes to greater transparency, which is crucial in a clinical environment where the decisions made can have life-altering consequences for patients (Žlahtič et al., 2024; Kelly et al., 2019; Alowais et al., 2023). With the persistent adoption of AI systems in pivotal healthcare processes and decisions, there is a dire prerequisite for such systems that can readily explain their logic. The relationship between explainability and responsibility is particularly important; physicians need to be able to answer ethical and trust obligations regarding patients with the necessary information about the AI's reasoning (Amann et al., 2020; Patel et al., 2024).

DOI: 10.1201/9781003605416-15

Equally important, XAI develops support mechanisms that improve patient comprehension of their diagnostic and therapeutic possibilities, thus aiding in the informed consent process – an explanation in essence, is based on a patient's autonomous decision (Abdullah et al., 2021; Mienye et al., 2024). Informed patients are more likely to manage their medical conditions, which leads to improved satisfaction and overall health outcomes (Chanda et al., 2024; Srinivasu et al., 2022). XAI resolves the issues of the gap in understanding sophisticated AI algorithms and user interfaces, fostering dialogue regarding AI's so-called "black box" mechanisms and fostering acceptance by healthcare professionals and patients (Hulsen, 2023; Reddy et al., 2024).

15.1.1 Empowering Patients through Explainable AI

The addition of explainable artificial intelligence in healthcare is important for increasing patients' knowledge and their active role in making decisions regarding their treatment. Traditional AI algorithms often function as "black boxes," meaning they issue predictions and recommendations with little to no explanation that a patient would understand (Antoniadi et al., 2021; Metta et al., 2024). This deficiency of clear frameworks limits the capability of patients to understand comprehensively, which makes it difficult for patients to engage thoughtfully in discussions regarding their healthcare plans (Stroud et al., 2024; Nelson et al., 2020). Metta et al. (2024) and Tiwari (2023) state that XAI attempts to solve these problems by providing interpretable answers that explain the processes of AI systems in regard to the provided diagnoses and aid outlined in treatment suggestions.

The use of XAI enhances decision support systems, which enables healthcare professionals to explain the critical medical reasons underlying the AI recommendations. For instance, Metta et al. (2024) and Mohseni et al. (2021) discuss how XAI tools are capable of explaining diagnostic imaging through specific biomarkers and imaging features as well as diagnostic genetic components. This is important when considering the confidence of patients in AI systems because those who understand the reasoning behind AI recommendations are more likely to take an active role in their treatment and adhere to medical recommendations (Stroud et al., 2024; Antoniadi et al., 2021). Evidence shows that patients who understand the reasoning behind the conclusions drawn by an AI system tend to have more confidence in the presented information, which further highlights the importance of XAI in healthcare systems designed for patients (Nelson et al., 2020; Antoniadi et al., 2021).

The participation of healthcare workers with XAI systems can aid in explaining intricate medical information to patients, which enhances the control of the patients over their health (Liao et al., 2020; Stroud et al., 2024). With increased comprehension of the reasoning behind AI-assisted choices, patients are more likely to actively engage in discussions with their physicians, fostering the ability to negotiate and come to a decision together (Nelson et al., 2020; Chakraborty et al., 2024). Therefore, the importance of XAI portraying patients as active participants in their health journeys is vital, demonstrating the need to attend to ethical issues and practical concerns in healthcare (Metta et al., 2024; Tiwari, 2023).

15.1.2 Enhancing Shared Decision-Making in Clinical Practice

The shift toward personalized medicine ensures an integrated approach to clinical decision-making involving the patient, the physician, and the AI-based system, collaboratively working to make healthcare decisions. The roles of explainable artificial intelligence (XAI) are significant for the shared decision-making (SDM) processes as AI-powered suggestions are tailored to suit patients' values and preferences along with their medical history and context (Noordman et al., 2022; Beach & Sugarman, 2019). In determining treatment options alongside patients within their defined autonomy, this collaboration is integral.

As an example, in oncology, AI models in combination with XAI frameworks are increasingly leveraged to develop and justify personalized treatment plans for patients based on their genomic data and other clinical characteristics. Oncologists, for instance, can explain the logic behind certain therapy recommendations, the reasoning for alternative choices, and detail the possible risks and benefits of each decision (Arrieta et al., 2020; Jungmann et al., 2022). Therefore, Noordman et al. (2022) explain XAI's role in that by enabling patients to actively participate in planning their treatment through sophisticated AI-based suggestions, patients are not rendered passive to authoritative medical decisions. The adoption of shared decision-making within oncology is essential to integrate patient preferences into treatment, thereby enhancing patient confidence in the entire healthcare system (Jungmann et al., 2022; Ozanne et al., 2020).

Moreover, XAI is important for improving patient education, especially with the visual explanation of the medical AI's assessments. In the field of radiology, for instance, explainable deep learning models apply heatmaps or attention maps to illustrate individual parts of the imaging, like MRI scans, that the AI was observed predicting a diagnosis (Yanagawa et al., 2023; Jin et al., 2022). This degree of visualization gives the patient a better comprehension of their ailment, motivating them to analyze and work with their clinical practitioners more actively (Yanagawa et al., 2023). Such improvements in communication offer a chance to capture information in a more sophisticated way during clinical consultations, which is very important for channeled SDM (Komatsu et al., 2021; Okada et al., 2023).

In addition, the dynamic interaction and iteration between patients and healthcare practitioners, with the assistance of XAI, strengthen patients' trust in AI recommendation systems. When patients can see how certain elements in their diagnostics impact an AI's outcome, they are more likely to comply with and follow the treatment plans (Sarwar et al., 2019; Ozanne et al., 2020). The combination of XAI and clinical practice causes a shift in focus from mere instruction to instruction accompanied by understanding for the patients, which leads to paradigm changes in the ethical use of medicine with respect to XAI-enabled transparency (Sukumar et al., 2020).

15.1.3 Promoting Ethical and Transparent AI Integration in Healthcare

The deployment of artificial intelligence (AI) within the medical decision-making paradigm certainly emphasizes ethical issues regarding patient autonomy, informed consent, and bias within AI algorithms. Explainable AI takes care of these ethical concerns by ensuring that patients do not simply receive AI-derived answers but actively engage with AI systems (Amann et al., 2020; Jungmann et al., 2022). This is critical for the ethics of medicine because it facilitates candor and the relationship between patients and medical professionals (Veer et al., 2021; Makubhai et al., 2023).

Both the General Data Protection Regulation (GDPR) and the Health Insurance Portability and Accountability Act (HIPAA) also highlight Shue's and Wang's claim about the need for transparency and upholding patient rights in AI-based healthcare. XAI's explainable, accountable, and logical pathway construction for auditable decisions ensures adherence to these regulatory requirements, introduces equity in the use of AI in medicine, and mitigates algorithmic discrimination (Jungmann et al., 2022; Shu et al., 2024). In particular, the regulations stress that patients need to comprehend the reasoning behind AI-enabled decisions, which strengthens consent (Wang et al., 2021; Gichoya et al., 2022).

XAI approaches are equally important in analyzing, assessing, and correcting biases within the algorithms of AI systems to guarantee fairness in attaining healthcare services (Kelly et al., 2019; Hulsen, 2023). When medical practitioners understand the rationale provided by AI systems regarding their recommendations, it is easier for them to notice discriminatory biases toward certain groups that are unique to certain patients (Ennab & Mcheick, 2022; Makubhai et al., 2023). With the explanation of AI processes, stakeholders can conduct analyses alongside other processes and correct any inequalities that are prejudicial, thereby reinforcing the confidence needed to engage with patients effectively (Žlahtič et al., 2024; Mienye et al., 2024).

Additionally, the application of AI in medicine triggers ethical concerns that necessitate a cross-disciplinary approach toward XAI, which embraces the ethics, law, and technology stakeholders. Such an approach is critical for the creation of instruments that meet the minimum requirements of legislation and the optimum standards of care (Makubhai et al., 2023). Thus, the scope of XAI logic goes beyond fulfilling particular technological requirements and extends to crafting an enabling environment of responsibility and confidence, which embodies patient self-governance and active participation in healthcare decision-making (Correra et al., 2023).

15.2 ETHICAL AND LEGAL CONSIDERATIONS IN AI-ASSISTED MEDICAL DECISION-MAKING

Artificial intelligence (AI) holds tremendous opportunities to transform the healthcare industry through integrating AI-assisted diagnostics, treatment planners, and patient outcome enhancers. This development, however, requires the assessment of the ethical and legal scrutiny related to the use of technology in the healthcare system. To build trust and accountability in AI-mediated medicine, it is critical that autonomous AI healthcare systems operate within ethical obligations, legal frameworks, and patient rights (Abdullah et al., 2021; Lee et al., 2021).

Abdullah et al. (2021) note that patients' ethical rights in the development and implementation of AI systems should be protected by key ethical principles as outlined in fundamental documents like the Belmont Report: beneficence, nonmaleficence, autonomy, and justice. An example is the building of an active partnership between healthcare practitioners and patients where key patient values are incorporated within AI recommendations geared toward optimal outcome AI solutions, thus enhancing shared decision-making. This solves the issue of dualism of consent and autonomy (Lee et al., 2021; Richardson et al., 2021).

As AI solutions are implemented in different industries, compliance with healthcare standards like GDPR and HIPAA emphasizes the need for explainability and data protection policies concerning AI-powered healthcare solutions. AI X Systems enhances regulatory compliance by maintaining audit-friendly, transparent decision-making paths that safeguard accountability structures designed to reduce algorithmic discrimination (Jobin et al., 2019).

Boundless frontiers of artificial intelligence can achieve transformative potential in the presence of robust ethical policies and frameworks tailored for training AI applicants in healthcare professions. Teaching clinicians about the application boundaries and ethical concerns surrounding AI technologies is fundamental to their moral use (Alanazi, 2023; Murphy et al., 2021). This not only fosters greater acceptance of AI technologies, but also helps ensure that the standards of care provided to patients remain uncompromised.

15.2.1 Ethical Responsibilities in AI-Driven Medical Decision-Making

The inclusion of artificial intelligence in the medical field poses new ethical challenges regarding AI's responsibility, the openness of its systems, and justice. A common issue with numerous AI algorithms is their "black box" configuration, which makes it difficult for both clinicians and patients to understand how a certain conclusion, diagnosis, or treatment was made. An absence of transparency would erode the trust patients have toward the system while leading to a lack of confidence by the physicians in the AI-generated results (Adam et al., 2022; Lukkien et al., 2024; Buchanan et al., 2020).

To confront these issues, explainable AI (XAI) approaches are being devised, concentrating on the interpretation, retrievability, and justification of AI-based decisions (Benjamens et al., 2020; Wang et al., 2022; Roller et al., 2022). In healthcare, ethical AI must advocate for the well-being and autonomy of the patients, actively involving them in the decision-making process whereby AI plays the role of aide to the doctor rather than replacing clinical judgment (Issa et al., 2024). The use of XAI also mitigates algorithmic discrimination that affects the most marginalized, thus promoting equity, inclusion, and ethical principles in medicine (Benjamens et al., 2020; Schwendicke et al., 2020).

One of the most pressing modern ethical issues revolves around the accountability for decisions made by AI systems. In a clinical context, a healthcare practitioner is routinely responsible for the pertinent choices they make in the delivery of services. The involvement of an AI system makes this liability less straightforward. Take, for example, an AI model that misdiagnoses a patient or suggests a treatment that is inappropriate for their condition. Who is to be held accountable, the healthcare practitioner, the AI's creator, or the organization employing the AI? Answering this question is not simple. The consequences of such a problem indicate a lack of ethical governance to determine the responsible parties and prevent damage, in this case to the safety of the patient, through erroneous AI interventions in healthcare (Vicente & Matute, 2023; Issa et al., 2024).

15.2.2 Patient Privacy and Informed Consent in AI-Assisted Healthcare

The use of AI technologies in automated medical diagnosis and treatment systems relies heavily on having patient data available at scale, which poses significant issues regarding privacy, data security, and the policy of informed consent. The construction of AI algorithms requires the use of large datasets, which often contain sensitive health data, and thus there are increasing needs to protect the privacy of patients and mitigate legal risks (Secinaro et al., 2021; Arigbabu et al., 2024). Legislative frameworks like the GDPR in Europe and HIPAA in the US have developed specific policies that guarantee patients' information is accessed, controlled, utilized, and disclosed only with their documented agreement (Hoseini, 2023; Lim et al., 2020).

As part of their healthcare processes, patients should agree to the use of AI after being educated on its role, which is a prerequisite of informed consent. Nevertheless, in many cases, patients do not appreciate how AI systems exploit their data or how their data alters clinical decisions (Jeelani et al., 2024). Ethically, patients need to be assured that they are in control of the decisions in their care, as healthcare institutions must educate patients on the benefits and risks AI has to offer while caring for them and the limits within which AI makes decisions recommended to patients (Burlina et al., 2020; Nguyen et al., 2022).

Furthermore, patient privacy is of the utmost importance, making anonymization and encryption of any data AI uses a prerequisite. Techniques like differential privacy and federated learning are fundamental – they permit the training of AI models on distributed sets of data without breaching patient confidentiality. These approaches meet privacy criteria while still offering strong protection for sensitive information (Guo et al., 2024; Kooli & Muftah, 2022; Yang et al., 2022). Secinaro et al. (2021) and Kooli and Muftah (2022) argue that there is a need for policy monitoring to ensure patient confidentiality is not compromised with the incessant technological advancement in medicine powered by big data.

15.2.3 Regulatory Compliance and AI Governance in Healthcare

With the incorporation of artificial intelligence (AI) within the medical field, an equally pressing concern has arisen to develop legal structures that clearly define the use, testing, and liability of AI systems. Legal governance for AI differs from one region to another. This diversity poses an added challenge for providers of healthcare and technology services who must deal with complicated regulatory compliance issues (Muralidharan et al., 2024; Santra et al., 2024).

In Europe, the General Data Protection Regulation (GDPR) captures wide-ranging AI privacy requirements and enforces the model to give a description, minimize data scope, and allow for an explanation of automated decisions made concerning patients. This compels AI developers to ensure that the models they build adhere to the principles of fairness, accountability, and explainability as dictated by the GDPR (Hoseini, 2023; Lim et al., 2020). From a US perspective, the Health Insurance Portability and Accountability Act (HIPAA) concentrates on the protection of patient health information data, restricting the manner in which AI models controlling sensitive medical data are allowed to handle the data and still comply with requirements for access control, transmission security, and data control (Jeelani et al., 2024; Burlina et al., 2020).

The EU's AI Act applies varying degrees of risk-based scrutiny for AI applications in healthcare, requiring greater oversight and regulatory approval for AI systems that incorporate clinical decision-making within their high-risk features (Joshi & Bhandari, 2022; D. Wu et al., 2024). Both the FDA and EMA impose robust testing, validation, and regulatory approval requirements on the deployment of AI-powered medical devices and software in clinical settings. These bodies emphasize the observation devoid of prejudice, the refreshing of AI models, and the need to perpetually change AI frameworks with regard to the framework model's efficacy and safety (Benjamens et al., 2020; Joshi et al., 2024).

Self-evidently, the growing international AI regulatory unification brings about multifarious complications, as countries have different interpretations and enforcement mechanisms for AI governance. To address this issue, healthcare companies must develop policies aligned with the distinct criteria of AI ethics regulations, set up AI governance boards, and deploy auditing systems aimed at ensuring adherence to shifting regulations (Muralidharan et al., 2024; Santra et al., 2024). With these measures, the risk of inappropriately addressing legal requirements will be reduced, thus enabling a much more effective and integrated application of AI technologies within healthcare settings.

REFERENCES

Abdullah, Y., Schuman, J., Shabsigh, R., Caplan, A., & Al-Aswad, L. (2021). Ethics of artificial intelligence in medicine and ophthalmology. *Asia-Pacific Journal of Ophthalmology*, 10(3), 289–298. https://doi.org/10.1097/apo.0000000000000397

Adam, H., Balagopalan, A., Alsentzer, E., Christia, F., & Ghassemi, M. (2022). Mitigating the impact of biased artificial intelligence in emergency decision-making. *Communications Medicine*, 2(1). https://doi.org/10.1038/s43856-022-00214-4

Alanazi, A. (2023). Clinicians' views on using artificial intelligence in healthcare: opportunities, challenges, and beyond. *Cureus*. https://doi.org/10.7759/cureus.45255

Alowais, S., Alghamdi, S., Alsuhebany, N., Alqahtani, T., Alshaya, A., Almohareb, S., … Albekairy, A. (2023). Revolutionizing healthcare: the role of artificial intelligence in clinical practice. *BMC Medical Education*, 23(1). https://doi.org/10.1186/s12909-023-04698-z

Amann, J., Blasimme, A., Vayena, E., Frey, D., & Madai, V. (2020). Explainability for artificial intelligence in healthcare: a multidisciplinary perspective. *BMC Medical Informatics and Decision Making*, 20(1). https://doi.org/10.1186/s12911-020-01332–6

Ansari, Z., Tripathi, M., & Ahmed, R. (2024). *Understanding the landscape: a review of explainable AI in healthcare decision-making*. https://doi.org/10.21203/rs.3.rs-4908320/v1

Antoniadi, A., Du, Y., Guendouz, Y., Wei, L., Mazo, C., Becker, B., … Mooney, C. (2021). Current challenges and future opportunities for XAI in machine learning-based clinical decision support systems: a systematic review. *Applied Sciences*, 11(11), 5088. https://doi.org/10.3390/app11115088

Arigbabu, A., Olaniyi, O., Adigwe, C., Adebiyi, O., & Ajayi, S. (2024). Data governance in AI - enabled healthcare systems: a case of the project nightingale. *Asian Journal of Research in Computer Science*, 17(5), 85–107. https://doi.org/10.9734/ajrcos/2024/v17i5441

Arrieta, A., Díaz-Rodríguez, N., Ser, J., Bennetot, A., Tabik, S., Barbado, A., … Herrera, F. (2020). Explainable Artificial Intelligence (XAI): concepts, taxonomies, opportunities and challenges toward responsible AI. *Information Fusion*, 58, 82–115. https://doi.org/10.1016/j.inffus.2019.12.012

Beach, M. and Sugarman, J. (2019). Realizing shared decision-making in practice. *JAMA*, 322(9), 811. https://doi.org/10.1001/jama.2019.9797

Benjamens, S., Dhunnoo, P., & Meskó, B. (2020). The state of artificial intelligence-based FDA-approved medical devices and algorithms: an online database. *NPJ Digital Medicine*, 3(1). https://doi.org/10.1038/s41746-020-00324–0

Buchanan, C., Howitt, M., Wilson, R., Booth, R., Risling, T., & Bamford, M. (2020). Predicted influences of artificial intelligence on the domains of nursing: scoping review. *JMIR Nursing*, 3(1), e23939. https://doi.org/10.2196/23939

Burlina, P., Paul, W., Mathew, P., Joshi, N., Pacheco, K., & Bressler, N. (2020). Low-shot deep learning of diabetic retinopathy with potential applications to address artificial intelligence bias in retinal diagnostics and rare ophthalmic diseases. *JAMA Ophthalmology*, 138(10), 1070. https://doi.org/10.1001/jamaophthalmol.2020.3269

Chakraborty, S., Misra, B., & Dey, N. (2024). *Explainable Artificial Intelligence (XAI) for air quality assessment*. https://doi.org/10.3233/faia231451

Chanda, T., Hauser, K., Hobelsberger, S., Bucher, T., Garcia, C., Wies, C., … Brinker, T. (2024). Dermatologist-like explainable AI enhances trust and confidence in diagnosing melanoma. *Nature Communications*, 15(1). https://doi.org/10.1038/s41467-023-43095–4

Correra, R., Jeong, J., Patel, B., Trivedi, H., Gichoya, J., & Banerjee, I. (2023). *A robust two-step adversarial debiasing with partial learning: medical image case-studies*. https://doi.org/10.1117/12.2647285

Ennab, M., & Mcheick, H. (2022). Designing an interpretability-based model to explain the artificial intelligence algorithms in healthcare. *Diagnostics*, 12(7), 1557. https://doi.org/10.3390/diagnostics12071557

Gichoya, J., Banerjee, I., Bhimireddy, A., Burns, J., Celi, L., Chen, L., … Zhang, H. (2022). AI recognition of patient race in medical imaging: a modelling study. *The Lancet Digital Health*, 4(6), e406–e414. https://doi.org/10.1016/s2589-7500(22)00063-2

Guo, C., Chen, Y., Ma, C., Hao, S., & Song, J. (2024). A survey on AI-driven mouse behavior analysis applications and solutions. *Bioengineering*, 11(11), 1121. https://doi.org/10.3390/bioengineering11111121

Hoseini, M. (2023). Patient experiences with AI in healthcare settings. *Aitechbesosci*, 1(3), 12–18. https://doi.org/10.61838/kman.aitech.1.3.3

Hulsen, T. (2023). *Explainable Artificial Intelligence (XAI) in healthcare.* https://doi.org/10.20944/preprints202303.0116.v1

Issa, W., Shorbagi, A., Alshorman, A., Rababa, M., Majed, K., Radwan, H., … Fakhry, R. (2024). *Shaping the future: perspectives on the integration of artificial intelligence in health profession education: a multi-country survey.* https://doi.org/10.21203/rs.3.rs-4396289/v1

Jeelani, O., Njie, M., & Korzhuk, V. (2024). *Methods and algorithms of ensuring data privacy in AI-based healthcare systems and technologies.* https://doi.org/10.3233/shti240640

Jin, W., Li, X., & Hamarneh, G. (2022). Evaluating explainable AI on a multi-modal medical imaging task: can existing algorithms fulfill clinical requirements?. *Proceedings of the AAAI Conference on Artificial Intelligence*, 36(11), 11945–11953. https://doi.org/10.1609/aaai.v36i11.21452

Jobin, A., Ienca, M., & Vayena, E. (2019). The global landscape of AI ethics guidelines. *Nature Machine Intelligence*, 1(9), 389–399. https://doi.org/10.1038/s42256-019-0088-2

Joshi, G., & Bhandari, M. (2022). *Fda approved artificial intelligence and machine learning (ai/ml)-enabled medical devices: an updated 2022 landscape.* https://doi.org/10.21203/rs.3.rs-2355147/v1

Joshi, G., Jain, A., Araveeti, S., Adhikari, S., Garg, H., & Bhandari, M. (2024). FDA-approved artificial intelligence and machine learning (AI/ML)-enabled medical devices: an updated landscape. *Electronics*, 13(3), 498. https://doi.org/10.3390/electronics13030498

Jungmann, F., Ziegelmayer, S., Lohoefer, F., Metz, S., Müller-Leisse, C., Englmaier, M., … Braren, R. (2022). Algorithmic transparency and interpretability measures improve radiologists' performance in BI-RADS 4 classification. *European Radiology*, 33(3), 1844–1851. https://doi.org/10.1007/s00330-022-09165-9

Kelly, C., Karthikesalingam, A., Suleyman, M., Corrado, G., & King, D. (2019). Key challenges for delivering clinical impact with artificial intelligence. *BMC Medicine*, 17(1). https://doi.org/10.1186/s12916-019-1426-2

Komatsu, M., Sakai, A., Dozen, A., Shozu, K., Yasutomi, S., Machino, H., … Hamamoto, R. (2021). Towards clinical application of artificial intelligence in ultrasound imaging. *Biomedicines*, 9(7), 720. https://doi.org/10.3390/biomedicines9070720

Kooli, C. and Muftah, H. (2022). Artificial intelligence in healthcare: a comprehensive review of its ethical concerns. *Technological Sustainability*, 1(2), 121–131. https://doi.org/10.1108/techs-12-2021-0029

Lee, J., Wu, A., Li, D., & Kulasegaram, K. (2021). Artificial intelligence in undergraduate medical education: a scoping review. *Academic Medicine*, 96(11S), S62–S70. https://doi.org/10.1097/acm.0000000000004291

Liao, Q., Gruen, D., & Miller, S. (2020). *Questioning the AI: informing design practices for explainable AI user experiences* (pp. 1–15). https://doi.org/10.1145/3313831.3376590

Lim, W., Luong, N., Hoang, D., Jiao, Y., Liang, Y., Yang, Q., … Miao, C. (2020). Federated learning in mobile edge networks: a comprehensive survey. *IEEE Communications Surveys & Tutorials*, 22(3), 2031–2063. https://doi.org/10.1109/comst.2020.2986024

Lukkien, D., Stolwijk, N., Askari, S., Hofstede, B., Nap, H., Boon, W., … Minkman, M. (2024). *AI-assisted decision-making in long-term care: qualitative study on prerequisites for responsible innovation* (preprint). https://doi.org/10.2196/preprints.55962

Makubhai, S., Pathak, G., & Chandre, P. (2023). Prevention in healthcare: an explainable AI approach. *International Journal on Recent and Innovation Trends in Computing and Communication*, 11(5), 92–100. https://doi.org/10.17762/ijritcc.v11i5.6582

Metta, C., Beretta, A., Pellungrini, R., Rinzivillo, S., & Giannotti, F. (2024). Towards transparent healthcare: advancing local explanation methods in explainable artificial intelligence. *Bioengineering*, 11(4), 369. https://doi.org/10.3390/bioengineering11040369

Mienye, I., Obaido, G., Jere, N., Mienye, E., Aruleba, K., Emmanuel, I., … Ogbuokiri, B. (2024). *A survey of explainable artificial intelligence in healthcare: concepts, applications, and challenges*. https://doi.org/10.20944/preprints202408.1702.v1

Mohseni, S., Zarei, N., & Ragan, E. (2021). A multidisciplinary survey and framework for design and evaluation of explainable AI systems. *ACM Transactions on Interactive Intelligent Systems*, 11(3–4), 1–45. https://doi.org/10.1145/3387166

Muralidharan, V., Adewale, B., Huang, C., Nta, M., Ademiju, P., Pathmarajah, P., … Olatunji, T. (2024). *Health disparities and reporting gaps in Artificial Intelligence (AI) enabled medical devices: a scoping review of 692 U.S. food and drug administration (FDA) 510k approvals*. https://doi.org/10.1101/2024.05.20.24307582

Murphy, K., Ruggiero, E., Upshur, R., Willison, D., Malhotra, N., Cai, J., … Gibson, J. (2021). Artificial intelligence for good health: a scoping review of the ethics literature. *BMC Medical Ethics*, 22(1). https://doi.org/10.1186/s12910-021-00577-8

Nelson, C., Pérez-Chada, L., Creadore, A., Li, S., Lo, K., Manjaly, P., … Mostaghimi, A. (2020). Patient perspectives on the use of artificial intelligence for skin cancer screening. *JAMA Dermatology*, 156(5), 501. https://doi.org/10.1001/jamadermatol.2019.5014

Nguyen, T., Dakka, M., Diakiw, S., VerMilyea, M., Perugini, M., Hall, J., … Perugini, D. (2022). A novel decentralized federated learning approach to train on globally distributed, poor quality, and protected private medical data. *Scientific Reports*, 12(1). https://doi.org/10.1038/s41598-022-12833-x

Noordman, J., Oosterveld-Vlug, M., & Rademakers, J. (2022). Shared decision making in clinical practice. *European Journal of Health Communication*, 3(1), 31–52. https://doi.org/10.47368/ejhc.2022.102

Okada, Y., Ning, Y., & Ong, M. (2023). Explainable artificial intelligence in emergency medicine: an overview. *Clinical and Experimental Emergency Medicine*, 10(4), 354–362. https://doi.org/10.15441/ceem.23.145

Ozanne, E., Noseworthy, P., Cameron, K., Schmidt, M., Cavanaugh, K., Pershing, M., … Fagerlin, A. (2020). Shared decision making in the era of telehealth: implications for practice and research. *MDM Policy & Practice*, 5(2). https://doi.org/10.1177/2381468320976364

Patel, A., Gu, Q., Esper, R., Maeser, D., & Maeser, N. (2024). The crucial role of interdisciplinary conferences in advancing explainable AI in healthcare. *Biomedinformatics*, 4(2), 1363–1383. https://doi.org/10.3390/biomedinformatics4020075

Reddy, S., Lebrun, A., Chee, A., & Kalogeropoulos, D. (2024). Discussing the role of explainable AI and evaluation frameworks for safe and effective integration of large language models in healthcare. *Telehealth and Medicine Today*, 9(2). https://doi.org/10.30953/thmt.v9.485

Richardson, J., Smith, C., Curtis, S., Watson, S., Zhu, X., Barry, B., … Sharp, R. (2021). Patient apprehensions about the use of artificial intelligence in healthcare. *NPJ Digital Medicine*, 4(1). https://doi.org/10.1038/s41746-021-00509–1

Roller, R., Mayrdorfer, M., Duettmann, W., Naik, M., Schmidt, D., Halleck, F., … Budde, K. (2022). Evaluation of a clinical decision support system for detection of patients at risk after kidney transplantation. *Frontiers in Public Health*, 10. https://doi.org/10.3389/fpubh.2022.979448

Santra, S., Kukreja, P., Saxena, K., Gandhi, S., & Singh, O. (2024). Navigating regulatory and policy challenges for AI enabled combination devices. *Frontiers in Medical Technology*, 6. https://doi.org/10.3389/fmedt.2024.1473350

Sarwar, S., Dent, A., Faust, K., Richer, M., Djuric, U., Ommeren, R., … Diamandis, P. (2019). Physician perspectives on integration of artificial intelligence into diagnostic pathology. *NPJ Digital Medicine*, 2(1). https://doi.org/10.1038/s41746-019-0106-0

Schwendicke, F., Samek, W., & Krois, J. (2020). Artificial intelligence in dentistry: chances and challenges. *Journal of Dental Research*, 99(7), 769–774. https://doi.org/10.1177/0022034520915714

Secinaro, S., Calandra, D., Secinaro, A., Muthurangu, V., & Biancone, P. (2021). The role of artificial intelligence in healthcare: a structured literature review. *BMC Medical Informatics and Decision Making*, 21(1). https://doi.org/10.1186/s12911-021-01488-9

Shu, L., Pandit, S., Tritsch, T., Levy, A., & Shoja, M. (2024). What goes in, must come out: generative artificial intelligence does not present algorithmic bias across race and gender in medical residency specialties. *Cureus*. https://doi.org/10.7759/cureus.54448

Srinivasu, P., Sandhya, N., Jhaveri, R., & Raut, R. (2022). From blackbox to explainable AI in healthcare: existing tools and case studies. *Mobile Information Systems*, 1–20. https://doi.org/10.1155/2022/8167821

Stroud, A., Minteer, S., Zhu, X., Ridgeway, J., Miller, J., & Barry, B. (2024). *Patient information needs for transparent and trustworthy artificial intelligence in healthcare*. https://doi.org/10.1101/2024.07.02.24309850

Sukumar, S., George, J., & Cataland, S. (2020). Shared decision making, thrombotic thrombocytopenic purpura, and caplacizumab. *American Journal of Hematology*, 95(4). https://doi.org/10.1002/ajh.25715

Tiwari, R. (2023). Explainable ai (XAI) and its applications in building trust and understanding in AI decision making. *International Journal of Scientific Research in Engineering and Management*, 07(01). https://doi.org/10.55041/ijsrem17592

Veer, S., Riste, L., Cheraghi-Sohi, S., Phipps, D., Tully, M., Bozentko, K., … Peek, N. (2021). Trading off accuracy and explainability in AI decision-making: findings from 2 citizens' juries. *Journal of the American Medical Informatics Association*, 28(10), 2128–2138. https://doi.org/10.1093/jamia/ocab127

Vicente, L. and Matute, H. (2023). Humans inherit artificial intelligence biases. *Scientific Reports*, 13(1). https://doi.org/10.1038/s41598-023-42384-8

Wang, W., Chen, L., Xiong, M., & Wang, Y. (2021). Accelerating AI adoption with responsible AI signals and employee engagement mechanisms in health care. *Information Systems Frontiers*, 25(6), 2239–2256. https://doi.org/10.1007/s10796-021-10154-4

Wang, X., Lu, Z., & Yin, M. (2022). *Will you accept the AI recommendation? Predicting human behavior in AI-assisted decision making* (pp. 1697–1708). https://doi.org/10.1145/3485447.3512240

Wu, D., Pen, O., Wang, Y., Stern, R., Bourland, J., & Mahesh, M. (2024). Embracing real AI: a call to action for medical physicists in healthcare. *Journal of Applied Clinical Medical Physics*, 25(9). https://doi.org/10.1002/acm2.14456

Yanagawa, M., Ito, R., Nozaki, T., Fujioka, T., Yamada, A., Fujita, S., … Naganawa, S. (2023). New trend in artificial intelligence-based assistive technology for thoracic imaging. *La Radiologia Medica*, 128(10), 1236–1249. https://doi.org/10.1007/s11547-023-01691-w

Yang, H., Lam, K., Xiao, L., Xiong, Z., Hu, H., Niyato, D., … Poor, H. (2022). *Lead federated neuromorphic learning for edge artificial intelligence*. https://doi.org/10.21203/rs.3.rs-1270383/v1

Žlahtič, B., Završnik, J., Kokol, P., Vošner, H., Sobotkiewicz, N., Schaubach, B., … Kirbiš, S. (2024). Trusting AI made decisions in healthcare by making them explainable. *Science Progress*, 107(3). https://doi.org/10.1177/00368504241266573

Index

B

C

D

E

H

I

J

K

L

R

S

T

U

V

W

Z